SOCIAL WORK
IN ONCOLOGY

SOCIAL WORK IN ONCOLOGY

Supporting Survivors,
Families, and Caregivers

Marie M. Lauria, MSW, LCSW
Elizabeth J. Clark, PhD, ACSW
Joan F. Hermann, MSW, LSW
Naomi M. Stearns, MSW, ACSW

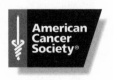

MANAGING EDITOR: Katherine V. Bruss, PsyD
PRODUCTION MANAGER: Candace Magee
PRODUCTION EDITOR: Tom Gryczan, MS
DESIGN: Shock Design, Inc., Atlanta, GA
PUBLISHER: Emily Pualwan

5 4 3 2 1   01 02 03 04 05

Library of Congress Cataloging-in-Publication Data
Social work in oncology : supporting survivors, families, and caregivers / Marie M.
Lauria ... [et al.].
    p.cm.
    Includes bibliographical references and index.
    ISBN 0-944235-30-1 (pbk.)
    1. Medical social work. 2. Cancer--Patients--Services for. 3. Social work with
the terminally ill. 4. Family social work. I. Lauria, Marie M.

HV687 .S588 2001
362.1'0425--dc21
                                                            00-054333

Published by
American Cancer Society
Health Content Products
1599 Clifton Road NE
Atlanta, Georgia 30329, USA
800-ACS-2345
http://www.cancer.org

Printed in the United States of America

TABLE OF CONTENTS

CONTRIBUTORS

Diane Blum, MSW, ACSW, is the Executive Director of Cancer Care, Inc. in New York, New York.

Nancy F. Cincotta, CSW, ACSW, CCLS, is a Preceptor in the Department of Social Work Services, Division of Pediatric Hematology-Oncology and Department of Community Medicine at Mount Sinai Medical Center in New York, New York.

Elizabeth J. Clark, PhD, ACSW, is the Executive Director of the New York State Chapter of the National Association of Social Workers in Albany, New York.

Michelle Fillios Cox, MSW, LMSW, is a Senior Social Work Counselor at the University of Texas M. D. Anderson Cancer Center in Houston, Texas.

Les Gallo-Silver, CSW, ACSW, is a Senior Social Worker in the Department of Social Work at New York University Medical Center in New York, New York.

Susan C. Hedlund, MSW, LCSW, is a Patient and Family Counselor in the Division of Hematology/ Oncology and Instructor in the School of Medicine at Oregon Health Sciences University in Portland, Oregon.

Joan F. Hermann, MSW, LSW, is the Director of Social Work Services at Fox Chase Cancer Center in Philadelphia, Pennsylvania.

Jennifer Keller, CSW, is a Clinical Social Worker at the Jewish Family and Children Services in Philadelphia, Pennsylvania.

Marie M. Lauria, MSW, LCSW, is an Oncology Social Work Consultant in Chapel Hill, North Carolina and Clinical Associate Professor, Department of Pediatrics, University of North Carolina.

Allen Levine, ACSW, is the Assistant Director of Social Services at Cancer Care, Inc. in New York, New York.

Ellen Levine, LCSW, is a social worker at the Cancer Institute of New Jersey in New Brunswick, New Jersey.

Carol P. Marcusen, LCSW, BCD, is the Director of Social Services at USC/Norris Comprehensive Cancer Center and Hospital in Los Angeles, California.

Lissa Parsonnet, PhD, ACSW, is the Director of Psychological Support Services and Cancer Program Management at Saint Barnabas Cancer Center in Livingston, New Jersey.

Philip A. Pizzo, MD, is Physician-in-Chief and Chair of the Department of Medicine at Children's Hospital in Boston, Massachusetts, and Thomas Morgan Rotch Professor of Pediatrics at Harvard University Medical School.

David S. Rosenthal, MD, is Director of Harvard University Health Services in Cambridge, Massachusetts; Henry K. Oliver Professor of Hygiene, Harvard University Professor of Medicine; and Medical Director, Zakim Center for Integrative Medicine, Dana-Farber Cancer Institute/Harvard Medical School.

John W. Sharp, MSSA, is the Web Administrator at the Cleveland Clinic Foundation in Cleveland, Ohio, a Lecturer in the Department of Social Work at Cleveland State University, and an Adjunct Instructor for the Mandel School of Applied Social Sciences at Case Western Reserve University in Cleveland, Ohio.

Naomi M. Stearns, MSW, ACSW, is an Oncology Social Work Consultant in The Woodlands, Texas.

Allison Stovall, MSW, LMSW, is an Oncology Social Work Consultant in Houston, Texas.

Amanda L. Sutton, CSW, is the Program Coordinator of Bereavement Services at Cancer Care, Inc. in New York, New York.

Mary E. Turney, MSW, LCSW, is Manager of Psychosocial Oncology at H. Lee Moffitt Cancer Center & Research Institute in Tampa, Florida.

Nancy L. Wells, MSW, LCSW, is Director of Patient Support Services at H. Lee Moffitt Cancer Center & Research Institute in Tampa, Florida.

Evaon C. Wong-Kim, PhD, LCSW, MPH, is an Assistant Professor in the School of Social Work at the University of Hawai`i at Manoa in Honolulu, Hawai`i.

INTRODUCTION

Marie M. Lauria, MSW, LCSW
Elizabeth J. Clark, PhD, ACSW
Joan F. Hermann, MSW, LSW
Naomi M. Stearns, MSW, ACSW

Oncology social work first gained recognition as a specialization in the early 1970s. Ruth Abram's book *Not Alone with Cancer* (1974) recounted her experiences and observations while working with cancer patients and their families at Massachusetts General Hospital. This was the first acknowledgment of the special psychosocial concerns of adult cancer patients, and it appeared around the same time that chemotherapy was beginning to show promise in adults. Massachusetts General Hospital was an apt setting for Abram's work since Ida Cannon started the first medical social work department there in 1919. In pediatric oncology, as the number of children surviving cancer increased, comprehensive care teams that included social workers were becoming the norm. Oncology social work steadily developed into a dynamic field with a strong theoretical and practical history.

Also in the mid 1970s, Marion Stonberg, a social worker at the Dana-Farber Cancer Institute in Boston, received a National Cancer Institute (NCI) grant to help social workers improve and refine their professional competence in oncology and to develop peer supports in this specialty. Ms. Stonberg formed a Social Work Oncology Group (SWOG) that served as a model for similar groups around the country. A survey resulting from the NCI grant attested to the effectiveness of such groups in validating and strengthening knowledge and skills, improving peer support, increasing access to information, and fostering leadership development, continuing education, and collaboration.

As new SWOGs developed in other locations, the success of these groups led to interest in forming national organizations of social workers. The Association of Pediatric Oncology Social Workers was established in 1977, followed by the National Association of Oncology Social Workers (NAOSW) in 1984. NAOSW later became the Association of Oncology Social Work (AOSW), reincorporating as a 501(C)(3), a charitable organization for educational purposes. The American Cancer Society (ACS) was instrumental in launching both organizations. It provided APOSW with seed money for initial operations, and convened a national oncology social work conference that made it possible for oncology social workers who worked primarily with adult cancer patients to plan formation of another organization.

Leaders of AOSW and APOSW recognized early the importance of educating social workers in oncology through training and publications. Again, the ACS offered critical assistance, initially by establishing training grants for oncology social workers. In 1993 the ACS published *Oncology Social Work: A Clinician's Guide*. It directed beginning practitioners, or those experienced but new to oncology, through the intricacies of social work practice with cancer patients and their families.

Today, providing cancer care is far more complex for all professionals and new and difficult issues have emerged. Information about cancer diagnosis and treatment options has exploded. Scientists have just mapped the human genome, promising a new era of disease prevention and treatment. Technology development, other new therapies, and treatment advances have changed the medical management of cancer. There is greater recognition of the importance of addressing social, emotional, and spiritual needs. Concern about escalating costs and the success or failure of managed care arrangements to contain them is raising new ethical issues about decision-making and consumer choice. There is heightened public and professional interest in prevention and early detection, new gene therapies, complementary treatments, survivors' rights, and quality of life and care. There is acknowledgment of the problems faced by family caregivers. Issues in palliative and end of life care are capturing widespread attention. The Internet has become a source of professional and consumer information and education, as well as a source of survivor and family support. There is renewed optimism about progress in finding more cures and controlling cancer more effectively. Clearly, the cancer experience now is more demanding and complicated for all involved. Given this complexity, social workers interested in oncology have a unique opportunity for a multifaceted, rich practice using a broad repertoire of professional skills.

Oncology social workers face daily challenges to ease the social and emotional burdens of cancer survivors, intervene in new and creative ways with fewer staff and shrinking resources, and demonstrate the efficacy of their work. Advocacy that extends beyond case advocacy has assumed even greater significance than it has in the past. Changes in the health care system since the publication of the initial oncology social work book also have had a dramatic impact on the setting, manner of practice, and roles of oncology social workers. More of our colleagues function as case managers or discharge planners and fewer as clinicians or counselors. More have expanded educational roles. Many are no longer in centralized social work departments. Some are affiliated with physicians' offices, freestanding clinics, or are finding a niche in community-based settings. Increased creativity, persistence, and flexibility have become necessary for all oncology social workers.

Much of the content of the earlier publication remains sound and relevant to current practice. The editors decided, however, that the numerous changes occurring in the field indicated the need for a different book rather than a revised edition of the previous one. *Oncology Social Work: Supporting Survivors, Families, and Caregivers* is not the definitive oncology social work text for clinicians but rather offers an overview of the field. It includes information about cancer diagnosis and medical treatment, the range of social work interventions applied in cancer care, professional issues in oncology social work, and the identification and access of resources. A new section on Internet use for patients and professionals should be of interest to the reader. It contains extensive information on oncology Web sites. The book also contains an educational piece for patients and families that explains the benefits of psychosocial support services (see Appendix A).

The editors hope that the book will provide a foundation on which to begin oncology practice. Both novice oncology social workers and those with years of social work experience should find useful and practical information in these chapters. Some information that is included in the chapters pertaining to children might well find application in work with adults and the reverse will also be true. While most chapters are meant to stand on their own, it is believed that there will be something of interest to all readers in each section. For example, the chapter on research should demystify the process for even the most non-research oriented reader.

For social workers interested in advancing their expertise in oncology, this text may be a first step. Equally valuable will be formal education experiences combined with significant patient and family contact, the best teacher for any specialization. Many local, regional, and national conferences for professionals are also available. The clinical and research literature is a rich source of both biomedical and psychosocial information. Much information is available via the Internet and listservs. Some hospitals and comprehensive cancer centers offer intensive courses for beginning and advanced practitioners in psychosocial oncology. AOSW and APOSW each offer annual educational conferences with extensive clinical content and the opportunity to network with colleagues.

Although challenging and intense, oncology social work offers tremendous rewards, primarily the opportunity to make a substantive, qualitative difference in the lives of patients and families. As always, social workers have much to contribute and are pivotal in helping people successfully navigate the entire illness experience. Social workers new to the field often are surprised to observe how effectively patients and families manage to deal with the stresses of the illness. Sharing in the patient's struggle and potential mastery of problems provides tremendous satisfaction for helping professionals. The work also generates a process of self-discovery and growth. Cancer challenges us to examine our philosophy of life, spirituality, and personal and professional attitudes and value systems. The social work commitment to self-exploration and insight in the service of client growth offers additional benefits to patients and professionals.

As the biology of cancer becomes clearer and advances in cancer treatment continue, realistic hope for successful management of the illness continues to grow. This hopefulness also extends to the quality of patient and family life and mastery of the challenges of cancer. Professional satisfaction will depend on clinical competence, strong advocacy skills, sensitivity to the human condition, and a belief in people and their capacity to grow. The practice of oncology social work is an opportunity to realize the value and richness of the human experience and of our profession.

CHAPTER 1

THE NATURE OF ADULT CANCER: MEDICAL DIAGNOSIS AND TREATMENT

David S. Rosenthal, MD

Cancer is not one disease state but rather many, all characterized by the presence of an uncontrolled (i.e., malignant) proliferation of a certain cell in the body. There are numerous types of cells, so there are many types of cancer. In the adult, cells that become malignant most frequently originate in the skin, prostate, breast, lung, colon, and rectum. This chapter will deal with the incidence, survival, and mortality of cancer, the risk or epidemiological factors associated with some of the common types of adult cancer, screening and early detection, establishing the diagnosis, staging, the modalities of therapy, the importance of clinical trials, the use of alternative and/or complementary therapies, and the issues of survivorship.

It is increasingly necessary to approach treatment of the cancer patient with all available medical and technological resources. The interdisciplinary approach to case management involves the participation of all members of the health-care professional team, including the primary care physician, the oncology specialist, the nurse specialist, the pharmacist, the nutritionist, the clergy, and others. The oncology social worker is a vital member of the team and must be aware of the many implications of the issues outlined above.

Mortality, Incidence, and Survival

Mortality

Cancer is the second leading cause of death in the United States, exceeded only by heart disease. In 1997, there were 539,577 deaths and in the year 2001, the American Cancer Society estimates that 553,400 will die of cancer in this country. While rates from most other causes of death have decreased in the last 40 years, cancer death rates increased (Greenlee, Murray, Bolden, & Wingo, 2000). The lung is by far the most common site of cancer deaths in men (31%), followed by the prostate (13%) and colon/rectal (10%). In women, lung (25%), breast (16%), and colon/rectum (11%) are the leading sites of cancer deaths. Trends in cancer death rates showed a steady annual increase until peaking in 1991 at 173 deaths due to cancer for every 100,000 people in the U.S. In March 1998, the American Cancer Society, the National Cancer Institute (NCI) and the Centers for Disease Control and Prevention (CDC) announced for the first time a decline in the cancer death rate in the U.S. From 1991 through 1995, there was an average annual decline of 0.5% in the death rate, with a decline of approximately 5.3% in men and 1.1% in women. Over the past 60 years, most of the increase in cancer deaths was related to lung cancer, but in men the increase slowed down beginning in the 1980s and the rate is now decreasing. In women, lung cancer death rates are now fivefold higher than what they were 30 years ago and the rate of death is still unfortunately increasing. The death rates for breast cancer began to decline in 1989. For men and women, the mortality rates for stomach and colon/rectal cancer have shown steady declines in the past decade.

In general, cancer death rates are higher in men than women (primarily due to the high rate of lung cancer), and black men and women have higher mortality rates than whites (secondary to many possible factors including advanced stage at diagnosis), especially in sites such as the lung, gastrointestinal tract, prostate, and breast. Figures 1 and 2 illustrate the age-adjusted cancer death rates from 1930 through 1997 for all sites and both sexes.

Figure 1

Age-Adjusted Cancer Death Rates,* for Males by Site, US, 1930–1997

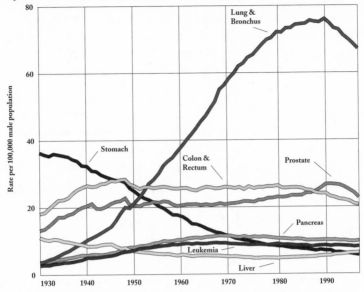

Figure 2

Age-Adjusted Cancer Death Rates,* for Females by Site, US, 1930–1997

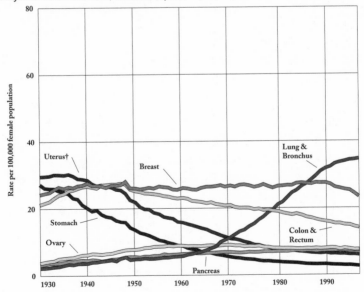

Note. From The American Cancer Society. (2001). *Cancer facts and figures* 2001 (pp. 2–3). *Atlanta, GA.*
‡ See endnotes on page 25.

Incidence

Almost every family will have at least one member in each generation become ill with cancer. The incidence of cancer increases with age. It is estimated that 1.268 million new cases of cancer will be diagnosed in the U.S. in 2001. In 2001, prostate, lung, colon/rectum, and urinary bladder cancers will occur most frequently in men and cancer of the breast, lung, colon/rectum, and uterus will occur most frequently in women. Cancer incidence rates (numbers of cases per 100,000 populations) peaked in 1992 and declined thereafter. During 1990–1996, incidence rates for all cancers combined decreased on average 0.7% per year after increasing 1.2% per year during 1973–1990.

Most of the cancer sites are decreasing in incidence or are stable; two cancers are continuing to increase: non-Hodgkin's lymphoma and malignant melanoma. Overall cancer incidence rates are higher in men than women. Black men have the highest incidence, followed by whites and then Hispanic men, and this has been true for over 20 years of data collection. Racial differences in women are not as extreme as in men.

The lifetime probability of a developing cancer is one in two in a man and one in three in a woman. The leading sites are prostate, lung, and colon/rectum in males and breast, colon/rectum, and lung in females.

Survival

Survival rates for certain cancers have improved significantly since the 1960s due to both earlier detection and treatment advances. Survival rates for cancers of the lung and prostate, and non-Hodgkin's lymphoma have increased by more than 50% over the 30-year period. Survival rates for cancers of the breast, colon, ovary, and pancreas, as well as leukemia and melanoma, have also shown marked improvement. However, 5-year relative cancer survival rates differ markedly among whites vs. blacks, with 10%–15% lower rates noted in blacks.

Cancer is still the second-leading cause of death in children under the age of 14, accounting for 11% of total deaths in this age group, with accidents being first. The major cancers in the pediatric population are leukemias, lymphomas, and brain tumors. In young adults, testicular tumors, ovarian malignancies, lymphomas, and leukemias are the most common forms of cancer. The 5-year relative survival rates have significantly increased from the early 1970s to the 1990s and range now from 76.6% for the 15-19-year-olds to 73.4% for the younger children.

EPIDEMIOLOGY AND ETIOLOGY

Several important observations can be made from the above statistics; most notably that lung cancer is the overall leading cause of cancer death, surpassing even breast cancer in women and prostate cancer in men. Of the almost 500,000 deaths due to cancer in the United States each year, tobacco use appears to be the single major etiologic factor, playing a role in lung, oral, gastrointestinal, and bladder cancer. Almost one-third of all cancers are tobacco related.

There is increasing evidence that nutrition and physical activity play significant roles and account for about 30% of cancer deaths (Schottenfeld & Fraumeni, 1996). High-fat diets are associated with a higher risk of colon, breast, endometrial, and prostate cancers. A low-fat, high-fiber diet appears to offer some protective effect against bowel cancer. The incidence of gastric cancer in native Japanese populations is high compared to other countries, although the incidence decreases in that population upon migration to the United States. Excessive alcohol consumption has been linked with liver and breast cancer and increases the incidence of other cancers when accompanied by tobacco use, such as nasopharyngeal, oral, esophageal, and gastric cancers. Increasing the intake of fruits and vegetables has been associated with reducing one's risk of developing cancer.

What makes a normal cell become malignant? This and similar questions have been the subject of intensive investigation throughout the past two centuries. Initial findings in the 1800s that there was a virtual absence of cervical cancer and a relatively high incidence of breast cancer in nuns led to the findings of the relationship of *hormonal* factors in modifying cancer risk. The finding of increased numbers of cancers in chimney sweeps led to the study of *occupational* carcinogenic exposures and then of course to the relationship of tobacco and cancer, first mentioned in the scientific literature in the 18th century. It is now recognized that certain viruses, total body irradiation, or exposure to chemicals can increase the risk of developing cancer. The Epstein-Barr virus (EBV) has been implicated in lymphomas and nasopharyngeal carcinoma, hepatitis B virus associated with liver cancer, human papilloma viruses (HPV) with an increased incidence of cancer of the cervix, and human T cell lymphotropic viruses (HTLV) linked to a type of acute lymphocytic leukemia.

Irradiation as an etiologic agent in cancer has been the subject of much controversy. Although high levels of total body irradiation can cause leukemias or lymphomas, low levels of radiation have not been proven to increase cancer incidence. Ultraviolet light (UVL) and excessive sun exposure are definite risk factors for skin cancers such as basal carcinoma and malignant melanoma. It has been demonstrated, for instance, that contact with asbestos and polycyclic hydrocarbons may result in lung cancer, while exposure to vinyl chloride and benzene have been linked to liver cancer and acute myelogenous leukemia (AML), respectively.

Gould, Piver, and Eltabbakh (1997) discuss the epidemiological evidence that has shown that many cancers occur at an increased rate among families (i.e., the influence of hereditary factors). For example, the chance of developing breast cancer is higher in a woman whose mother or sister (first degree relative) has had the disease. Many cancers begin with genetic defects that may be passed on from generation to generation. The discovery of genes such as BRCA1 and BRCA2 that can cause some breast cancers represents considerable promise that individuals can be identified as susceptible to cancer, although at the same time it represents difficult ethical issues. This group of patients still represents only a very small subset of people who will get breast cancer. The vast majority of breast cancer patients so far have not been found to have a specific gene marker. Other genes have been discovered that are associated with familial cancers of the colon, rectum, kidney, ovary, thyroid, and others. Genetic factors probably account for 15% of all cancers. All health care providers should be aware of a patient's family history and the potential effect this information has on the individual's cancer risk.

PREVENTION, SCREENING, AND EARLY DETECTION

As we learn more about epidemiology, we gain insight into prevention of some cancers. Some cancers that are otherwise potentially deadly can be treated with great success if detected early. Early detection measures are available for several cancers and ongoing research is aimed at developing and testing new and more sensitive methods. The American Cancer Society together with other voluntary health organizations, the NCI, and the CDC emphasize cancer control programs with guidelines for reducing ones risk of developing cancer. Knowledge-based evidence suggests that there is a great deal that the individual can do for himself or herself to reduce their risk of developing cancer (Willett, 1999). First, avoid tobacco, tobacco-related products, and environmental tobacco smoke. Second, eat well. Existing evidence suggests that about one-third of the cancer deaths that occur in the U.S. each year are due to dietary factors. Cancer risk can be reduced by an overall dietary pattern that includes a high proportion of plant foods (fruits and vegetables) and limited amounts of meat, dairy, and high fat foods, and limited alcohol intake. The American Cancer Society revised its nutrition guidelines in 1996 based on new scientific evidence. Third, be physically active. Physical activity can help protect against some cancers, either by balancing caloric intake with energy expenditure or by other mechanisms. An imbalance can lead to overweight, obesity, and increased risk for cancers such as colon/rectum and breast.

The guidelines for early detection are aimed at detecting the disease at an early, potentially curable stage. Table 1 summarizes the 2001 American Cancer Society recommendations for the early detection of cancer in the asymptomatic individual. Newer research technologies are being developed that will allow cancers to be detected when molecular changes first occur, even before cells show microscopic signs of malignancy.

TABLE 1

Summary of American Cancer Society Recommendations for the Early Detection of Cancer in Asymptomatic People

SITE	RECOMMENDATION
Cancer-related Checkup	A cancer-related checkup is recommended every 3 years for people aged 20-40 and every year for people age 40 and older. This exam should include health counseling and depending on a person's age, might include examinations for cancers of the thyroid, oral cavity, skin, lymph nodes, testes, and ovaries, as well as for some nonmalignant diseases.
Breast	Women 40 and older should have an annual mammogram and annual clinical breast exam (CBE) by a health care professional, and should perform monthly breast self-examination (BSE). The CBE should be conducted close to and preferably before the scheduled mammogram. Women ages 20-39 should have a clinical breast examination by a health care professional every three years and should perform monthly BSE.
Colon & Rectum	Beginning at age 50, men and women should follow one of the examination schedules below: 1) A fecal occult blood test (FOBT) every year or 2) A flexible sigmoidoscopy every five years* or 3) FOBT every year and flexible sigmoidoscopy every five years,* **(of these three options, the American Cancer Society prefers option 3, annual FOBT and flexible sigmoidoscopy every five years)** or 4) A double-contrast barium enema every five years* or 5) A colonoscopy every 10 years.* * A digital rectal exam should be done at the same time as sigmoidoscopy, colonoscopy, or double-contrast barium enema. People who are at moderate or high risk for colorectal cancer should talk with a doctor about a different testing schedule.
Prostate	Beginning at age 50, the prostate-specific antigen (PGA) test and the digital rectal exam should be offered annually to men who have a life expectancy of at least 10 years. Men at high-risk (African-American men and men who have a first-degree relative who was diagnosed with prostate cancer at a young age) should begin testing at age 45. Patients should be given information about the benefits and limitations of tests so they can make an informed decision.
Uterus	**Cervix:** All women who are or have been sexually active or who are 18 and older should have an annual Pap test and pelvic examination. After three or more consecutive satisfactory examinations with normal findings, the Pap test may be performed less frequently. Discuss the matter with your physician. **Endometrium:** Beginning at age 35, women with or at risk for hereditary non-polyposis colon cancer should be offered endometrial biopsy annually to screen for endometrial cancer.

Note. From The American Cancer Society. (2001). *Cancer facts and figures 2001* (p. 35). Atlanta, GA.

ESTABLISHING THE DIAGNOSIS

A biopsy or a fine needle aspiration of an organ or suspected mass via computed tomography (CT) or ultrasound is usually the first step in establishing a diagnosis. Once obtained, all tissue specimens are analyzed by microscopy, but further investigative studies such as immunologic studies, electron microscopy, and in some cases chromosomal and gene analysis may be required. The role of the surgeon is to assure that there is sufficient material to establish a diagnosis, and if cancer, being able to differentiate it from disorders masquerading as a malignancy such as infections or benign tumors. Often a second opinion or a second biopsy of a tissue may be necessary in difficult cases. Although routine methods of examination may be adequate, frequently the biopsy material may not resemble any normal tissue and the pathologist will require additional studies such as histochemistry, receptor studies, and immunologic and/or cytogenetic studies to determine the site of origin of the cancer.

The pathologist also "grades" the cancer according to the tumor's virulence or rapidity of growth. In addition, the microscopy studies will determine whether the surgical excision was complete. For example, after the surgeon removes a localized cancer of the bowel, it is important to know if the resected margins are free of cancer. Persistent tumor might signify a poor prognosis with both immediate and delayed complications.

After a biopsy, the patient often experiences extreme anxiety while awaiting the final results. Although a "quick look" or "frozen section" may differentiate a benign tumor from a cancer, rarely will a pathologist make any final diagnosis on these rapid studies. It is strongly recommended to have the complete pathology report in hand before discussing the diagnosis with the patient.

Staging

Three important determinants of prognosis in cancer are the size and local spread of the tumor, the number and location of lymph nodes involved, and the presence or absence of distant metastases. For each cancer there are internationally recognized criteria for staging. Staging is an extremely important component of care of the cancer patient and will determine treatment and prognosis. For example, Hodgkin's disease spreads in a very orderly fashion. Knowing how far the disease has spread at the time of diagnosis makes it possible to treat the known disease as well as the next site of potential involvement. Similarly, with localized breast cancer, the involvement of axillary lymph nodes significantly changes the prognosis, and this will have an impact on treatment options. Staging systems offer little help in some malignancies, such as acute leukemia. Because it is essentially widespread at the time of diagnosis, staging offers no added prognostic help.

A staging system is a standardized way in which the cancer multidisciplinary team describes the extent to which the cancer spread. Completion of staging the cancer may require studies in addition to the primary surgery. Radiologic studies, such as CT scans, magnetic resonance imaging scans, and ultrasound; nuclear medicine studies using various radioisotopes that are sensitive for minimal disease; and further surgical procedures may be necessary to complete the staging.

The standardized staging system most used is the American Joint Committee on Cancer (AJCC) also known as the TNM system. The letter T followed by a number (0–4) describes the tumor's size and local spread. The higher the T number the larger the tumor size. The letter N followed by a number 0–3 indicates whether the cancer has spread to lymph nodes (N) and if so whether they are fixed to the underlying structures. The letter M followed by a 0 or 1 indicates whether or not the cancer has spread to distant organs (i.e., metastasized to distant sites). Once a patient's cancer has been staged by the T, N, and M categories, this information is combined in a process referred to as "stage grouping" to determine the disease stage. The "Stage" is expressed in Roman numerals 0, I, II, III, or IV, with Stage 0 being the least advanced and Stage IV the most advanced stage.

The staging of breast cancer, for example, requires knowing the size of the primary mass in the breast, involvement of regional lymph node sites, and presence of organ involvement such as the lung, bone, or liver. With this information, the physician and patient can make an informed decision regarding therapy and also be able to give prognostic information as 5-year survival statistics are reported on a stage-by-stage basis.

The staging work-up could also include blood studies with various serum markers that are correlated with active disease, such as carcinoembryonic antigen (CEA) in colon cancer, prostate-specific antigen (PSA) for prostate cancer, and CA 125 for ovarian cancer.

TREATMENT

Major advances continue to be made in surgery, radiation therapy, and chemotherapy. New therapeutic modalities have also been developed, such as biologic immune modifiers, high-dose chemotherapy with marrow or stem cell transplantation, use of growth factors, monoclonal antibodies, vaccines, gene therapy, and angiogenesis inhibitors. Results from basic research continue to offer new technologies that allow more and better tools to treat and cure cancer.

Surgery

The surgeon plays a role not only in the diagnosis of cancer but also in its treatment. Cancers are sometimes cured by removal of the primary tumor, such as a simple mastectomy, without any further intervention. A radical resection for a localized cancer may also be indicated, for example, in localized prostate cancer, certain stages of breast cancer, or head and neck cancer. Palliative surgery is employed when a cancer is incurable by resection, but removal of the tumor mass may alleviate suffering by removing an obstruction or prevent bleeding. Cytoreductive surgery is the removal of a large tumor mass (debulking), a procedure that may enhance the effectiveness of a second therapeutic modality such as radiation therapy or chemotherapy. Photodynamic therapy employs a combination of drugs and lasers to destroy cancer cells. A drug that concentrates in certain types of cancer cells, but not in healthy cells, is injected into the patient. A laser operating at a specific light wavelength is then directed at the area of the tumor where it selectively destroys the drug-containing cancer cells. This type of therapy may be very effective in some bladder cancers.

Laser surgery involves the use of a laser focused on a specific tumor site to relieve obstruction, aid in further surgical removal, or combine with chemotherapy or radiation therapy. Extreme thermal changes, or cryoablation, may be applied via probes to symptomatic metastatic lesions in the liver or other sites. The surgeon is also involved in assisting in the staging process, second-look procedures, and reconstruction. Second-look surgical procedures are used in evaluating the responses to therapy and are appropriate for diseases such as advanced ovarian cancer.

Reconstructive surgery may be indicated after mastectomy, head and neck surgery, or other physically disfiguring procedures to improve appearance or function. Indirect surgical procedures refer to the placement of Hickman lines or portacatheters to provide easy access for infusions of chemotherapy or blood products. Disfiguring or mutilating radical surgical procedures largely have become a thing of the past because of new knowledge about the effectiveness of less radical surgical procedures and the increased efficacy of both radiation therapy and chemotherapy. For example, with better chemotherapy, limb sparing surgery for osteosarcoma and Ewing's sarcoma is recommended.

Radiation Therapy

Beams of energy produced by orthovoltage and cobalt via linear accelerators target high-energy x-rays or subatomic particles (such as electrons) directly to the malignant tumor. This treatment is referred to as external beam radiation therapy. Alternatively, pellets of radioactive material placed into or next to a cancer are used for brachytherapy. There are a variety of radiation procedures that are used to destroy cancer cells. The newer radiotherapy techniques are less likely to damage skin and are only effective in the direction of the beam. Thus, radiation therapy is applicable for localized tumors in its curative attempt. The use of the energy from the cyclotron (proton beam) allows the clinicians to treat isolated brain tumors and other unresectable cancers while minimizing damage to adjacent normal tissue.

Hodgkin's disease and non-Hodgkin's cells are more sensitive to radiation therapy than are the cells of melanoma or most soft tissue sarcomas. An important consideration in radiation therapy is the ability of normal tissues adjacent to the malignant disease to tolerate radiation. In treating lymphomas, for example, the trade off between the damaging effect on lymphoma cells and adjacent normal cells is very acceptable. In the treatment of lung cancer, however, the amount of radiation needed to control and eliminate the disease is extremely high, and this causes significant damage to adjacent normal cells. The kidney and liver are extremely sensitive to radiation and are excluded from most radiation fields.

Curative radiation therapy is possible in Hodgkin's disease; non-Hodgkin's lymphomas; and cancers of the testis, cervix, prostate, and bladder. As with surgery, other forms of radiation therapy can be palliative or used as neoadjuvant therapy. Palliative (i.e., non-curative) radiation therapy is used locally to reduce bone pain caused by bone metastasis or an obstruction that cannot be approached by surgery. In Hodgkin's disease, for example, a mass in the chest may hamper blood flow by obstructing the superior vena cava. Blood is unable to return to the right side of the heart and the patient's arms, neck, and face swell. Focused irradiation therapy will alleviate the obstruction and normal blood flow will resume. Neoadjuvant radiation therapy uses less than curative doses to decrease the tumor size; neoadjuvant therapy is treatment to improve the potential for local control by other therapeutic modalities such as surgery and/or chemotherapy. Similarly, combined modality therapy joins chemotherapy with radiation therapy in an attempt to cure. For example, in Hodgkin's disease patients with widespread or advanced-stage disease, chemotherapy would be the treatment of choice. However, after chemotherapy, radiation therapy to previous sites of bulk disease would ensure a better outcome by potentially preventing recurrence at the sites.

Certain chemical agents are available that will improve tumor responsiveness to radiation therapy and decrease normal tissue damage. These agents are referred to as radiation sensitizers and radiation protectors, respectively. Hyperthermia (induced increase in body temperature) is sometimes employed to increase local effectiveness of radiation therapy.

In some cancers, clinical trials combine radiation with immunotherapy to improve specificity of radiation's killing capability. This involves the preparation of a monoclonal antibody against a specific type of cancer cell, which is then linked with a radiation-emitting substance injected into the bloodstream. The radiation-emitting substance will only be released once the monoclonal antibody has attached itself to the cancer cell.

Many tumors that develop resistance to radiation therapy have been associated with the development of radiation-resistant genes. With progress in gene therapy it may be possible to increase a cancer's radiosensitivity by altering these genes, allowing radiation to become a more effective treatment modality.

Chemotherapy

In 1940, chemotherapy drugs first became available to treat cancer. Since then, chemical agents made from plants, bacteria, and other sources have been used to destroy tumors by inhibiting cell division and selectively destroying proliferating cells. Different drugs work in different parts of the cell life cycle. For example, methotrexate (used as a single agent) can result in a 30% remission rate in childhood acute lymphocytic leukemia (ALL) by acting at a particular phase of DNA synthesis, interfering with synthesis, repair, and cellular replication. Similarly, alkylating agents (such as chlorambucil, cyclophosphamide, and nitrogen mustard) destroy malignant cells by producing an effect in dividing cells diffusely throughout the body similar to the effects caused by radiation. By combining medicines that work in different phases of the cell cycle, response rates increase dramatically in diseases such as childhood ALL, Hodgkin's disease, and non-Hodgkin's lymphoma. This combination approach is also employed in a number of other cancers including breast cancer, ovarian carcinoma, and testicular germ cell tumors.

There continues to be a dramatic increase in chemotherapeutic classes of agents, such as topoisomerase inhibitors, such as anthracyclenes, microtubule-targeting agents, such as plant alkaloids, and taxanes, platinum compounds, etc.

Since most chemotherapy drugs follow first-order kinetics (i.e., a fixed percentage of tumor cells are killed with each course of therapy), the larger the cancer, the less effective the chemotherapy. If the tumor burden is first reduced by surgery and irradiation, the chemotherapy is more likely to result in potential cure because the chemotherapy will be more effective against a smaller burden of cancer cells. This combined-therapy approach has made it possible to replace the radical amputation of limbs, performed for osteogenic sarcoma, with limb preservation surgery and intensive chemotherapy to eradicate any systemic disease.

The use of chemotherapy prior to any local treatment modality is referred to as neoadjuvant chemotherapy, in which the therapy is aimed at reducing the size of the primary tumor with the intent to cure the disease. Chemotherapy can create local control, followed by subsequent curative surgery and radiation therapy. In head and neck cancer, for example, chemotherapy will not be curative but can reduce the extent of the cancer and may significantly improve survival following surgery and radiation therapy.

In animal and human studies, it has been demonstrated that dose intensity can be a critical factor in the outcome of chemotherapy. However, the toxic effects of chemotherapy limit the amount of chemotherapeutic drugs that can be given. In some cases, growth factors and/or marrow transplantation has facilitated fivefold to twentyfold increases in chemotherapy doses, and these higher doses have effected substantially higher cure rates for some leukemias and lymphomas.

Combined modality therapy refers to the use of serial courses of chemotherapy and radiation therapy to treat the cancer, as in management of certain stages of Hodgkin's disease, or a combination of surgery and radiotherapy and chemotherapy, as in the treatment of various solid tumors.

Besides dose-limiting toxicity, another major problem in chemotherapy is the development of drug resistance, which may be acquired during chemotherapy or may be inherent in the patient's physiology. Many cancers can develop multidrug resistance (MDR), which has been associated with increased expression of some gene products. Overcoming MDR is likely to be difficult, but it is expected that using combination chemotherapy and exploring techniques to reduce or inhibit the drug-resistant genes will play a role. Finally, combining monoclonal antibodies (see below) with toxins or chemotherapeutic agents may also be a way to effectively target cancer cells and attain reduced side effects.

Hormonal Therapy

Less toxic than chemotherapy, hormonal therapy offers the possibility of significant objective responses in breast and prostate cancer, but may not be curative. The administration of pharmacological doses of gonadal hormones may impair cancer growth. Certain malignant cells are known to have hormone receptors, making the selection of patients for such therapy possible. The presence of the estrogen receptors on breast cancer cells, for example, is correlated with a good response to hormonal therapy. However, non-endocrine tumors (such as those in colon cancer) that are found to have hormone receptors do not respond to this form of therapy.

It is important to keep in mind that 50 years of chemotherapy is a relatively short period in the long history of cancer. Newer agents and newer techniques using older agents continue to be developed.

Immunotherapy and Biologicals

One of the most exciting advances in the approach to cancer over the past two decades has been the development of immunotherapies such as monoclonal antibodies, immunotoxins, and biological agents such as interferon, interleukins, and growth factors.

Monoclonal antibodies, as mentioned previously, have been used as diagnostic tools in tumor imaging and in detecting serum markers for the presence of some cancer types. These antibodies can also be used as anticancer agents when a tumor-specific antigen can be identified. It is now possible in many cancers to identify more specific molecular proteins on the surface of cancer cells, neither on normal cells nor on the normal cells of origin. In breast cancer, approximately 1 in 5 patients overexpress the HER-2/neu oncoprotein on their malignant cells for which monoclonal antibodies can be made. Trastuzumab is such a product with demonstrable antitumor effect. Similarly in non-Hodgkin's lymphoma, monoclonal antibodies have been made against a common protein on the malignant lymphocyte, the "B1" antigen, and the resultant monoclonal antibody (Bexxar or Rituximab) has been very effective in therapy.

Cytokines are proteins that send messages from one group of cells to another. Three subtypes of these proteins have been used in cancer research and show effectiveness in cancer therapy: interleukins, interferons, and other growth factors. Interleukins (numbered 1–6) transmit messages between leukocytes and are important molecules normally involved in the body's response to an infection or inflammation. Interferons have an antiviral effect and suppress certain tumor cells both in vitro and in vivo. Most notably, these agents have been responsible for causing a high complete remission rate in hairy cell leukemia. Promising outcomes with interferons also have been reported with chronic myelogenous leukemia, renal cell carcinoma, and malignant melanoma.

Other growth factors can stimulate hematopoietic or blood stem cells to grow, mature, and differentiate. The growth factors granulocyte-macrophage colony stimulating factor (GM-CSF) and granulocyte colony stimulating factor (G-CSF) act on primitive marrow precursors, causing them to proliferate, and differentiate to mature white blood cells. The potential is to improve marrow reserve and prevent marrow suppression due to chemotherapy and radiation therapy, allowing the use of higher doses of conventional therapies.

Gene, Vaccine, and Antiangiogenesis Therapies

Many genes are formed in a cell either as a result or as the cause of a cancer. One such acquired gene product is the "BCR-ABL" protein in chronic myelogenous leukemia, a result of a translocation of part of the 9th chromosome to the 22nd chromosome. Therapies are now being aimed at this molecular target gene or protein and proving effective. As more and more defective genes become associated with cancer, there will be newer and more specific targets to which investigators can address the therapy. In non-Hodgkin's lymphomas, there is progress in treating some patients with vaccines designed specifically against their tumors. This is accomplished by a multi-step process that helps the patient's immune system recognize and attack an abnormal protein or substance on the surface of the cancer cell that is not found on normal cells.

Angiogenesis, in cancer, refers to the formation of new blood vessels that provide a tumor with nutrients and oxygen needed for growth. In most cancers, the tumor cannot grow without its own blood supply. Angiogenesis inhibitors or antiangiogenesis therapies interfere with the development of new blood vessels that support the cancer cells and thus can limit their growth or destroy them by "starvation." Many current chemotherapeutic agents have antiangiogenesis activity in addition to their primary method of action (e.g., the anthracyclenes and taxanes).

Marrow Transplantation

Marrow or stem cell transplantation (TP), for many years an investigational treatment, is now considered standard therapy for several diseases. For a growing number of patients, TP offers the best possibility for long-term remission. The purpose of TP is to allow high-dose chemotherapy to be administered that would otherwise cause potential fatalities because of severe myelosuppression. TP provides donor marrow cells or peripheral blood stem cells to replace the destroyed marrow cells and allow full and quick hematological recovery after high-dose chemotherapy. Some of the diseases treated with TP are leukemia, non-Hodgkin's lymphoma, and Hodgkin's disease. TPs are also used to treat certain solid tumors such as those of the breast and ovary, and germ cell tumors. It has also been used as treatment for other medical problems such as aplastic anemia, severe combined immunodeficiency disease, thalassemia, and Gaucher's disease.

There are several types of marrow/stem cell transplantation:

allogeneic, syngeneic, and autologous. In *allogeneic* TP the marrow comes from a person other than the patient. Usually, the donor is a sibling, but donors other than relatives are sometimes used. The goal is to find the closest match between donor and recipient, which lessens the chance that the donated cells will cause damage to normal recipient's cells. This situation, known as graft-versus-host disease, occurs in nearly one-half of all allogeneic transplants. Graft-versus-host disease may have both acute and chronic effects and requires prophylaxis as well as concurrent treatment to control symptoms. "Matching" is based on the human leukocyte antigens (HLA antigens); cell-surface proteins found on lymphocytes that match between donor and recipient. About 30%–40% of patients have an HLA-matched sibling. Through a cooperative national marrow donor program, it is now easier to find excellent HLA-matched donors.

A *syngeneic* transplant occurs between identical twins, which provides a perfect match.

Autologous TP is when the patient (in remission) is his or her own donor. With this type of TP, HLA matching is not necessary and the risk of graft-versus-host disease is eliminated. Peripheral stem cell TP refers to the harvesting of blood precursors from the peripheral blood rather than the marrow through an apheresis machine. There are enough stem cells obtained in this procedure from the peripheral blood that could be stimulated by growth factors to result in a product similar to a marrow harvest.

CLINICAL TRIALS

Before a new treatment is introduced into direct cancer care, it is carefully researched and evaluated in the laboratory. Clinical trials are those studies which lead to new and improved ways of preventing, detecting, treating, or curing cancer. Preclinical research identifies potential useful therapies and demonstrates that they are safe and effective. Once a new treatment technology is identified and shown to be effective in an animal or test tube model, it then moves on to be tested as a clinical trial. Clinical trials are studies that will determine if the new treatment or technology is an improved way of preventing, detecting, or treating a patient.

There are three important phases of a clinical trial. A **Phase I** study is structured to answer the question whether a new technology or treatment can be given safely. It usually involves a small number of patients and the results determine the highest amount of the agent that could be given safely. A **Phase II** study takes the "safe" amount of the drug and applies it to a series of patients with different cancers to determine the beneficial effects. If the drug is relatively safe and there is a significant number or degree of responses, the treatment moves on to a **Phase III** study. Phase III studies involve large numbers of patients with a specific cancer to determine the response rates and often have a control group of patients that are receiving the current "gold standard therapy." During Phase II and III, the investigators continue to monitor side effects and weigh the risks and the benefits of the therapy. Most cancer clinical trials are approved and funded by the NCI. Patients should be well informed about them and whenever possible, be urged to take part in these studies when it is appropriate (e.g., a cancer with a poor prognosis). Professionals and patients can acquire the most up-to-date information about clinical trials by contacting the American Cancer Society or the National Cancer Institute.

Clinical trials are critically important to our ability to treat, control, or cure cancer. Every standard treatment regimen, whether it be a surgical approach or one using chemotherapy or radiation therapy, has been tested in a clinical trial and proven to be effective to a greater or lesser degree. This is not a random process but one which depends on scientific rigor and a steady progression of knowledge and insights leading up to the conclusion that this particular drug is better than what has gone before it and should be offered to patients. Without the benefits of clinical trials, doctors would have no scientific way of knowing which treatments are better, for which patients, and against which diseases.

A comparison between pediatric and adult cancer management highlights the importance of clinical trials. The survival data for children with cancer is today, far better than that possible for many adult cancer patients. While children are as a rule healthier than adults upon a cancer diagnosis, there are two other factors which account for their better rates of survival. These are the following: 1) The number of children with cancer is far less that the incidence for adults, and 2) most children in this country are treated in or in conjunction with a pediatric cancer program, meaning that most of them have been treated on a clinical trial. This has made it possible to accrue valuable data about treatment advances far more quickly than is possible for adults who are treated in just about every hospital in the country. Clinical trials represent the "gold standard" for children with cancer.

In spite of the advances made in these state of the art treatment approaches, many health care professionals are ambivalent about their use. Clinical trials mandate that a very rigorous research protocol be utilized in terms of the accuracy of the results obtained, creating a burden for the busy community physician. Sometimes physicians without a strong research orientation to their practice believe they know better than an experimental protocol what is best for their patients. The more compelling barrier, however, has to do with the experimental nature of the trial and the perception that the patient is a "guinea pig" and not getting the best that medicine has to offer.

For social workers, with their commitment to quality of life, the question often comes down to an ethical one. Is it fair to subject patients to treatment with an unknown result and which will cause physical and emotional stress? Certainly, attention must be paid to quality of life and informed consent so that patients know exactly what is involved in a clinical trial. Oncology social workers are often the professionals who have the ability to help patients examine all of their options. Because clinical trials represent the answer to future cures of cancer, any social worker involved in oncology needs to examine this issue carefully so that their own possible biases do not interfere with advances in cancer management.

COMPLEMENTARY AND ALTERNATIVE METHODS OF THERAPY

Complementary and alternative methods (CAM) for cancer patients, according to Cassileth (1999), are "actually a vast collection of disparate, unrelated regimens and products, ranging from adjunctive modalities that enhance quality of life and promising antitumor herbal remedies now under investigation, to bogus therapies that claim to cure cancer and that harm patients not only directly but also indirectly by encouraging them to avoid or postpone effective cancer care" (p. 362).

Complementary therapies generally are used by cancer patients as an accompaniment to the specific therapy recommended and administered by the oncology specialist. Therapies such as the relaxation response, yoga, meditation, massage, and music improve the patient's quality of life by reducing pain, nausea, stress, and other side effects of the entire diagnostic and treatment process. Most of these therapies have been shown to be scientifically effective in reducing symptoms, decreasing pain, and improving well-being.

Alternative therapies have been defined as unproven or questionable and of no proven scientific benefit. Some are dangerous with potential life-threatening side effects, while others are used in place of standard therapy of known benefit. Often alternative therapies are expensive. They include "metabolic therapies," essiac, and iscador (Cassileth, 1998). For more in-depth information on this topic, readers can contact the American Cancer Society (800-ACS-2345; www.cancer.org) to order a copy of the *American Cancer Society's Guide to Complementary and Alternative Cancer Methods* (2000).

SUPPORTIVE THERAPY

The health professional dealing with a cancer patient must realize that he or she is not working in a vacuum. Although the primary doctor-patient relationship is central, both patient and physician

need strong support from the entire multidisciplinary health professional team: specialists, members of the tumor board of the
hospital, nurses, social workers, nutritionists, clergy, pharmacists,
physical and occupational therapists, dentists, etc. At times,
home-health and chronic-care professionals may be involved. The
supportive therapy team should be formed early in the diagnostic
phase and should be available throughout the course of illness
rather than only in response to an acute crisis. This kind of preventive approach helps patients and families anticipate and handle treatment-related problems. However, some social workers
that are working in an isolated setting may not have the advantage
of a strong multidisciplinary team, but might be the catalyst to
formulate one.

LATE EFFECTS OF TREATMENT AND LONG-TERM FOLLOW-UP

Each year there are increasing numbers of survivors of cancer, now
estimated at approximately 8.4 million people. Aggressive treatment
and improved survival have resulted in greater need for attention to
the psychosocial and physical effects of cancer treatment. The
short- and long-term effects may be medical (e.g., the late occurrence of toxicity) or psychological (e.g., the failure to cope effectively with the disease). Much is known about the immediate physical side effects of the various therapeutic modalities and more is
becoming known about their long-term effects. Many years after
completing therapy, a childhood cancer survivor may have diminished growth or the potential for a second malignancy. Young adults
treated with both chemotherapy and radiation therapy for
Hodgkin's disease are at a higher risk for developing a second malignancy such as acute non-lymphocytic leukemia or malignant lymphoma of a non-Hodgkin's type. Young men aggressively treated
with certain chemotherapeutic agents may develop gonadal dysfunction and permanent infertility. Likewise, women may also expe-

rience infertility or an increased risk of breast cancer secondary to chest irradiation. Children receiving cranial radiation along with systemic chemotherapy are at risk for dyslexia and other learning disabilities.

In addition to the therapy-related late effects, there may be numerous psychosocial effects, such as problems with employment, insurability, and ability to get back in the mainstream of life. Both the physical and the psychosocial late effects may require continuing intervention by the supportive therapy team.

SUMMARY

The cancer patient's need for integrated team care does not end with complete remission of disease or with achievement of 5-year disease free survival. Health professionals are still in the learning phase of cancer management. It is already clear that long-term routine follow-up, both medical and psychological, is necessary for an optimal outcome. Further research on long-term effects will enable team members to better predict psychosocial outcomes and needs and to offer more effective support to cancer patients and their families.

REFERENCES

American Cancer Society 1996 Advisory Committee on Diet, Nutrition, and Cancer Prevention. (1996). Guidelines on diet, nutrition and cancer prevention: Reducing the risk of cancer with healthy food choices and physical activity. CA–A Cancer Journal for Clinicians, 46, 325-341.

American Cancer Society's guide to complementary and alternative cancer methods. (2000). Atlanta, GA: American Cancer Society.

Cassileth, B. R. (1998). The alternative medicine handbook. New York: W. W. Norton & Co.

Cassileth, B. R. (1999). Evaluating complementary and alternative therapies for cancer patients. CA–A Cancer Journal for Clinicians, 49, 362-375.

Gould, R. L., Piver, M. S., & Eltabbakh, G. H. (1997). *Cancer and genetics. Answering your patients' questions.* Melville, NY: PRR.

Greenlee, R. T., Murray, T., Bolden, S., & Wingo, P. A. (2000). Cancer Statistics, 2000. *CA–A Cancer Journal for Clinicians, 50*, 7-33.

Schottenfeld, D., & Fraumeni, J. F. (1996). *Cancer epidemiology and prevention.* Oxford, England: Oxford University Press.

Willett, W. C. (1999). Goals for nutrition in the year 2000. *CA–A Cancer Journal for Clinicians, 49*, 331-352.

‡ Endnotes for Figures 1 and 2 (page 3).

Figure 1
*Per 100,000, age-adjusted to the 1970 US standard population. **Note:** Due to changes in ICD coding, numerator information has changed over time. Rates for cancers of the liver, lung & bronchus, and colon & rectum are affected by these coding changes.

Source: US Mortality Public Use Data Tapes 1960-1977, US Mortality Volumes 1930-1959, National Center for Health Statistics, Centers for Disease Control and Prevention, 2000.

American Cancer Society, Surveillance Research, 2001

Figure 2
*Per 100,000, age-adjusted to the 1970 US standard population. †Uterus cancer death rates are for uterine cervix and uterine corpus combined. **Note:** Due to changes in ICD coding, numerator information has changed over time. Rates for cancers of the uterus, ovary, lung & bronchus, and colon & rectum are affected by these coding changes.

Source: US Mortality Public Use Data Tapes 1960-1977, US Mortality Volumes 1930-1959, National Center for Health Statistics, Centers for Disease Control and Prevention, 2000.

American Cancer Society, Surveillance Research, 2001

CHAPTER 2

COMMON ISSUES FACING
ADULTS WITH CANCER

Nancy L. Wells, MSW, LCSW

Mary E. Turney, MSW, LCSW

The diagnosis of cancer is a universally feared phenomenon due to its associated risk of mortality and the potential impact the disease can have on all spheres of life. Research since the 1970s supports the belief that significant levels of distress are found among patients, their families, and significant others when faced with cancer, and that the disease can have immediate and long-term emotional, psychosocial, and behavioral consequences (Kornblith et al., 1992). In 1996, as an effort to recognize the psychosocial dimension of cancer among oncology professionals and improve this domain of care, a panel of representatives from the National Comprehensive Cancer Network (NCCN) developed standards of care for the management of distress (NCCN, 1999). To reduce the stigma of psychological problems and recognize the normalcy of the psychosocial aspect of the cancer experience, the panel recommended the use of the term "distress." The panel defined the term "distress" as it applies to cancer patients and their family members as the following: "Distress is an unpleasant experience of an emotional, psychological, social, or spiritual nature that interferes with the ability to cope with cancer treatment. It extends along a continuum, from common normal feelings of vulnerability, sadness, and fears, to problems that are disabling, such as true depression, anxiety, panic, and feeling isolated or in a spiritual crisis" (NCCN, 1999, p. 115).

A Framework for Understanding the Psychosocial Response to Cancer

The nature and sources of distress among cancer patients, their family members, and significant others are understood by utilizing the framework of identifying common issues at different stages in the disease: the cancer diagnosis, treatment, post-treatment, recurrence, and terminal illness (Christ, 1993). These stages of illness are recognized as potential crisis points in the lives of those affected by the disease, and often require mastery of adaptational tasks specific to the stage of illness in order to cope effectively.

In addition to recognizing the common issues at each stage of illness, it is also important to take into consideration other factors that affect an individual's or family member's psychosocial response and adaptation to the cancer experience. These include the following factors:

- *The type of cancer, including its stage and prognosis.* Those forms of cancer associated with a high risk of mortality and more intensive treatment have the potential of eliciting a higher level distress and more serious consequences to the patient's and family's lifestyle and quality of life.
- *The degree of disability the disease and treatment cause.* Individuals who experience loss of limbs or function, or who are disfigured as a result of the cancer or its treatment, face additional challenges in coping.
- *The intensity of treatment.* The length and aggressiveness of treatment and the severity of side effects are factors that can significantly affect physical and emotional functioning and sense of well-being.
- *The person's age and stage in the life cycle.* Tasks at one stage of the life

cycle can be disrupted with less impact than at another stage. For example, a young adult with cancer may face obstacles in performing important life tasks such as receiving an education, starting a career, and being independent. Delaying or not achieving these important life tasks can have detrimental consequences for successes in future years, impacting self-esteem, career achievements, and personal financial resources.

- *The person's past experience with cancer.* The degree of optimism and emotional and physical reserves available for employing coping strategies can be affected by the nature of previous experiences with cancer. Negative or positive past experiences can create additional challenges to individuals despite the diagnosis, treatment plan, and prognosis. Expecting similar experiences and outcomes can cause the individual or family member to have unrealistic feelings of hope or pessimism.

- *The person's current situation.* The individual's current status as it relates to quality of life, personal relationships, financial stability, access to health care, quality of health care insurance, concurrent stresses, life expectations, and existential outlook can affect one's psychosocial response to cancer.

- *Each person's unique emotional makeup.* Pre-morbid functioning and personality characteristics can affect the individual's response and ability to cope with the experience of cancer. Strong problem solving and communication skills, high self-esteem, success in personal relationships, trust in others, and spiritual beliefs are predictors of positive coping.

- *The degree of social support and caregiver availability.* The amount and quality of social support that is perceived by the cancer patient and family can affect the degree of distress. Support from friends, family, medical personnel, and other cancer survivors can provide a buffer against the harmful effects of stress.

- *Typical ways of coping with stressful situations.* A person's response to a previous crisis is often predictive of the coping strategies and skills which will be employed when facing the cancer experience.

POSITIVE CHANGES FROM THE CANCER EXPERIENCE: A THEME THROUGHOUT THE CONTINUUM

Individuals who have gone through cancer diagnosis and treatment often report that in addition to being harmed, they were positively changed by the experience (McMillen, 1999; Curbow, Somerfield, Baker, Wingard, & Legro, 1993). Recognition of the phenomena that there can be some gains that result from adversity is found in Frankl's classic publication on suffering and the search for meaning as a result of living through the Holocaust (Frankl, 1962). However, it was not until the 1990s that researchers began looking at what growth may occur from the cancer experience. In two studies of cancer survivors it was found that positive and negative changes were common, with positive changes more frequently reported than negative changes (Curbow et al., 1993). Researchers in several different fields have studied the effects of adversity as it relates to a spectrum of experiences including but not limited to cancer. The results of these studies revealed that several positive categories were proposed consistently and independently: changed life priorities, increased sense of self-efficacy, enhanced sensitivity to others, improved personal relationships, and increased spirituality (McMillen, 1999). Finding meaning in the experience, and thus recognizing the positives, is commonly reported by cancer patients. As a result of one's search for meaning, an individual's existential outlook may be affected. Beliefs related to life, death, and religion may change, bringing different world views and life structures. The search for meaning and other experiences related positively to cancer are not limited to one stage of illness, but are commonly reported throughout the continuum of experiences. Of course for many patients, the cancer experience will not bring about these positive changes. For some, it will be a permanent, negative, and life-altering experience.

THE CANCER DIAGNOSIS

When confronted with a cancer diagnosis, the patient and family often experience feelings of disbelief, shock, and panic. Depending on the individual's general sense of physical well-being and the degree and chronicity of symptoms leading to the medical work-up, the diagnosis may come as a startling surprise or it may be the confirmation of a dreaded fear. In either case, degrees of denial may occur, ranging from a healthy and naturally protective response to allow assimilation of the information and acceptance of the new reality to a pathological level of denial, which prevents successful coping and decision making about treatment options. Patients and family members often experience a sense of shock, report feeling dazed, not able to think clearly, have trouble remembering phone numbers and other routine information, feel a sense of being out of control, and feel vulnerable and afraid. Fears of dying, pain, mutilation or disfigurement, loss, and harm to loved ones through abandonment or burden are common regardless of the diagnosis, due to the common association of these outcomes with cancer in today's society. Guilt is often present, ranging from rational to irrational ideas about one's role in the causation of the disease. Some feel guilty about lifestyle choices that are known to be high risk factors for the development of cancer, such as smoking or sun exposure. Others feel responsible for their plight due to lack of routine screening or delay in seeking medical care. For some, guilt is related to irrational thoughts about why they developed cancer such as sinful or wrongful acts.

Cancer, like many illnesses, can elicit a sense of helplessness that makes the individual feel controlled by external forces. Individuals with a diagnosis of cancer become acutely aware of not being able to control or predict one's future or destiny. They fear loss of autonomy as a result of the disease, and often experience loss of independence in the health care setting.

Anger and hostility are common reactions. With some individuals, feelings of anger about having the illness are projected onto others. In these situations, hostility is often directed at family members or individuals in supportive or helping roles. This can lead to avoidant behavior by those who can potentially provide social support, causing the individual with cancer to feel isolated.

An existential crisis can occur with the diagnosis of cancer. A sense of being alone in life's journey can be evoked by the experience, causing feelings of isolation, alienation, and despair. However, existential exploration precipitated by the crisis can also lead to a greater sense of spirituality, providing some benefits to the patient in coping with the disease.

Concerns for family are often paramount, especially for those with children or aging parents. Newly diagnosed cancer patients worry about family members' emotional reactions and their wellbeing. They are concerned with how to communicate the news, what emotional and financial effects the cancer will have on family members, and whether they will be a burden to others. When cancer diagnoses are associated with heritable risk factors, the patient often worries about family members' chances of developing the disease and feels guilt for potentially passing along the genetic risk to loved ones.

Communication about the diagnosis is a common concern. There are questions about whom to tell and level of disclosure in relation to family, employer, and social network. Age appropriate information is important when explaining the diagnosis to children. Patients and family members are faced with decisions about communication, as well as many other important issues during the diagnostic stage of illness. These decisions may include: whether to seek a second opinion; choice of facility, physician, and treatment option; whether to complete an advance directive; genetic testing and counseling; participation in clinical trials; whether to seek alternative forms of treatment; and participation in integrative and complementary medicine programs.

Patients and families are confronted with many challenges during the diagnostic stage of illness. Mastery of these challenges fosters effective adaptation to the disease.

CANCER TREATMENT

Those embarking on cancer treatment may approach the initiation of treatment with a sense of ambivalence. It is a time frequently mixed with the relief of actively combating the illness while also experiencing distress regarding the uncertain immediate consequences and the final long-term outcome.

Several factors affect the impact of cancer treatment on patients, family members, and caregivers. The aggressiveness of the treatment regimen, side effects experienced, general physical health, disruption to routine and lifestyle, level of understanding about the treatment plan, age and point in the life cycle, tolerance of uncertainty, problem-solving capacity, relationship with the health care team, and availability of social support will collectively influence the ability of each person to manage the rigors of therapy.

Physical Reactions

While the range of physical symptoms will vary for each individual based on treatment modality and body constitution, there are several reactions that are common to many who undergo cancer therapies. This spectrum of symptoms may include fatigue, hair loss, mouth and digestive tract ulcerations, nausea and vomiting, diarrhea or constipation, weight loss or gain, susceptibility to infection, sexual dysfunction, decreased libido, pain, skin rashes, blood clotting problems, and sleep disruption.

Throughout the continuum of care, fatigue is the symptom most frequently reported by cancer patients in descriptive studies (Cella, Peterman, Passik, Jacobsen, & Breitbart, 1998). Its impact is felt on many levels (quality of life perception, self-esteem, and productivity) and numerous barriers often restrict its management. These can range from the oversight of the medical team to inquire about patients' fatigue to the acceptance by patients of fatigue as an inevitable and untreatable side effect. When properly evaluated, fatigue may be diminished by a variety of appropriate interventions aimed at treating its root causes or manifestations including administration of anemia therapies, energy conservation strategies, or restorative energy attempts.

Many treatment side effects can be essentially eliminated or minimized with the recent advances made in the development of new pharmacological agents for nausea and vomiting, neutropenia, and cachexia. These and other symptoms are treated most effectively when a trusting, productive partnership, formed between the patient/caregiver and health care team, aims to ensure the well-being of the patient under treatment.

As denoted in the NCCN (1999) guidelines for assessment and treatment of cancer-related distress, the range and degree of cognitive, emotional, and behavioral symptoms experienced by those living with cancer is wide. Certainly, pre-morbid personality traits and predisposition to mental health disorders influence the extent to which individuals manifest such reactions and require careful exploration prior to any intervention. Other variables such as treatment modalities, social supports, prognosis, intellect, and past experiences with serious illness will impact the capacity of those affected by cancer to cope psychologically with treatment.

Emotional Responses

The period of treatment presents many emotionally laden challenges to patients and their loved ones. Comprehending and monitoring the cumulative amounts of information necessary for informed participation and clear decision-making can be anxiety provoking for all involved. Mood swings and emotional lability caused by steroids and hormonal medications often prove unsettling even when attributed to the therapy received. Feelings of loss of control are not unusual as the treatment regimen dictates daily schedules, restrictions, and limitations. For some individuals, self-doubt or disillusionment may occur when the side effects of treatment are perceived to be more ravaging than the illness itself. Anxiety, depression, and fear, to varying degrees, can present difficulties for those affected by cancer throughout the treatment course.

Changes in Daily Life

The period of treatment poses many changes in lifestyle, routine, roles, and perspective for the person with cancer and the family and caregivers. Hospital and clinic visits as well as the administration of treatment at home by home health agencies dominate the lives and routine of cancer patients. Disruption or termination of employment and infringement on recreational activities is not unusual during this time. Increased dependence upon caregivers and family members inevitably changes the equilibrium within families and temporarily, at least, reverses roles that have been long established. Changed routines can evolve from the re-examination of lifestyle choices such as diet, exercise, and alternative therapies. Similarly, reflection while undergoing treatment for cancer can lead to an exploration of life-time goals and a resetting of priorities in life. Many cancer survivors discuss their shift in perspective regarding values and relationships as a result of the cancer experience made real by the treatment course. For some, this shift means a concern about burdening family and caregivers; for others, it strains or enhances intimacy and the search for connectedness. There is frequently a heightened appreciation of life and its many gifts as a result of the treatment experience.

Spiritual Issues

Recent psychosocial literature reflects increased attention to the significance of one's spiritual beliefs and faith system in coping with the cancer experience (Smith, 1995). For some, the reality of the cancer is brought home by the intensity of treatment and, as a result, reliance on a spiritual foundation for finding meaning and solace can be instrumental in coping. Prayer, rituals, sense of community, and a belief in the grand plan of a higher power can be very comforting to many. At the same time, the difficulties presented by treatment can challenge even the most firmly held beliefs and many individuals may feel conflicted as they face a perceived test of faith. Others may have strayed from a religious upbringing and feel guilt and self-blame about their illness because of this.

Practical Matters

The time of treatment is intense not only on an emotional, spiritual, and physical level but also in very practical ways as well. The cost of treatment and adjuvant out-of-pocket expenses can be financially perilous for even the most fiscally astute in the population. A constant hardship for many individuals is presented by the difficulty of understanding and managing the myriad number of medical bills and related insurance negotiations that are inevitable. Managed care intricacies, reduced income, and limited available resources can be very burdensome and frustrating. Frequent or long-distance trips to the treatment center pose transportation challenges for those unable to drive or without a network of persons able to assist with this need. Distance from the treatment site may require lodging away from home that can incur significant expense and deprive the individual of the corps of support available to them in their own community. Young families face separation from children during treatment courses or the hospitalizations that are necessitated by the complications of treatment. Invariably, childcare arrangements must be made that can be costly and problematic to arrange for consistency.

In addition to this disruption in family life, those who are employed face decisions and negotiations within the workplace. In collaboration with their oncologist, patients must determine their ability to work at all or on a flexed schedule, if permitted by the employer. Discrimination due to illness is unfortunately a factor that many persons must contend with in the workplace. Organizations such as the National Coalition for Cancer Survivorship (www.cansearch.org), Cancer Care (www.cancercare.org), the American Cancer Society (www.cancer.org), and the National Patient Advocate Foundation (www.npaf.org) can provide information and guidance to individuals who experience job discrimination. These practical issues can be the source of significant stress for patients, their caregivers and families throughout the treatment course.

POST-TREATMENT

The completion of prescribed treatment holds great significance for cancer survivors and their families. It is a milestone to be celebrated in the cancer experience, an event that symbolizes for many their successful victory over the cancer and expectation of resuming normal routines and lifestyles. Others view this time predominantly with dread, fearful that without the continuation of therapy they are unprotected from the likelihood of cancer recurrence. Frequently, it is a combination of both perspectives that influences the re-entry of the survivor.

Survivors are challenged after the successful completion of treatment to resume activities, employment, and relationships as before their diagnosis despite the possible existence of lingering physical and emotional sequelae from the experience. Individuals with permanent disabilities and intense side effects from cancer therapies (incapacitating fatigue, decreased libido, diminished cognition) must deal with a new reality as they shift focus from coping with treatment to adapting to life that is, perhaps forever, changed. Dissonance with family members and friends regarding expectations within this new reality can exacerbate an already frustrating situation.

A more daunting challenge for some survivors centers around the uncertainty and ambiguity that can persist following the completion of treatment. Referred to as the "Damocles syndrome" (Koocher & O'Malley, 1981), it is the nagging and, for some, disabling fear that cancer will reappear at some point. Blended with the relief of no longer having to endure the rigors and hardship of therapy is the apprehension of not knowing what to expect and dreading that recurrence is what awaits. Adding to this insecurity may be the perceived loss of the health care team in their pivotal supportive role as briefer and less frequent visits are scheduled. Those with low tolerance for ambiguity or with pre-existing anxiety disorders or other emotional problems are likely to be most vulnerable and suffer ongoing distress following the ending of cancer treatment.

RECURRENCE

The experience of cancer recurrence, while debated in the psychosocial literature as being more or less traumatic than the diagnosis phase, is clearly one of great distress for patients and their families (Zabora et al., 1997). Dashed hopes and dreams for long-term survival ensue. Sadness and anger are often expressed that despite every effort to comply with prescribed, often arduous treatment, it has failed to obliterate the cancer. Recrimination and, at times, mistrust of the medical team may occur as patients struggle to make sense of why the unthinkable has happened. Parallel to the period of diagnosis, patients are once again thrust into a situation of being presented overwhelming information in order to make critical decisions while feeling most out of control and emotional. It is at such times that individuals and their families feel highly vulnerable and are more likely to seek out alternative or "last-ditch" kinds of care.

Recurrence, as with all phases of the continuum, carries very individualized associations for each patient who must adjust to the news of progressive cancer. Certainly some forms of cancer are quite treatable and even curable despite recurrent episodes. However, in the vast majority of situations, the reappearance of cancer at the primary site or metastatic disease signifies the resistance of the malignancy to front-line treatment and the lessening of chances for survival. How this is perceived and accepted by patients and their families can vary drastically and will influence their adjustment to the crisis of recurrence.

For some individuals, learning of a cancer recurrence precipitates a realignment of priorities. If their length of survival is to be curtailed, they wish to place greater importance on certain relationships, activities, goals, and beliefs in the time ahead. Frequently, in their quest for some meaning out of the cancer experience, patients will turn to, rediscover, or initiate a spiritual connection to help with coming to terms with advancing disease and threatened mortality. Some individuals, however, experience a sense of alienation rather than connection with their spirituality or with those around them. Patients with recurrent cancer often struggle for a balance between hopefulness and realism in facing this phase of their illness. It is not unusual for some patients to maintain a stance of denial regarding the implications of recurrence for their long-term survival. Depending upon the quality of relationships and communication styles within families, serious strain can occur as family members struggle to support the patient without certainty of how hopeful or realistic to be. Similarly, some individuals view a recurrence in a most pessimistic and fatalistic way. Their ability to maintain any hope is limited and severely impacts their quality of life and that of those around them. The challenge for patients with recurrent illness is striving to achieve and maintain a balance in perspective about their future for whatever time there may be.

Familiarity with various forms of treatment and their side effects may alleviate some anxiety about resuming cancer therapy if the decision is made, in consultation with the physician, to pursue further treatment options. However, patients who have already experienced therapy are well aware of the many other hurdles (insurance complexities, child care, caregiver needs, employment or school absence) that must be faced in order to receive the best care. On several levels, the time of recurrence presents a series of existential, physical, emotional, and practical challenges to the cancer patient and the family.

TERMINAL ILLNESS

The terminal phase of cancer has been reported to be the most distressful to patients of all phases through the disease continuum (Zabora et al., 1997). Several factors can be attributed to this. Primary for most patients and their families is anxiety about pain and concern about the availability of pain relief during their limited time. Patients fear abandonment when cure is no longer the goal and need reassurance from the health care team that they will not be left to contend alone with intractable pain. Fears about the actual death and the circumstances surrounding and preceding it are prevalent. Concerns about the time frame in which the death is likely to occur, level of physical and cognitive incapacity in the period prior to death, actual conditions of the death, and the degree of pain and suffering to be expected are predominant. In a society in which the subject of death is avoided and often viewed as taboo, many myths and anxieties exist which can exacerbate the distress of the patient and family. On an existential level, questions about death itself, the concept of non-existence, and the quandary regarding life after death abound. For many patients, diminished functioning and imposed dependence on others for vital needs is a very distressing and frightening outcome. Intermingled with their fears of loss of control is a genuine concern about the well-being of caregivers who must assume a heavy load of responsibility, sometimes for prolonged periods of time. Additionally, patients face distress in feeling burdened by unfinished business that may or may not be possible to rectify prior to death.

As in any other phase of the cancer experience and undoubtedly even more so, the amount of social support available to the dying person is critical. Having caring, non-judgmental family, friends, and health care professionals in attendance alleviates many of the fears of the terminal cancer patient. Reliance also upon spiritual beliefs and rituals can provide great comfort and peace. Opportunities for life review with loved ones and staff brings closure and satisfaction for many.

Even at the terminal phase of cancer, patients or family are faced with decisions. These may include whether to enroll in an experimental clinical trial, receive palliative care only, whether to die at home or in the hospital, and whether or not to initiate hospice care. The role of hospice in providing in-home services, emotional, and spiritual support and assistance with managing the dying process cannot be overemphasized.

ADAPTATIONAL CHALLENGES

Throughout the course of the cancer experience, those affected by the illness are faced with many challenges. These challenges require mobilization of resources, use of problem solving skills, and the mastery of multiple tasks.

At diagnosis, the patient and family are faced with a life crisis that topples equilibrium and emotional balance. It requires sustained and deliberate effort over time to restore a sense of stability and well-being. In this early phase, patients and family members are confronted with the need to understand and integrate complex information about the disease and options for treatment. Additionally, the health care system is often an unfamiliar environment and requires new knowledge and skills to effectively navigate the maze. Frequently, care is received in more than one setting, requiring good communication, coordination, and organization of time. Negotiation skills are needed when interacting with billing, insurance, and managed care representatives. Common to all stages of illness is the challenge of living with uncertainty and the quest for meaning that a life-threatening diagnosis presents.

Cancer treatment thrusts those affected into a new realm of awareness and responsibility. As treatment progresses, patients are faced with the indisputable chronicity of the disease and the need to modulate their energy, interests, and emotions for the long haul. High-tech skills are being increasingly demanded of patients and caregivers within their own home and some may find these expectations to be beyond their capabilities. They are challenged day after day by the need to problem-solve and navigate the health care system in the manner that best ensures the well-being of the patient.

Maintaining healthy, supportive relationships with those most significant is crucial on many levels. The emotional support received can sustain a sense of hopefulness that is essential while experiencing the rigors of therapy. Practically speaking, no person can manage aggressive treatment regimens without the hands-on care of helpful caregivers. The ability of a support network in which open communication exists enables patients to balance the competing needs of self and family. During the treatment phase, the patient is often challenged with the resumption of work and leisure activities. In response to both the relief and fear of ending treatment, the patient often rejoices that treatment has been completed while attempting to manage anxiety and fear about possible recurrence. Normal life is resumed and new goals and aspirations are established. Family priorities are realigned and altered values and perspectives are integrated into family and social lifestyles. Information is sought about long-term side effects, risk of secondary malignancies, and genetic risks for family members. For some, adjustment to late effects of treatment is required.

At a time of recurrence the patient and family are confronted with decisions which need to be made about treatment options, including clinical trials. They need to understand and make choices about these alternatives as it relates to intensity of treatment, potential for cure, possible consequences, palliation of symptoms, and quality of life. Hope needs to be re-established, and sometimes reframed. If the expectation of a cure is not realistic, the patient and family can focus on other issues to find hope and inspiration.

Terminal illness brings many challenges to the patient and family. They are faced with the mourning of actual and anticipated losses, savoring and separating from loved ones, getting things in order personally and financially, living until death occurs, managing pain and other symptoms, finding meaning in life, and accepting the impending death.

SUMMARY

Individuals and their families face myriad issues and challenges when confronted with cancer. Each stage of illness carries its common concerns and stresses; however, many issues ebb and flow or remain constant throughout the continuum of the illness. Important to note is the uniqueness of each person's perception and psychosocial response to the experience. Distress at some level is expected universally; however, the intensity and degree of this distress is dependent on many variables. Challenges, as well, can be expected, and are mastered with differing levels of competency and skill for effective coping.

REFERENCES

Cella, D., Peterman, A., Passik, S., Jacobsen, P., & Breitbart, W. (1998). Progress toward guidelines for the management of fatigue. *Oncology, 12,* 369-377.

Christ, G. (1993). Psychosocial tasks throughout the cancer experience. In N. M. Stearns, M. M. Lauria, J. F. Hermann, & P. R. Fogelberg (Eds.), *Oncology social work: A clinician's guide* (pp. 79-99). Atlanta, GA: American Cancer Society.

Curbow, B., Somerfield, M. R., Baker, F., Wingard, J. R., & Legro, M. W. (1993). Personal changes, dispositional optimism, and psychological adjustment to bone marrow transplantation. *Journal of Behavioral Medicine, 16,* 423-443.

Frankl, V. E. (1962). *Man's search for meaning: An introduction to logotherapy.* Boston: Beacon Press.

Koocher, G. P., & O'Malley, J. E. (1981). *The Damocles syndrome: Psychosocial consequences of surviving childhood cancer.* New York: McGraw-Hill.

Kornblith, A. B., Anderson, J., Cella, D. F., Tross, S., Zuckerman, E., Cherin, E., Henderson, E., Weiss, R. B., Cooper, M. R., Silver, R. T., et al. (1992). Hodgkin's disease survivors at increased risk for problems in psychosocial adaptation. *Cancer, 70,* 2214-2224.

McMillen, J. C. (1999). Better for it: How people benefit from adversity. *Social Work, 44(5),* 455-468.

National Comprehensive Cancer Network. (1999). Practice guidelines for the management of psychosocial distress. *Oncology, 13 (5A),* 113-147.

Smith, E. D. (1995). Addressing the psychospiritual distress of death as reality: A transpersonal approach. *Social Work, 40 (3),* 402-413.

Zabora, J. R., Blanchard, C. G., Smith, E. D., Roberts, C. S., Glajchen, M., Sharp, J. W., BrintzenhofeSzoc, K. M., Locher, J. W., Carr, E. W., Best-Castner, S., Smith, P. M., Dozier-Hall, D., Polinsky, M. L., & Hedlund, S. C. (1997). Prevalence of psychological distress among cancer patients across the disease continuum. *Journal of Psychosocial Oncology, 15 (2),* 73-87.

CHAPTER 3

ONCOLOGY SOCIAL WORK
IN THE 21ST CENTURY

Diane Blum, MSW, ACSW
Elizabeth J. Clark, PhD, ACSW
Carol P. Marcusen, LCSW, BCD

Cancer patients and their families are found not only in medical and other health care settings, but also in their homes, offices, schools, places of worship, and other community settings. Social workers, regardless of their practice setting, will be presented with people struggling with cancer's impact. Cancer is characterized by both acute and chronic phases. Social workers will be intervening during periods of acute stress and disorganization as well as providing services designed to have an impact on long-term quality of life.

Psychosocial needs have become increasingly complex in recent years as treatment has shifted to the outpatient area, as patients are presented with more treatment choices, and as the patient and family bear increasing responsibility for managing care. Patients and families spend significantly less time with health care providers than in the past, and are expected to manage complicated treatment regimens on their own. With the improvement in symptom management, patients hope to continue to work and maintain consistency in their daily routines. This progress in lessening the debilitating aspects of cancer is one of the success stories of cancer treatment in the last decade, but it has created new challenges and burdens for the family.

The dramatic shifts in insurance reimbursement also have psychosocial impact. The movement to managed care has created situations in which recommended treatments may be postponed or denied. Patients frequently must become strong advocates for their own needs (Walsh-Burke & Marcusen, 1999), and at times even engage in legal battles to receive a certain treatment. Some managed care policies have helped patients and families improve their medical care with the inclusion of procedures such as regular cancer screenings. A decrease in complicated insurance filings has also relieved stress, but may be countered by delays in scheduling appointments with specialists. A significant change of recent years has been the explosion of outpatient drugs, many of which are not reimbursable under insurance plans, and the financial burden that this shift in costs has created.

As it always has, cancer continues to differ from other chronic illnesses in that it evokes our deepest fears about death and questions related to the meaning of life. Although increasing numbers of patients are surviving cancer, almost half will die from it. The impact of this reality on patients and professional caregivers cannot be minimized. Since professionals struggle with the same existential issues as patients, they can experience reluctance or ambivalence regarding involvement with this population. While personal feelings must certainly be addressed, social work with oncology patients offers significant opportunities to profoundly influence the quality of a family's experience with chronic illness. This potential to truly strengthen and enrich patient and family coping engages us in the practice of oncology social work.

SCREENING AND ASSESSMENT

Cancer patients are a diverse group whose pre-existing strengths and problems have significant impact on their abilities to cope with the disease process. Screening and assessment of individual psychosocial needs are crucial to developing a care plan that meets the specific concerns of patients and their families.

Screening

Since the 1970s, a body of social work literature has been developed describing screening mechanisms to determine who would benefit from social work services. Patients who are identified as high risk by a variety of criteria are contacted and evaluated by a social worker at the time of hospital admission. Because of the shift to outpatient care in the 1990s, there have been a number of studies to evaluate the effectiveness of screening which enables the social worker to assess needs in the outpatient area and to initiate service. Through both inpatient and outpatient screening, social workers can identify persons with cancer, chronic illness, or terminal illness as high-risk individuals who require routine assessment and intervention.

For the social worker who works exclusively with cancer patients, screening becomes more complicated; it may be impossible to routinely evaluate all patients. Since cancer patients receive most of their care as outpatients, both patient volume and setting make universal screening difficult. There are several methods of screening cancer patients that allow for the identification of patients in need of social work services.

UNIVERSAL CHART SCREENING

Universal chart screening involves routine screening of the demographic data and admission work-up recorded in inpatient and outpatient medical records. Factors such as age, marital status, insurance coverage, stage of disease, and type of treatment can all be indicators of high risk during the diagnosis and treatment of cancer.

> **Example:** A 35-year-old man, married and the father of two small children, with a new diagnosis of leukemia, and who lives two hours from the medical center, meets the criteria for a high-risk admission. The combination of aggressive treatment, predictable transportation, and lodging problems, and having young children indicates that he should be offered social work services.

Example: A 72-year-old man with recurrent colon cancer who lives alone following the death of his wife six months previously, meets the criteria for a high-risk admission. His recurrent disease and relatively new bereavement indicate that he should be offered social work services.

Example: A 42-year-old single woman is being treated as an outpatient with adjuvant chemotherapy for her newly diagnosed breast cancer. The medical work-up indicates two psychiatric hospitalizations in the past eight years for depression. Although this patient probably will not require hospitalization for her chemotherapy, her prior psychiatric history puts her at high risk for problems related to coping.

These examples indicate how routine chart screening targets patients who may benefit from counseling, education, and other services. In each setting, social workers can identify factors in the patient's environment that may cause the patient to be vulnerable to psychological and social problems. A systematic assessment of these factors by chart screening helps to identify these patients early in the treatment process. The obvious disadvantage of this screening method is that a review of demographic and medical data does not describe an individual patient's coping skills or resources outside of the immediate family. It also gives a picture of the patient at one particular point in time and does not predict adjustment to the disease over a period of months or years.

MULTIDISCIPLINARY ROUNDS

A weekly conference attended by representatives of the various disciplines involved in the patient's health care is an excellent screening method. It is an opportunity for discussion by the team members who have interacted with the patient and for the social worker to discuss the characteristics that may make an individual at risk for psychosocial problems. The disadvantage of this method is that it is difficult to ensure regular attendance by all members of the health care team. Multidisciplinary rounds that are sanctioned and approved by the various departmental administrations will be an effective format for setting priorities. Successful multidisciplinary rounds that have give-and-take among all the staff are both a cause and result of effective team functioning.

PATIENT SELF-SCREENING TOOLS

Several methods allow patients and family members to pinpoint their own needs. Checklists of needs can be distributed to patients through the admitting office or through any registration process, and completed manually or electronically. Patients can use checklists to describe their individual needs for help in areas such as transportation, home care, communicating with physicians, communicating with family members, or work concerns. Use of these checklists also allows patients to become aware of social work services. The social worker's prompt follow-up response to requests for service is crucial to the success of this kind of screening.

The disadvantages of this method are that many patients do not take the time to complete a checklist, the data must be collected and stored by a staff person in the medical facility, and the checklist describes needs at only one particular time. The checklist, however, can include information that tells the patient that social work services are available at any time. Such information should include the social worker's name and telephone number.

PSYCHOLOGICAL DISTRESS SCREENING

The literature suggests that there are three crucial points of high distress for cancer patients over the disease continuum. These occur at initial diagnosis, at recurrence or progression of the disease, and at the terminal stage. Studies indicate that screening patients for psychological distress at these points using a brief distress screening tool and a problem list can be an effective way of identifying those patients most in need of the services of a social worker (Zabora et al., 1997). To fully appreciate the value of this screening method, a review of the National Comprehensive Cancer Network practice guidelines for distress management is helpful (www.nccn.org). Again, the disadvantages of this method are that data must be collected and scored by a staff person in the facility and the screens must identify needs at the crucial points.

Assessment

Psychosocial assessment is the process by which the oncology social worker evaluates the particular needs of the cancer patient and those of the patient's family. Assessment involves a psychosocial history, a beginning treatment plan, and communication of needs and the plan to other health care team members. The strength of social work lies in the ability of its practitioners to assess people within the context of their environment. This is particularly crucial in oncology social work, where cancer has an impact on the patient not only in the medical setting, but also at home and at work. Social workers in a medical setting frequently must obtain psychosocial information in an environment of interruptions, space constraints, and lack of understanding of the social worker's role. Often, information is gathered from several sources. The oncology social worker must be flexible, must have knowledge of the disease process, and must possess an understanding of how illness and treatment can affect an individual's psychosocial well-being.

In a classic book, Weisman (1979) presented seven questions that remain excellent assessment tools for the social worker:

1. What problems, if any, do you see this illness creating?
2. How do you plan to deal with them?
3. When faced with a problem you must do something about, what happens? What do you do?
4. How does it usually work out?
5. To whom do you turn to when you need help?
6. What has happened in the past when you have asked for help?
7. What kinds of problems usually tend to get you down or upset?

These questions elicit information about the patient's priorities, usual coping skills, and sources of support that is used to determine patients' concerns about treatment, work, insurance, family issues, and ability to cope. The answers are not always predictable. A patient, for example, may say that her major problem is her husband's recent stroke and her own diagnosis of cancer is something she must get through so she can resume care of her husband. A patient may identify a friend or co-worker as a source of support rather than a family member. Answers may indicate that a person is not accustomed to talking about feelings or problems, or that professional help for problem solving has typically been sought. The information gathered from this assessment process, along with the social worker's knowledge of the patient's cancer diagnosis and the method or methods that will be used to treat it, help the social worker to:

- Place the patient at a particular developmental stage
- Make a clinical prediction about how the patient and family will fare in this particular system
- Evaluate the priority that should be given to the patient in the context of many other referrals
- Evaluate what the particular health care system offers the patient and family
- Evaluate what resources are available outside of the setting to meet the needs of the patient and family.

Often, the oncology social worker may feel rushed in carrying out this evaluation and developing an intervention plan. Despite the short time that may be available for the process, the plan should be as specific as possible, describing steps that the social worker will undertake in assisting the patient and the family in dealing with their needs. The social worker's responsibility is to help other professionals understand how a patient will cope with the diagnosis and treatment and what interventions will be helpful to the patient. An articulate assessment and a clear-cut plan enhance patient care and clarify the important role of the social worker on the oncology team.

Understanding the Disease

Cancer encompasses many different diseases and rapidly changing theories of treatment. The social worker may have difficulty keeping up with new information, but an understanding of concepts such as stage of disease, local versus systemic treatments, and risks and benefits of treatment is important. Vocabulary that describes specific cancers, the terms to explain dosages of chemotherapy, radiotherapy, and hormonal therapy, and knowledge of diagnostic tests are also valuable to the social worker whose caseload includes cancer patients. The social worker who is knowledgeable about the treatment for and prognoses of specific types of cancer is better able to help patents set priorities, make choices, and experience a greater sense of control.

Learning about cancer can be accomplished in many ways. In a hospital setting, patient charts, multidisciplinary rounds, and conferences all provide the social worker with opportunities for understanding the disease. The social worker's participation in patient and family meetings in which medical information is being delivered is also quite useful. In a nonmedical setting learning may be more difficult, but opportunities are available. Excellent patient education and professional education materials produced by organizations such as the American Cancer Society (www.cancer.org), the National Cancer Institute (www.nci.nih.gov), and the Leukemia and Lymphoma Society (www.leukemia.org), all available online, may be useful learning tools. Interaction with physicians and nurses, field trips to hospices and day hospitals, and observations of procedures are all methods of learning medical information. The oncology social worker must be able to understand the reality of the patient's physical needs. Administrative staff involved in establishing social work services for cancer patients should also provide the social worker with opportunities for learning.

Accessibility of Services

Most of the requests for oncology social work services stem from a person who is experiencing crisis. In 1967, Oppenheimer wrote, "The diagnosis of cancer with all of its implications can be counted on to precipitate a state of crisis of varying intensity and duration for nearly every patient." More than 30 years later, social workers see many crisis points during the course of cancer. For example, moving away from treatment and intense medical scrutiny can be as unsettling as starting treatment. Certain individuals may cope effectively with cancer at first but will experience a crisis as they begin to deal with a side effect such as hair loss. Other patients and families cope well with every need and demand until the patient requires intense physical care.

A social worker should be accessible when the patient experiences a crisis. Access to social work services can be built into well-designed assessment tools. Orientation sessions for new cancer patients are useful for letting patients and their families know about the availability of social work services. Geographic location of the social worker in relation to where patients are, a visible office, good telephone coverage, Internet access, and continuity of care all work to make services available to the patient when they are needed.

The effectiveness of an oncology social work program will be realized only if the services are well publicized. Patients and the health care staff must have knowledge about a social worker's function. Brochures, needs-assessment checklists, videotapes, and educational presentations all inform the patient about potential problems that may be alleviated by a social worker's intervention. As patients become knowledgeable about predictable problems and available services, they are helped in identifying their own needs and in seeking timely social-work intervention.

INTERVENTIONS

Basic Principles of Oncology Social Work Interventions

Social work services for cancer patients and their families must reflect the following principles:
- Social work interventions must be based on an understanding of the patient's specific cancer diagnosis and treatment plan, as well as on the patient's emotional and social situation.
- Social work services for cancer patients and their families should be accessible. Most individuals with cancer need help during a time of crisis and they should be able to have direct access to a social worker.
- Oncology social work services are designed to help patients and their families feel more in control of a situation that predictably makes them feel helpless and out of control. Interventions should be focused on helping people cope with

the medical, emotional, and social problems they encounter at different points in the cancer experience.

The diverse population of cancer patients has needs that vary over time. A comprehensive program encompassing counseling services, resource utilization, and education will be most effective in meeting the changing needs.

Social workers offer a range of social work services, or interventions, to cancer patients and their families. Clinical experience with cancer patients has shown that the entire range of human behavior is reflected in individuals who develop this disease (Christ, 1993). The choice of interventions depends on the particular needs and issues identified through screening or assessment. Some, such as referral to financial assistance programs, may occur only once. Others, such as counseling, may continue throughout treatment or be provided periodically around crisis points or when specific issues must be addressed, such as planning for discharge or for continuity of care in the patient's home community. Social work interventions are likely to be most effective when patients and health care professionals are knowledgeable about the comprehensive nature of needs and when the social worker is flexible and capable of using various clinical strategies (Fawzy, Fawzy, Arndt, & Pasnau, 1995).

Individual Counseling

Social workers in oncology spend considerable time with patients or family members discussing responses to the cancer diagnosis and problems created by it. At each stage of the disease, the patient may be faced with difficult decisions, with feelings of being overwhelmed, with communication problems at home or at work, or with personal feelings of helplessness and hopelessness. Injuries to self-esteem, feelings of dependence, and fear of pain and death are commonly experienced by the person with cancer. Through individual counseling the social worker can help the patient to focus on specific concerns and to set priorities.

An important part of the individual counseling session is that it may allow the person with cancer to express feelings and ideas that close family members have been unable or unwilling to hear or discuss. Many cancer patients feel that their psychological stress is a sign of weakness that makes them less competent in coping with cancer. Realistic reassurance and what social workers call universalization are important therapeutic techniques. The ability to tolerate and accept the patient's intense emotions (e.g., anger, hostility, bitterness, severe anxiety, profound sadness, depression) is an important therapeutic skill, especially when those emotions are associated with dying.

When working with cancer patients, the social worker must be aware that time is short, whether limited by the setting or the patient's physical condition, and counseling needs to be tailored to the patient's energy and the progression of the illness. It is important to understand that traditional psychotherapy may not be appropriate for all settings. Counseling is provided to help patients and their families manage the problems associated with chronic illness. While this process is therapeutic, the goal of social work intervention more frequently is not intrapsychic change. In many settings, social workers have the qualifications to provide psychotherapy. When this is not the case, those social workers should be knowledgeable about clinicians who are capable of providing psychotherapy to meet the unique needs of cancer patients. Individual counseling in oncology social work has much to do with asking questions that elicit feelings and concerns and listening carefully to the patient's answers. The following are examples of specific questions:

- What is your understanding of what is happening? What are your ideas about what will happen over the next few days?
- How have you been feeling emotionally through all of this? How can I be helpful to you?

These questions encourage patients to describe what they are experiencing and allow them to express whatever feelings they are having. Useful responses by the social worker include:

- I see you look at things cheerfully. Do you ever have dark moments?
- The way you feel is so understandable. Many people in your situation express similar feelings.
- You have been through so much recently. This would be difficult for many people. How has it been for you?

Individual counseling sessions frequently elicit a sense of the patient's despair and the social worker, as well as the patient, can be overcome by feelings of sadness and futility. Trying to maintain or redefine hope is an important goal of social work counseling. Oncology social workers have many resources for helping patients manage their despondency and distress and to feel that life is still worth living. Clinical experience teaches that most patients and families possess a natural inclination to retain hope (Farran, Herth, & Popovich, 1995). The following are general guidelines for structuring individual counseling for the oncology social worker:

- Choose a place to talk where there is some privacy, perhaps over the telephone or online
- Ask questions that are broad enough to elicit emotions
- Listen carefully to answers, paying specific attention to feelings, and observe nonverbal behavior
- Try to focus on one issue at a time
- Convey hope without creating unrealistic expectations
- Select interventions that are purposeful and address mutually agreed upon goals
- Review what has been discussed and set up a time for another contact.

Group Counseling

PURPOSE OF GROUPS

Group counseling can be an effective social work intervention for cancer patients and their families. People with cancer frequently express a sense of isolation and feelings of being unprepared for coping with this unexpected crisis in their lives. The ability to meet others in similar circumstances, to share methods of coping, and to develop new relationships at a time of perceived isolation are all factors that encourage people to attend groups. Groups also play an important role in increasing the participant's knowledge of cancer and in offering specific techniques to deal with a complex health care system. Support groups, which are useful at all stages of the disease, focus on coping with, adapting to, and living with cancer

(Cella & Yellen, 1993).

ROLE OF THE GROUP LEADER

Leading a cancer-related support group is a demanding, challenging experience. The leader always plays a vital role as the provider of support and guidance to all group members. In essence, the leader has the primary responsibility for setting the tone for the group, beginning with a screening interview and continuing throughout the group sessions.

Within the constraints of efficient use of staff, co-leadership of groups provides some advantages. If one leader is unavailable, the co-leader can provide continuity. It also enables the leaders to share and process emotionally difficult information more effectively. Co-leadership with other disciplines provides a blending of skills. For a population struggling with both the physical and emotional impact of illness, co-leadership by a social worker and a nurse provides one such example.

The most important task for the group leader is to create a safe atmosphere in which members feel free to participate, without fear of judgment or ridicule. To accomplish this, leaders must be active forces in the group and consistently demonstrate, by verbal and nonverbal behaviors, that they can be trusted. No real work begins toward problem resolution until such a climate is established.

GROUP STRUCTURE

Support groups may be open-ended, with constantly changing membership, or they may be time-limited, from 6 to 12 sessions. The open-ended group is harder to lead because new members are constantly changing the group composition and there may be no opportunity for screening. The open-ended group, however, is sometimes the only practical format in inpatient settings or in communities with limited resources. Consideration should be given to the use of the telephone or Internet to provide support groups since these methods may overcome the barrier of physical attendance. The leader of the open-ended group, whether the group is offered in person or through technology, must actively integrate new members into the group and prevent undue repetition. Both open-ended and time-limited formats may provide education, using written materials, speakers, or videotapes. The educational component is useful in both recruiting members and in maintaining the interest of participants, who often come to the group looking for answers to questions.

GROUP START-UP AND COMPOSITION

Support groups provide a cost-effective service to a large number of patients and families. The start-up time of organizing a group and recruiting members is often lengthy, however, and months may pass before the social worker sees the timesaving advantages of a group.

Groups can be organized by stage of disease, diagnosis, age, or other common factors such as treatment modality. As a group becomes more homogenous, it becomes easier for the leader to focus its work. An 8-session group composed of people who have Hodgkin's disease, for example, will deal with a more consistent set of issues than a group made up of people with a range of diagnoses. Similarly, patients with newly diagnosed cancers may be reluctant to participate in a group with patients who have metastatic disease. Other groups may be developed on the basis of age or relationship to the person with cancer, for example, adult children or spouses of cancer patients. The social worker, however, may want to include a more diverse population in order to launch the group. Although this is a practical approach, particularly if the social worker is just beginning a group program, it is more difficult to focus a group with a diverse composition and to ensure that its members feel a sense of accomplishment.

EVALUATION

The completion of a group series that has had steady attendance and participation by members is exhilarating for the social worker and justifies the preparatory work. Objective evaluation of the group, however, is helpful in planning another group and also in convincing administration and other staff that groups are an appropriate intervention. Evaluation need not be complicated or elaborate, but should provide some objective measure. (See end of this chapter for a sample evaluation questionnaire.) For additional, in-depth information about support groups, readers can contact their local ACS office to order the publication entitled *Cancer Support Groups: A Guide for Facilitators* (ACS, 2001; Code #4660).

Family Counseling

Abrams (1974) was an early pioneer in recognizing the effect of cancer on the entire family. Spouses, parents, children, and siblings are affected by the disease, particularly when it becomes a chronic illness, and the equilibrium of the family is disrupted for extended periods.

Family members frequently express concerns that are remarkably similar to those of the patient. These feelings include helplessness, confusion, and anger. Spouses and children may experience feelings of guilt because they may become impatient with the person who is sick. Grown children may have difficulty dealing with a parent's illness, especially if the relationship has been troubled. Also, caring for the cancer patient may burden a family financially and exhaust them physically, a problem that is more and more common with decreased hospitalizations and extended survival. Family systems or their individual members may bring dysfunctional coping systems to the cancer experience. Social workers need to recognize these situations and tailor their expectations and interventions accordingly.

The following is an example of a situation in which family functioning is disturbed by the mother's cancer.

> **Example:** A 48-year-old woman with widespread cancer is the mother of three girls, ages 13, 16, and 18, and the wife of a 50-year-old postal worker who works the night shift. Both parents individually report heavy drinking by the oldest daughter, school problems for the 16-year-old, and serious problems in managing household responsibilities. The patient and her husband both express to the social worker, but not to one another, their wish that "the illness would not drag on much longer" because they are exhausted. They have never discussed the prospect of the mother's death with the daughters.

This example demonstrates the need for comprehensive social work services. The family had home care needs, each parent expressed hopelessness and guilt, and the children were reported to be engaged in maladaptive behavior. The social worker used a variety of resources and interventions to help the family manage their difficult situation: holding counseling sessions with the parents and children, making the children aware of programs and materials for their specific needs, advocacy for the children in their schools, and offering homemaker assistance. The social worker also encouraged the couple to share their feelings about the wife's eventual death with one another and with their daughters. This helped to decrease the isolation each family member had experienced. Most significantly, by viewing the family as a unit and involving all of them in planning, the social worker offered them the opportunity to share their mutual distress and regain some of the closeness they had before the mother's illness.

Direct support of family members, both individually and in groups, is based on principles similar to those used to offer support to the patient. Specific educational programs and written materials for spouses, children, and parents are valuable in addressing and focusing attention on their particular needs. Resource utilization such as assistance in transportation and home care directly benefits family members, and volunteer visitor programs offer the family a respite from caregiving. When providing support to the family, the social worker must view the family as a unit, communicate with them as an entity, and help them to communicate with one another.

Behavioral Interventions

Social workers have successfully incorporated behavioral techniques into their repertoire of skills and have used these interventions with individual patients and in groups (Behar, 1999). In this era of shrinking health care resources, behavioral methodologies may represent more cost-efficient service delivery. Another advantage of these modalities is that patients are less dependent on the professional staff for help. They can be taught the techniques to use whenever they experience difficulty with emotional reactions to the illness or treatment.

Social workers may also use a relaxation or guided-imagery exercise as part of their group sessions. The group leader asks the members to concentrate on specific parts of the body and to relax each one until the whole body feels relaxed. Visualization of scenes or activities that are restful and create pleasurable thoughts is another technique that works well in groups. These exercises promote a sense of relaxation and calmness and allow the members to feel more in control of their feelings. Using this kind of imagery requires training, which can be accomplished by attending conferences or workshops on the subject.

Hypnosis, imagery, meditation, relaxation training, and music therapy have all been used in the management of cancer pain. Knowledge of these techniques and skill in using them are helpful to the social worker on the multidisciplinary team. Training in hypnosis is required and is now available to the social worker in many settings. The ability to help patients control their pain and enhance their sense of control over the illness is a significant clinical intervention.

Behavioral techniques are now an established part of comprehensive cancer treatment. Patients, families, and other staff members are often appreciative of behavioral interventions that have a positive impact on the patient's behavior or mood. As social workers in oncology define and broaden their roles, behavioral techniques will continue to emerge as an area for training and professional activity.

Bereavement Counseling

Bereavement counseling is another intervention about which social workers should be knowledgeable (Clark, 1997). The availability of such counseling will vary depending on the type of setting and staff resources. Hospice programs, for instance, are mandated to provide bereavement care if they are accredited by the Joint Commission for the Accreditation of Health Care Organizations (JCAHO). In settings such as comprehensive cancer centers, social work intervention for family members is often included in the package of available services. At the very least, social workers should be knowledgeable about community resources that offer bereavement care to offset the effects of long-term illness and death upon survivors.

In dealing with an illness such as cancer, it is important to realize that grieving occurs at many points in the illness experience for both patients and their families. People often begin this experience grieving for the loss of predictability and certainty in their lives. Normally, people do not require mental health intervention to deal with serious loss. Most people, however, do not know what to expect in the immediate acute phase and in later stages of bereavement. Social workers can provide this kind of education and should take advantage of the many excellent resources available to educate themselves (Worden, 1991; Rando, 1993). (See Chapter 13 for more information regarding end of life issues.)

In terms of services, individual bereavement counseling is perceived as a luxury that many acute care hospitals are unable to provide. If this is the case, social work departments might want to develop a standard bereavement protocol designed to assess how a family is resolving its loss. For instance, routine telephone contacts at one, three, and six months might give the social worker enough information to determine whether bereavement is proceeding normally or if complications have arisen. Hospitals or community agencies might experiment with time-limited bereavement support groups as a way of offering a more cost-efficient service. Groups are particularly helpful for the bereaved due to the normalization experience that occurs. Bereavement groups help to lessen the impact of patient loss and provide a way for families and staff to begin again.

Resources, Information, and Advocacy

The cancer patient faces many potential needs: financial assistance, transportation, home care, prostheses, insurance coverage, and medical equipment. Interventions that focus on providing these services directly or information about them not only assist patients in obtaining the medical and nursing care they require but also have beneficial psychological and social impact. Examples might include:

- The provision of an attractive wig will have a positive impact on body image and self-esteem
- Facilitating the process of securing supplemental income fosters independence
- Assisting patients who need transportation to and from treatment relieves one burden of anxiety about the ability to comply with the regimen.

Oncology social workers must be knowledgeable about guidelines for assistance programs in various communities and must have an understanding of how laws are applied to the rights of cancer patients (Hoffman, 1998).

DISCHARGE PLANNING

Discharge planning is the process of putting advocacy, information programs, and direct service together. It is a clinical social work activity in which psychological, social, and specific interventions are combined to develop a treatment plan that meets the needs of the patients. Hospital-based social workers who are responsible for discharge planning assess the individual patient's needs, identify the most significant problems, and develop a treatment plan with the patient that uses family and community resources. Discharge planning begins with a psychosocial diagnosis of the patient and extends over the entire period of hospitalization. The event of discharge is simply the culmination of these earlier processes.

EDUCATION

Education is effective in helping cancer patients and their families understand the cancer diagnosis, use medical care effectively, and obtain access to the resources of their community. Education has also been identified as a method to help patients cope psychologically with their cancer and it complements other interventions. Individual counseling includes helping the patient to learn about the disease and teaching communication skills. This knowledge can be imparted as part of the counseling process and supplemented by written materials. Group treatment, as well, can incorporate specific educational components using speakers, videotapes, and brochures. Highly structured groups with preplanned topics help patients deal with the enormous amount of information presented to them when they are treated for cancer. These educational groups are effective in both inpatient and outpatient settings.

Workshops that focus on topics such as coping with chemotherapy, communicating in the health care system, and using community resources can be offered to large numbers of people. Patients and families who are reluctant to attend a group or to use individual counseling may be comfortable participating in a workshop that has a didactic format. After specific information is presented, discussion groups offer the attendees an opportunity to present their own problems. This type of workshop helps individuals become more knowledgeable and also helps participants to realize that their questions and concerns are not unique to them.

PROGRAMS THAT REACH THE UNDERSERVED

Poverty, a lack of adequate health care coverage, and limited access to available resources can have a devastating impact on those diagnosed with cancer (Haynes & Smedley, 1999). Underserved families generally have fewer resources and limited access to information, basic health care, and screenings. Those with cancer are often diagnosed at advanced stages, and have more difficulty coping with their illness effectively, sometimes leading to a lack of treatment compliance and a diminished quality of life. Social workers are committed to the underserved and, in oncology, take leadership roles in developing programs that meet the special needs of patients and families with fewer resources.

Program development for the underserved should include literature reviews, needs assessments, multidisciplinary and community collaboration, and an evaluation of existing patient education materials. Multicultural and bilingual programs must be offered that reach actively into the community and solicit input and support from identified community leaders. Concerns as varied as transportation, competing financial needs for everyday obligations such as rent, and discomfort in a large medical setting all can interfere with quality medical care. This role is a challenging one as there are many people who are uninsured or underinsured, and entitlements have become more difficult to utilize and more limited in scope. The social worker is the key member of the team to recognize these barriers to care and the professional who can best mobilize resources to overcome the impediments to diagnosis and treatment.

USING TECHNOLOGY TO EXTEND SERVICES

Despite the development of many excellent and comprehensive psychosocial support programs that are consistent with the goals described in this chapter, there continue to be formidable barriers to psychosocial services. People with cancer often remember little of what they are told in medical settings; they spend brief periods of time in a clinic or physician's office, and often then may be isolated from resources in their community; and they have many demands on their time as they strive to maintain routine in their lives. As a result of these factors, social workers have looked to the telephone and Internet to provide patients and families with the information and support that they need (Bucher, Houts, Glajchen, & Blum, 1998). (See Chapter 14 for more information on accessing oncology resources through technology.)

SUMMARY

A broad range of social work services is necessary to address the many psychosocial concerns of cancer patients and their families. With knowledge, experience, and creativity, the social worker has a pivotal role in patient care. Social workers offer comprehensive services through effective screening; sound psychosocial assessment; carefully designed and implemented interventions such as individual, family, and group counseling; use of behavioral techniques; linkage to community resources; program development; assistance with bereavement; discharge planning; and consultation, teaching, and research.

Advances in treatment offer prolonged survival and mandate increased attention to the quality of that survival. This is the challenging arena in which social workers, with their expertise, can make a significant contribution in the health care setting as well as in the community.

SAMPLE GROUP EVALUATION QUESTIONNAIRE

Group Leader: _____Date:_____

In an ongoing effort to improve our services, we evaluate each group series and invite comments from group members. All questionnaires are confidential and no names are requested.

Please take a few minutes to think about your group experience. Answer each question by placing a check next to the response that best applies to your experience in the group.

1. What made you decide to join this group?
____(a) To learn how to deal more effectively with my family member's illness
____(b) To acquire more information about cancer and its treatment
____(c) To talk with other people in a similar situation
____(d) To meet new people
____(e) To help others by offering information, suggestions, or support
____(f) Other (please explain)_____
_____
_____
_____

2. What has been most helpful to you about the group?
____(a) Learning that others experience thoughts and feelings similar to my own
____(b) Obtaining information about cancer and its treatment
____(c) Sharing my experiences and problems with other group members
____(d) Learning how to express my feelings
____(e) Belonging to and being a part of a group
____(f) Helping other group members
____(g) Obtaining suggestions and advice
____(h) Improving my communication skills
____(i) Other (please explain)_____
_____
_____
_____

3. During the group discussions, which topics were most relevant to you?
____(a) Communicating with physicians
____(b) Making decisions about cancer treatment
____(c) Dealing with uncertainty about the illness

_____(d) Dealing with feelings of guilt and anger
_____(e) Dealing with life-style changes
_____(f) Relationships with family and friends
_____(g) Stress management
_____(h) Financial planning
_____(i) Concerns about the future
_____(j) Other (please explain)_____

_____

_____

_____

4.   What were the most helpful methods used by the group leader?
_____(a) Providing information
_____(b) Offering direct suggestions
_____(c) Encouraging general discussion
_____(d) Providing written materials
_____(e) Sharing anecdotes and examples
_____(f) Encouraging role-playing
_____(g) Drawing out thoughts and feelings
_____(h) Other (please explain)_____

_____

_____

_____

5.   What aspects of the group would you suggest changing?
_____(a) Number of group members
_____(b) Number of group sessions
_____(c) Group meeting room
_____(d) Style of group leader
_____(e) Mix of group members
_____(f) Topics of group discussion
_____(g) Time of day group was held
_____(h) Other (please explain)_____

_____

_____

_____

6.   Which changes, if any, have you experienced as a result of your participation in this group?
_____(a) A greater ability to reach out to others for help and support
_____(b) An improvement in social responsibilities
_____(c) An improvement in communications with others

____(d) An improvement in family relationships
____(e) A greater sense of self-confidence
____(f) An improved ability to adapt to changes in my life
____(g) An improvement in work relationships
____(h) A greater trust in groups and other people
____(i) Other (please specify)_____
_____
_____
_____

7.   If you had friends in a similar situation, would you recommend this group to them? Yes_____ No_____ If not, why?_____
_____
_____
_____

8. What suggestions/additional comments do you have?
_____
_____
_____
_____
_____
_____
_____
_____
_____
_____
_____

Thank you for your time and comments. We greatly appreciate your suggestions.

REFERENCES

Abrams, R. D. (1974). *Not alone with cancer.* Springfield, IL: Charles C. Thomas.

American Cancer Society (2001). *Cancer support groups: A guide for facilitators.* Atlanta, GA: American Cancer Society.

Behar, L. C. (1999). Social work with adult cancer patients: A vote-count review of intervention research. *Social Work in Health Care, 29*(2), 39-67.

Bucher, J., Houts, P., Glajchen, M., & Blum, D. (1998). Telephone counseling. In J. Holland (Ed.). *Psychooncology* (pp. 758-766). New York: Oxford Press.

Cella, D.F., & Yellen, S. B. (1993). Cancer support groups: The state of the art. *Cancer Practice, 1*, 56-61.

Christ, G. H. (1993). Psychosocial tasks throughout the cancer experience. In N. M. Stearns, M. M. Lauria, J. F. Hermann, & P. R. Fogelberg (Eds.), *Oncology social work: A clinician's guide* (pp. 75-99). Atlanta, GA: American Cancer Society.

Clark, E. J. (1997). The end of the continuum. *Cancer Practice, 5*(4), 252-254.

Farran, C., Herth, K., & Popovich, J. (1995). *Hope and hopelessness: Clinical constructs.* Thousand Oaks, CA: Sage Publications.

Fawzy, F., Fawzy, N., Arndt, L., & Pasnau, R. (1995). Critical review of psychosocial interventions in cancer care. *Archives of General Psychiatry, 52*,100-113.

Haynes, M. A., & Smedley, B. D. (1999). *The unequal burden of cancer.* Washington, DC: National Academy Press.

Hoffman, B. (1998). *A cancer survivor's almanac: Charting your journey.* Minneapolis, MN: Chronimed Publishing.

Oppenheimer, J. R. (1967). Use of crisis intervention in casework with the cancer patient and his family. *Social Work, 12* (2), 44-52.

Rando, T. A. (1993). *Treatment of complicated mourning.* Champaign, IL: Research Press.

Walsh-Burke, K., & Marcusen, C. (1999). Self-advocacy training for cancer survivors. *Cancer Practice, 7*(6), 297-301.

Weisman, A. D. (1979). *Coping with cancer.* New York: McGraw-Hill.

Worden, J. W. (1991). *Grief counseling and grief therapy: A handbook for the mental health practitioner* (2nd ed.). New York: Springer Publishing.

Zabora, J., Blanchard, C. G., Smith, E. D., Roberts, C. S., Glajchen, M., Sharp, J. W., BrintzenhofeSzoc, K. M., Locher, J. W., Carr, E. W., Best-Castner, S., Smith, P. M., Dozier-Hall, D., Polinsky, M. L., Hedlund, S. C. (1997). Prevalence of psychological distress among cancer patients across the disease continuum. *Journal of Psychosocial Oncology, 15(2)*, 73-87.

CHAPTER 4

CHILDREN OF CANCER PATIENTS: ISSUES AND INTERVENTIONS

Joan F. Hermann, MSW, LSW

Social work intervention with the families of young and adolescent children is one of the most exciting areas of oncology social work. Children facing a serious or life-threatening parental illness may be at high risk for adjustment reactions during a cancer experience, and for many years afterwards if the parent should die (Worden, 1996). Intervention with this group of families represents an opportunity for preventive work that is well within the social work practitioner's repertoire of skills.

For social workers new to the field, it can also create significant anxiety as professionals learn to feel competent with this population. This anxiety is related to three issues. One is an almost primitive fantasy that children can be protected from such a devastating reality as the potential loss of a parent. Unfortunately, this is not possible, but children do possess the capacity to learn to deal with this threat to their daily lives and to their futures. A second source of anxiety is a perceived lack of knowledge or skills in working with children. Social workers without direct experience with children may fear that they might unwittingly damage a child if their intervention is incorrect. Fortunately, children are not that fragile and they do not suffer permanent damage because of an ill-conceived explanation or use of language. The third source of anxiety centers on parental resistance to intervention, especially if the parent is newly diagnosed and does not yet have a trusting relationship with health care staff. Most often this resistance is based on anxiety and uncertainty rather than unwillingness to deal with the issues. The task confronting the social worker is to enable parents, as the child's best source of security, to help their children cope. A child's adjustment to catastrophic illness is intimately connected to the quality of parental coping. Most social work intervention will focus on parental coping rather than on direct work with children.

This chapter offers social workers new to oncology basic knowledge upon which to develop intervention skills applicable to this population of vulnerable children and their families. The material is discussed in relation to the predictable phases of the cancer experience: diagnosis, cure or survivorship, progressive and terminal illness, and bereavement.

ISSUES AT DIAGNOSIS

Providing Information

Giving correct information about the diagnosis of cancer and how it will be treated is the first and most important step in helping a child deal with a parent's diagnosis.[1] For many parents, this is an extremely difficult task to master as it threatens them at their most vulnerable point. Parents can become overwhelmed, as they incorrectly assume the imagined reactions of their children to be identical to theirs. Social workers need to reassure parents that young children do not have the same intellectual awareness of or emotional reaction to cancer as do adults. For this reason, children usually will not demonstrate the shock, anxiety, and fear of death characteristic of

---

[1] Videotape describing how patients can talk to their children about cancer entitled, "Talking About Your Cancer: A Patient's Guide to Helping Children Cope." Call the Fox Chase Cancer Center at 215-728-2668 for a brochure and order form.

the diagnostic phase. Parents often think that they may be able to shield their child from knowledge of the diagnosis as long as they can continue to behave normally. This is not possible because life is far from normal for a family grappling with a cancer diagnosis. Children absorb the unspoken anxiety of their parents and intuitively know that something is very wrong. The energy used in trying to keep cancer a secret is an enormous strain. At a minimum, children should be told the name of the disease (cancer), the site (part of the body affected), and how the disease will be treated. The child's most immediate psychological need is for security, so the uncertainties in the child's world need responses. The child's concerns such as "Who will cook dinner if mom's in the hospital?" or "Who will take me to baseball practice?" must be addressed. The child must be given the message that even though the family is faced with a serious problem, parents are still in charge and are planning for the disruption in family life associated with the initial treatment course.

Obviously, the explanation of cancer will differ, depending on the child's age and developmental stage. For young children, a parent may say something like the following: "Cancer is a growth that is usually called a tumor. A tumor is something that shouldn't be there. The tumor is made up of thousands of cells that grow too fast and eventually grow into other parts of the body where they don't belong. By treating the tumor, the doctors will try to make the bad cells go away." Older children need more information; they are exposed to cancer via the lay press, health education classes in school, people in the community or their peer group or perhaps the experience of cancer in a grandparent or other relative. The principle of giving children appropriate information is sound regardless of prognosis. The focus should be on living with a chronic illness, unless treatment is known to have failed and the focus must shift to dealing with progressive disease and palliation.

Because of the egocentric nature of childhood, children also need to be told that it is not anyone's fault that cancer has happened. As in divorce situations, children often think they are the cause of family problems but rarely will ask directly if they are to blame. Children need to know that it is extremely unlikely that the other parent will get sick and that they themselves will not get cancer. Parents are universally afraid of being asked if they or the patient will die. If this question is asked, parents need to respond with something with which they are comfortable. A social worker may help parents rehearse their answer to this question so that the parents feel prepared and in control. Possible answers might be, "Many people are cured of cancer these days, that's why I'm getting treatment" or "We are all going to die one day. I'll tell you if that is something you should be worrying about."

While questions about death are extremely threatening, parents will feel more in control of themselves and their lives if they are able to deal with their children's questions and fears. Since the primary task of parenthood is to help children cope with life, parents and their children will experience relief in tackling problems together with the implicit message being, "As a family we can cope with this." Social workers can be extremely useful in helping parents to sort out overwhelming feelings and to find appropriate ways to communicate with their children.

It is important for a child to understand how cancer is to be treated and what side effects the parent is likely to experience. Surgery can be explained as an operation in which the doctor removes the tumor; the parent will not be awake so it will not hurt. Because the idea of a parent being "cut open" can produce powerful fantasies in a young child, it is important that children be permitted to visit in the hospital as soon after surgery as possible. They should be prepared for what they may see: the parent with bandages, intravenous (IV) bottles, feeling and looking sick. The trappings of hospital care are often fascinating to children, not horrifying as some adults expect. As long as a parent is able to communicate with a child, a hospital visit offers powerful reassurance that the child has not been abandoned.

The side effects of chemotherapy should be explained before they occur so that children know what to expect. Hair loss and nausea can be explained as temporary and a sign that the drugs are working. Children should know that their parent under treatment may be "grouchy," tire and have less patience, and that it is not the child's fault if the parent is more irritable. If radiation therapy is planned, children can be told that side effects will vary, depending on the area of the body being treated. Depending on their age, children should be told that the parent is not "radioactive." It is extremely useful for children to visit the outpatient setting on a day when treatment is not planned. Children should meet the treatment staff (e.g., chemotherapy nurses, radiation therapy technologists), see where the treatment will take place, and be reassured that what is to happen is in the parent's best interest.

Preserving Family Routines

A child's ability to master the impact of parental illness will be greatly enhanced by preserving the child's routine as much as possible. Extended family and friends can be called upon to enable the child to continue extracurricular activities and lessons so that life remains as much the same as is possible. Young children should not be removed from the family environment, if at all possible. It may be tempting to suggest a visit to a grandparent if a parent is having difficulty with the demands of parenting, but this often reinforces the child's fantasies of abandonment. School age and adolescent children should continue their studies, with the message that parents expect the same behavior and attention to lessons as before. Social workers can suggest that a parent communicate with the child's teacher or guidance counselor so that they may be alert to a child who is having difficulty at school.

During this period, it is useful to assign children specific, age-appropriate tasks to accommodate the necessary changes in household routines. This helps the child feel included in the family's experience. Adolescents may take on more responsibilities than younger children, as is age appropriate. Teenagers should be helped to know that parents are not abdicating their responsibilities, only postponing them for a period of time.

Likewise, parents should adhere to the same guidelines on discipline and other issues as before the illness. This may impose more stress on the well parent, but most children will feel out of control if suddenly the usual family rules no longer apply. Social workers can be helpful during this time by helping parents establish priorities, reach out to extended family (especially for single parents), suggest "family meetings" in which parents and children can discuss issues (Harpham, 1997), and offer support during this very stressful time. Community agencies may be useful for homemaking assistance, help with transportation, and/or other services.

Support groups for children whose parent has cancer can be extremely effective in teaching children about cancer and helping them to verbalize their anxieties about a parent's illness. While there are many models of how these groups can be organized (Bedway & Smith, 1996), it is the author's belief that any support program for children should always be planned with a parent's groups happening concurrently. Children should be grouped with others at a similar developmental stage and engaged in activities designed to help them express feelings and worries (e.g., art, working with clay, games, medical equipment, and journaling[2]).

Adolescents may feel especially burdened during periods of active treatment because they realistically can assume many parental duties (Harpham, 1997). Although parents can expect more of adolescents, they should be aware that the teenager needs relief from family responsibilities, special "thank you's," and time to be with peers and carry on usual activities. A social worker working with several families may offer group meetings for teens as a means of reducing the isolation that teenagers may be feeling. Social workers can be very helpful in enabling families to make family life accommodations to serious illness. The social work role is one of anticipation and education; parents usually know their children best, but they cannot know the potential effects of serious illness until it is experienced.

Developmental Considerations

A child's developmental needs continue in spite of parental illness, so social workers need to be aware of some general principles.

---

[2] Kid's Night Out. (1998). A workbook to be used by children and their parents to express how they feel about a family member's experience with cancer. It uses art, games, and storytelling to help parents and children communicate. Call the Fox Chase Cancer Center at 215-728-2668 for a brochure and order form. Bulk rates are available.

Helping seriously ill parents support their children's developmental needs can be challenging but ultimately reassuring to parents struggling to cope. The way a child reacts is most often reflected in his or her behavior. Young children may appear to lose ground or regress if their world is threatened. For instance, children who are fully toilet trained may start having accidents. Two- and 3-year-olds, who normally are very adventuresome in exploring their environments, may become unusually clingy. First-graders who have adjusted well to starting school may resist going to school and display exaggerated separation anxiety. For children who cannot articulate their worries, parents will know by their child's behavior if they are anxious about changes in the household or in their relationship to their parents. During these times, parents may need to offer extra attention to their children. If a parent is feeling too ill, other family members may be called upon to manage the situation temporarily.

School-age children have the advantage of being able to verbalize their feelings and have more resources outside of their immediate families to help them cope. School personnel should be informed of parental illness so the child's responses can be understood within that context.

Parental illness can be particularly difficult for adolescents, who are in a developmental stage of separation from parental figures (Hilton & Elfert, 1996). Teens achieve this separateness by gradually testing their limits until they feel safe and more confident in who they are and where they are going. When this process is interrupted precipitously by illness, young people may remain "stuck" in the ambivalent relationship, feeling resentful and having trouble achieving independence. This is especially true if teens are asked to take over parental responsibilities temporarily. Social workers, by helping parents anticipate the developmental needs of their children in relation to chronic illness, can make a substantial difference in how parents can continue to support age-appropriate independence for their teenage children.

SURVIVORSHIP

Unanticipated Complications

Nearly 50% of cancer patients treated today will achieve long-term survival or cure, so it is important to consider the impact of this on developing children and adolescents. For the parent, believing that the disease is under control or cured is often difficult. Many people describe the pervasive anxiety that characterizes medical follow-up appointments. Fortunately, most children react to what they experience and if a parent looks and feels well, they often cease to feel threatened. There are situations, however, in which children can have difficulty. Depending on age, some children may have made significant gains in assuming more responsibilities and feel resentful if the parent is not able to appreciate their growing independence. Children can also experience anger toward the recovered parent, as it is now psychologically safe to express such feelings. If a parent has been idealized during illness, children can feel tremendously guilty about angry feelings and need reassurance that it is normal to have such negative thoughts. No family is ever the same following a cancer diagnosis, so children will have had to adjust to whatever changes were necessary in family routines and roles. Children who assumed responsibilities of the sick parent can develop a pseudo-maturity that is inappropriate to the parents' recovery. This situation needs monitoring in order to prevent "parentification" of the child. ("Parentification" means a reversal of roles in which the child seems to be caretaking the parent.) One study of the adjustment of young breast cancer patients reported that these women often turned to their children as a source of support (Lewis, Zahlis, Shands, Sinsheimer, & Hammond, 1996). The impact of extended long-term treatment may have financial and social implications. A troubled marital relationship may worsen or dissolve and children may have to endure that threat to their identities and security.

Interventions

Because of the nature of the health care delivery system, social workers are less frequently consulted about the problems associated with cancer survivorship. Social work departments in hospitals need to consider what the absence of such services will mean to children and their families. Other models of intervention might be considered if staffing does not permit reaching out to cancer survivors. These models include the following:

1. distributing psychosocial information routinely through ambulatory care departments or pediatricians' offices
2. integrating content concerning children into support/educational groups
3. reaching out to educators and school counselors, an often overlooked source of help in the community
4. helping parents access the Internet as long as people are warned about outdated or incorrect information
5. contacting the American Cancer Society and other national or community agencies which offer specific information about the needs of children with a sick parent. The American Cancer Society can be accessed by calling 1-800-ACS-2345 or at their web site at www.cancer.org, Children and Cancer section. Call 1-800-4-CANCER (www.cis.nci.nih.gov) to reach the National Cancer Information Service.

ISSUES OF PROGRESSIVE ILLNESS

Engaging Families

The ability of a social worker to be truly helpful to families facing progressive disease will depend on many factors, not the least of which is the social worker's skill in connecting with a family in crisis. Families are often more amenable to help during crisis points and social workers should take advantage of this in assessing the needs of children. Even if children have been told very little about the parent's condition, they often know a great deal based on the parent's appearance, behavior, and interaction with medical caregivers (Mireault & Compas, 1996). The social worker's role at this point in the illness is an enabling and educational one. Parents need suggestions as to how they will facilitate the child's coping. Social workers are sometimes uncomfortable with such an active role, fearing that the clients' right to self-determination will be undermined. However, it is important for social workers to realize that most parents have no way of knowing about how children best cope with this experience. It is the social worker's responsibility to share information about how other families have coped, so parents can make an informed choice about how to best help their children.

Providing Clear Information

Children should be given information gradually, and it should be tailored to the reality of the medical situation. For instance, if a parent has experienced a first recurrence of the disease and will require more aggressive treatment, children can be told that the doctors will be using "stronger medicines" to control the situation. If a parent has widely metastatic disease, children can be told that the doctors are worried that the medicines are not working as well as they did in the past. Children most often take their cues from what they physically experience. If a parent looks well, as some people with advanced disease do, a child may not realize the meaning of disease progression. In such situations, it is even more important that communication continue to occur. It is always useful to solicit a child's perception of what is happening with a sick parent so that information can then be tailored to that reality rather than something which the child has not even considered. For example, a simple "What have you thought about how Mom is doing?" can be the starting point in the dialogue.

For adolescents, this can be a particularly trying time because they realistically can be given more responsibilities around the house but still need to meet school and social responsibilities. Teenagers still need to maintain boundaries between themselves and a sick parent and should be encouraged to participate in as much of their outside activities as possible. Parents need to be watchful of inadvertently putting the teen in the position of "parent substitute."

In contrast to other illnesses, cancer usually occurs over a prolonged period of time. Children and adults will have a period of time in which to prepare for the eventual loss. For a child, the loss begins when the parent is no longer able to interact with the child in the usual way. If a father is too sick to go to a ball game, an uncle might substitute. If a mother is not able to shop for a prom dress, another relative may offer to do so. While it is healthy for a child to be able to adapt to these parental substitutions, they engender feelings that must be acknowledged. The well parent might say, "It is great that Uncle Harry likes baseball too, but I know you would rather be going with your Dad. It makes me angry too that he is so sick." Children sometimes need permission to be angry. While it is not a "rational" response to he angry at someone who is ill, it is nevertheless a very common and human response. Children who are unable to express these feelings bear a far greater burden and the potential for psychological damage is more likely.

Preserving Positive Memories

A child or adolescent may begin to withdraw from parental relationships, especially if a parent is unable to physically respond to his or her needs. At this point, it can be useful to give the child certain tasks that will help in the care of the sick parent. This enables the child to stay connected to his or her parent, albeit in a different manner, and it supports the child's mourning process with positive memories of the relationship. Some children are reluctant to be involved in actual physical caretaking. Depending on their age, it may be too "intimate" a relationship for the child to deal with, in which case there may be other roles they may fulfill like reading to a parent, helping to open the mail or any number of similar jobs. Sometimes children who help bring medications to the bedside for instance might be upset and feel responsible for the medicines "not working." Some might also have underlying worries about "catching" cancer or misunderstand their parent's irritability or withdrawal as directly related to something the child has done rather than advancing disease. So, if a child is reluctant to be involved in actual caretaking activities, it will be important to accept that reality but explore the resistance so the child is not left with the burden of inappropriate guilt or regrets.

ISSUES OF TERMINAL ILLNESS AND BEREAVEMENT

Talking About Impending Death

A child or adolescent must he prepared for the expected death of a parent. This preparation will be much easier when the child has been included in the illness experience from the beginning. If this has not been the case, parents usually realize at this point that this information needs to be communicated. Many parents find this conversation too painful to have and need the help of a relative or the social worker to facilitate. For ill parents who feel guilty about their inability to take on this very difficult task, the social worker might suggest that they write letters to their children expressing their love and hopes for them. Some dying parents can communicate with their children by making an audio or videotape. These kinds of activities can do much to help children retain a positive memory of a parent they have lost.

For the well parent or relative faced with telling the child about their mother or father's eventual death, the anxiety will be substantial. If possible, parents should be encouraged to do this themselves, as they will achieve a tremendous sense of mastery by doing so. A parent may need a social worker's help to prepare for the conversation, but the social worker should not attempt to take over this responsibility unless the parent is totally unable to do so and requests assistance. The social worker may help the parent to role-play how the dialogue may go, so the parent feels as prepared as possible. Depending on age, the course of the illness, and family circumstances, a child may have already begun the process of withdrawal from the sick parent. If this has happened, it is useful to use that reality in the service of the child's understanding. For example, saying "You know that Daddy has not been able to play baseball with you for a while" may help reinforce the child's understanding of what will happen.

The reactions of children to impending parental death depend on several factors including age, how much preparation they have received since the initial diagnosis, their relationships to both the sick and well parent, their own coping mechanisms, and the availability of social support. Some important concepts for parents to know include the following:

- Prior to age 5 or 6, children are unable to comprehend the finality and universality of death. Children will often ask when "Mommy is coming back."

- Death can be explained as not being able to see, hear, feel, or be with us anymore. For example, "We will not see Mommy anymore, but we will be able to remember her through pictures and stories."

- Illness and death are not anyone's fault. "We did not cause Dad to be sick (or die) when we were angry with him" and "It is okay to be angry that Dad died. He loved you very much and did not want to leave" may be appropriate responses.

- It should not be assumed that adolescents need less by way of information or will be more able to resolve the loss because they are more mature. Because of their developmental struggles and conflicted or ambivalent relationship with a parent, they may in fact need more monitoring than younger children who might be more accessible in terms of feelings and reactions to a dying parent.

Bereavement Rituals & Issues

Social workers can be enormously helpful to parents facing the bereavement phase of the illness. The most pressing need is to give information in anticipation of the actual event and family bereavement rituals. The issue of a child's attendance at the parent's funeral is a useful example, as this is typically controversial. This is an area, however, where social workers can share their knowledge about children's reactions to funerals, so that parents can make a decision that is right for them. While children need preparation for a funeral, they receive considerable benefit from attendance. Funerals can be explained as, "The way we say goodbye to someone we love." It can be useful to explain who will be there, what the service will be like, that people will be upset, and how the child is expected to act.

The younger a child is, the harder it will be to understand death. A funeral is a tremendous help in the child's reality testing of that event. When the 5-year-old cannot understand that Mommy will not be there for Christmas, the memory of the funeral can be reinforced as a way to help the young child understand. Although parents may be tempted to exclude children from the funeral ritual, feeling that it may be too emotional, confusing, or upsetting, it should he pointed out that children may interpret this to mean that death is so dreadful that it is not possible to cope with it. Parents unwittingly may also give the message that the child is not part of the family and that their relationship to the deceased is unimportant. Families will do what they can tolerate, but the exclusion of children from this significant event can have lasting, long-term repercussions (Christ, 2000).

Obviously, death will be explained to children according to a family's cultural and religious beliefs. For families with a strong spiritual life, the combination of death with afterlife is a more comforting association than for families for whom such an idea is less certain or unacceptable. For those families, children are better able to tolerate an honest "I don't know" than explanations that do not fit into a family's belief system. The social worker's belief system is immaterial, but it can be useful to point out some of the areas of conflict that some religious beliefs can produce for children. Examples are "God chose Mommy to be with Him in Heaven" (resulting in anger at God) or "Daddy is watching you from Heaven" (which can interfere with spontaneity and the natural experimentation of childhood). Children should also be offered the opportunity of talking with the family minister, priest, or rabbi in their attempts to make sense out of a loss as profound as that of a parent.

Children are often quite sensitive to incongruities in the way adults deal with death. They wonder about the family gathering that often occurs following the burial, since this event can look to them like a party. Likewise, adults may misunderstand the grief of a child and incorrectly assume that it will follow the same pattern as that of an adult. Young children express their grief in abbreviated doses and are incapable of the intensity or depth of expression characteristic of adults. Children for example, may cry for brief periods of time but will typically use the safety of play activity to manage their feelings. Children's sadness and grief will be manifested in their behavior, which can become regressed or provocative as a way of signaling their distress.

Parents know their children best, but it is useful to help a parent put their child's behavior into the perspective of what is usual in understanding how to respond effectively. Parents may need to be reminded to model their own feelings for their children, such as by saying, "I feel so sad today that Mom isn't with us anymore," especially if a child is not sharing his or her feelings with anyone. The surviving parent should remember to tell the children that death is no one's fault, and that specifically, the children did not cause their parent to die. This is one of the most common thoughts reported by children dealing with the death of a parent. Social workers can do much to help parents prepare for this uncharted territory.

Parents also need to be educated about the typical course for childhood mourning. Children often seem to have a more protracted grief experience than do adults due to developmental changes and the child's changing ability to understand and process the death as they mature. Children can experience feelings of intense grief during periods of their lives in which the parent's participation would be significant such as a graduation, wedding, holidays, or upon the anniversary of the parent's death.

Specialized Referrals for High Risk Children

There will be some children who are not able to successfully resolve the loss of a parent without specialized help. Worden (1996) has identified ten specific "red flag" behaviors that, if they persist for several months, signal the need for a professional evaluation by a child therapist. These behaviors are:

- persistent difficulty in talking about the dead parent
- severe aggressive behavior
- serious anxiety which is inhibiting of the child's normal activities
- somatic complaints like stomach or headaches or the development of psychosomatic disorders

- sleeping disturbances
- eating disturbances such as overeating or not eating well
- marked social withdrawal
- school difficulties or serious academic reversal
- persistent self blame or guilt
- self-destructive behavior or expressions of wanting to die.

Social workers also need to realize that surviving parents will be unable to facilitate the children's mourning process if their own bereavement needs are unmet. A parent who has no outlet for feelings will be unable to respond to the needs of his or her children. Therefore, the social worker who is offering bereavement services facilitates a resolution for the entire family.

INTERVENTIONS

Many interventions are available to social workers involved in the management of serious loss for children. These include individual and family counseling, support groups, complementary therapies, the use of educational materials, and the use of the hospital environment to reinforce the reality of a parent's death. The nature of those services will depend on the nature of the contract between client and social worker.

Support Groups

Support groups are extremely helpful in all stages of the cancer experience, but especially so with the bereaved. While social workers can educate about what to expect, that information coming from someone who has experienced it may be more meaningful. The person who believes that his or her loss will never be resolved can discover that many different kinds of resolution are possible. Bereavement groups are also quite helpful for children. For young children, they typically take the form of play or art therapy and offer the bereaved child an acceptable way to move through the feelings of aloneness and abandonment that the loss of a parent produces. Information about such groups can be obtained by contacting the social work departments of major cancer centers, hospice programs, the Association of Oncology Social Work (www.aosw.org), and the American Cancer Society (www.cancer.org).

In addition to such traditional services, social workers can be helpful in utilizing the available medical environment to help children understand the terminal illness of a parent. Family meetings with the physician can be arranged to provide children an opportunity to learn what to expect. Hospital visits to sick parents can be arranged without fear of damage to children. As long as a parent is able to communicate, such visits are extremely useful to the child and reinforce reality in a very concrete way. If a parent is not conscious, a visit can still be a powerful way for a child to test reality, as long as the child is prepared for what to expect (McCue & Bonn, 1996).

Help-Rejecting Families

Many families will use the help offered by social workers but some families will be uninterested in what is available. While this is frustrating, parents generally do the best they can; social workers who are too aggressive in their desire to help will most likely, incur a negative response. If we somehow communicate that families are not living up to our expectations, they will feel judged and reject our efforts to help in order to protect themselves from the implied criticism. Families may isolate themselves and a relationship that might be less threatening after a death has occurred is thwarted. Families who are resistant to intervention during the illness might accept reading materials, contact with another parent who has successfully dealt with the experience, and may be more responsive to a social worker's outreach following a death.

Hospice programs offer routine bereavement follow-up. If a patient has not had hospice services, social work follow-up should certainly be offered. This may be difficult in many hospital environments in which services are being restricted rather than expanded, thus making knowledge of community resources important.

It is also very useful for social workers to experience directly how families are able to work through the bereavement process and successfully resolve a loss. That perspective actually represents the "hope" in the practice of oncology social work and should be experienced first hand in order to enrich and balance the professionals' experience. It also gives the professional a perspective against which to judge the "normal" bereavement process in contrast to a more pathological process.

SUMMARY

Only in recent years have the needs of children of adult patients been recognized and given attention. Much remains to be learned, especially in the area of research designed to demonstrate the effectiveness of intervention with this group of children. What is known from clinical experience is that social workers have the opportunity to positively influence the quality of the families' experience with catastrophic illness. In dealing with the impact of cancer, social workers usually have the advantage of a process that occurs over time. During that experience, with its predictable crisis points, parents can be helped to monitor and engage their children in ways of coping with the potential of serious loss. Families bring their own internal resources to the experience. Within the context of a supportive relationship, they can often begin to utilize these strengths in helping children understand the reality of serious illness.

Social workers can sometimes feel immobilized by the challenges faced by these young families and the ultimate unfairness of life. However, it is in helping families meet the challenges that the unfairness becomes tolerable and the impact of cancer is reduced to problems that are amenable to solutions. The loss of a parent in childhood is a devastating reality, but social workers have much to offer in helping families confront the tasks of illness and move toward healing and resolution.

REFERENCES

Bedway, A. J., & Smith, L. H. (1996). "For kids only": Development of a program for children from families with a cancer patient. *Journal of Psychosocial Oncology. 14(4),*19-28.

Christ, G. H. (2000). *Healing children's grief: Surviving a parent's death from cancer.* New York: Oxford University Press.

Harpham, W. S. (1997). *When a parent has cancer: A guide to caring for your children.* New York: Harper Collins.

Hilton, B. A., & Elfert, H. (1996). Childrens' experiences with mothers' early breast cancer. *Cancer Practice, 4,* 96-104.

Lewis, F. M., Zahlis, E. H., Shands, M.E., Sinsheimer, J.A., Hammond, M. A. (1996). The functioning of single women with breast cancer and their school-aged children. *Cancer Practice, 4,* 15-24.

McCue, K., & Bonn, R. (1996). *How to help children through a parent's serious illness.* New York: St. Martin's Press.

Mireault, G. C., & Compas, B. E. (1996). A prospective study of coping and adjustment before and after a parent's death from cancer. *Journal of Psychosocial Oncology, 14(4),* 1-18.

Worden, J. W. (1996). *Children and grief.* New York: Guilford Press.

CHAPTER 5

THE MEDICAL DIAGNOSIS AND TREATMENT OF CHILDHOOD CANCER

Philip A. Pizzo, MD

OVERVIEW OF PEDIATRIC MALIGNANCIES

Fortunately, childhood cancer is uncommon. In the United States, approximately 8,600 new cases of cancer are diagnosed in children younger than 15 each year, or fewer than 1% of all malignancies. During the past decades, major strides in the treatment of children with cancer have been made. The overall 5-year relative survival rate for cancers diagnosed before age 20 has risen to 74.9%, and 10-year survival is approaching 70%. There is every reason to believe that further advances will occur as a result of ongoing research.

Nonetheless, a diagnosis of cancer has devastating implications for the child, the family, and the community. Many children diagnosed today face a potentially fatal outcome and nearly all experience side effects of therapy. These side effects can be acute, chronic, extremely incapacitating, and detrimental to growth and development. All persons involved in the care and treatment of children with cancer should be aware of the rationale behind current therapeutic strategies and understand their risks and benefits. While the future might bring ways to lessen toxicity and improve treatment efficacy, the current approaches to therapy, though highly successful, place tremendous demands upon the patient, the family, and the medical team. The insights gained from research and the development of effective therapies for pediatric malignancies have formed the foundation for the principles of pediatric oncology, as well as guideposts for the treatment of adults with cancer.

Epidemiology

The cancers that occur in children differ significantly from those that arise in adults. The most notable difference is the initial response of most childhood cancers to current therapeutic modalities, resulting in a significant number of cures (Pizzo & Poplack, 1996). This encouraging aspect of treatment relates to the nature of the cancers that occur in children. Cancers of epithelial or differentiated cells predominate in adults, and cancers of embryonal or developing cells and tissues predominate in children. Pediatric malignancies are characterized by a high growth fraction or a higher rate of tumor cell multiplication, enabling the tumors to increase in size more quickly than in many adult malignancies. Unlike in adults, pediatric malignancies tend to be generalized or systemic illnesses at the time they are diagnosed. A tumor in a child that appears to be localized to bone or to a soft tissue nearly always involves microscopic spread to other body organs, although this may be undetectable at the time of initial diagnosis.

Age, sex, race, and geography are important factors in defining pediatric malignancies. Table 1 presents the cancers that predominate in children by age and site. Some cancers that are observed soon after birth (e.g., neuroblastoma or retinoblastoma) suggest a genetic basis for their occurrence. Other malignancies appear to peak during early childhood (e.g., acute lymphoblastic leukemia), or others tend to arise during the periods of growth and development associated with adolescence (e.g., osteosarcoma, Ewing's sarcoma, and rhabdomyosarcoma). Age can also influence the outcome for the child with a malignancy. For example, children younger than 1 year of age with neuroblastoma tend to fare well, whereas the prognosis is much poorer for children with the same tumor who are older than 2 years of age. The incidence of pediatric malignancies appears to be slightly higher in males, for reasons that are not clear.

TABLE 1

Predominant Pediatric Tumors by Age and Site

TUMORS	NEWBORNS (<1 yr)	INFANCY (1-3 yr)	CHILDREN (3-11 yr)	ADOLESCENTS & YOUNG ADULTS (11-21 yr)
HEMATOLOGIC MALIGNANCIES				
Leukemias	Congenital leukemia AML AMMoL	ALL AML CML, juvenile	ALL AML	AML ALL
Lymphomas	Very rare	Lymphoblastic	Lymphoblastic Burkitt's	Lymphoblastic Burkitt's Hodgkin's
SOLID TUMORS				
Central Nervous System	Medulloblastoma Ependymoma Astrocytoma Choroid plexus papilloma	Medulloblastoma Ependymoma Astrocytoma Choroid plexus papilloma	Cerebellar astro- cytoma Medulloblastoma Astrocytoma Ependymoma Craniopharyngioma	Cerebellar astro- cytoma Astrocytoma Craniopharyngioma Medulloblastoma
Head & Neck	Retinoblastoma Rhabdomyosarcoma Neuroblastoma	Retinoblastoma Rhabdomyosarcoma Neuroblastoma	Rhabdomyosarcoma Lymphoma Multiple endocrine neoplasia	Lymphoma Rhabdomyosarcoma Multiple endocrine neoplasia
Thorax	Neuroblastoma Teratoma	Neuroblastoma Teratoma	Lymphoma Neuroblastoma Rhabdomyosarcoma	Lymphoma Ewing's sarcoma Rhabdomyosarcoma
Abdomen	Neuroblastoma Mesoblastic nephroma Hepatoblastoma Wilms' tumor (>6 mos)	Neuroblastoma Wilms' tumor Hepatoblastoma Leukemia	Neuroblastoma Wilms' tumor Lymphoma Hepatoma	Lymphoma Hepatocellular carcinoma Rhabdomyosarcoma
Gonads	Yolk sac tumor of testis (endodermal sinus tumor) Teratoma Rhabdomyosarcoma (sarcoma botryoides) Neuroblastoma	Rhabdomyosarcoma Yolk sac tumor of testis	Rhabdomyosarcoma	Rhabdomyosarcoma Dysgerminoma Teratocarcinoma, Teratoma Embryonal carcino- ma of testis Embryonal carcino- ma & endodermal sinus tumors of ovary
Extremities	Fibrosarcoma	Fibrosarcoma Rhabdomyosarcoma	Rhabdomyosarcoma Ewing's sarcoma	Osteosarcoma Rhabdomyosarcoma Ewing's sarcoma

ALL, acute lymphocytic leukemia; AML, Acute myelogenous leukemia; AMMoL, acute myelomonocytic leukemia; CML, chronic myelogenous leukemia

Note. Adapted from Pizzo, P. A., Horowitz, M. E., Poplack, D. G., Hays, D. M., & Kun, L. E. (1993). Solid tumors of childhood. In V. T. DeVita, S. Hellman, & S. A. Rosenberg (Eds.), *Cancer: Principles and practice of oncology* (4th ed., p. 1740). Philadelphia: Lippincott, Williams, & Wilkins.

Race is also an important factor in childhood cancers. For example, the incidence of cancer in African-American children is 80% that of the incidence in white children, largely because of lower incidence of acute leukemia, lymphoma, Ewing's sarcoma, and malignant melanoma. Notable geographic differences in the rate of childhood malignancies have also been observed. For example, although retinoblastoma (a tumor of the eye) accounts for only 4% of childhood cancers in the United States, it is far more common in India. Burkitt's lymphoma accounts for nearly half of the childhood cancers in Uganda, but is relatively rare outside of the so-called "Burkitt's Belt" of central Africa. Some of these differences are due to genetic and/or environmental factors (ecogenetics) that may interact and contribute to the development of a malignancy. Over the next several years, the relevance of both genetics and ecogenetics to childhood cancer is likely to become increasingly defined and understood.

Leukemias and lymphomas are the most common childhood cancers, accounting for over 40% of cases. Tumors of the central nervous system make up over 20% of childhood malignancies, followed by tumors of the sympathetic nervous system (neuroblastoma), kidney, soft tissues, bone, liver, eye, and germ cells.

Biology of Childhood Cancer

The understanding of the biology and molecular biology of pediatric cancers has exploded in the past decade. The ability to grow tumor cells in vitro (in the test tube) and to study their metabolism and the factors that control their growth and differentiation is providing researchers with enormous insights into the basic mechanisms of cancer. The recognition that certain genes (called oncogenes) can transform normal cells into tumor cells whereas others (called tumor suppressor genes) can suppress the malignant phenotype has set the stage for understanding the fundamental aspects of tumor formation. This knowledge base will likely take a quantum leap with the complete mapping and sequencing of the human genome.

Some cases of childhood malignancies (e.g., retinoblastoma, Wilms' tumor) are known to be genetically transmitted (Malkin, 1997). Molecular biology has given researchers the tools to identify specific genes that appear to account for the connection between cancer and genetics. This degree of knowledge will likely unlock principles that might lead to more selective and effective mechanisms for tumor control and prevention.

A careful evaluation for any genetic basis for malignancy must always be considered in the initial evaluation of the child in whom cancer is diagnosed. Such an evaluation would enable the health care providers to assist the parents with their concerns about siblings and future offspring. A careful environmental exposure history should also be taken as part of the overall evaluation of the child with a newly diagnosed malignancy. Environmental factors are increasingly being implicated in the development of tumors in adults, and the possible impact of changes in the environment cannot be overlooked in the pediatric population.

Children with congenital immune deficiency disorders are known to be at increased risk for developing certain malignancies, particularly leukemias and lymphomas. Congenital immunodeficiency diseases (e.g., ataxia telangiectasia, Wiskott-Aldrich syndrome) occur infrequently. In the 1990s, however, the number of pediatric patients who were becoming immunodeficient as a consequence of infection with the human immunodeficiency virus (HIV) expanded rapidly. An increased incidence of lymphomas and other malignancies is being observed in adult patients with acquired immunodeficiency syndrome (AIDS) who are living longer because of improved supportive care and treatments directed against the HIV virus, such as zidovudine (AZT), an antiretroviral drug. As with the adult AIDS population, children with AIDS are benefiting from highly active antiretroviral therapies (HAART) with combinations of drugs that include nucleoside and non-nucleoside reverse transcriptase inhibitors along with protease inhibitors. Children infected with HIV are thus expected to live longer, albeit perhaps, becoming more vulnerable to the development of tumors. The interaction of the immune system in controlling cancer expression thus becomes another piece of the puzzle of how cancer develops and is regulated.

Principles of Diagnosis

The first step in the diagnostic process is to determine whether a cancer is present. This requires using a combination of the child's medical history, physical examination, and laboratory measurements, including x-rays and nuclear scans. With rare exceptions (e.g., retinoblastoma) it is virtually always necessary to perform a biopsy to obtain a tissue sample in order to confirm the diagnosis of cancer.

Because cancer is rare in children, it is not frequently considered in the diagnostic evaluation of a child with general system complaints. However, clinical suspicion should be heightened when a child is brought to the physician's office because of the presence of a new mass or lump, unexplained bruising or bleeding, or constitutional symptoms that affect the child's ability to carry on his or her normal activities. These can include fatigue, fever, pallor, weakness, or evidence of lengthy or recurrent infection. Pain at the site of a tumor mass or generalized bone pain due to the invasion of the bone marrow cavities by cancer cells are other signs suggestive of malignancy.

When signs and symptoms suggest a possible malignancy in a child, the first step for the examining pediatrician or physician is to determine how far to proceed with the diagnostic evaluation. If the diagnosis of cancer seems likely, prompt referral to a pediatric oncologist is most appropriate. However, if there is only a suspicion of cancer, further diagnostic evaluation including radiographs, computed tomography (CT) or magnetic resonance imaging (MRI) scans, a nuclear scan, and perhaps a biopsy might be undertaken before a referral is made. Once a diagnosis of cancer is confirmed, it is in the best interests of the child and family to assure that treatment will be provided in a center where pediatric cancer specialists and a multidisciplinary team are available to provide the comprehensive care that is necessary to maximize the chances for cure.

Staging

Even when a cancer appears to be localized to a specific body site, it is highly likely that cancer cells have already spread to distant portions of the body. This process, referred to as micrometastasis, is the rule rather than the exception for nearly all pediatric malignancies. It is important in defining the therapeutic approach, to recognize that pediatric cancer is generally a systemic process. The child undergoing diagnostic evaluation for malignancy should be evaluated extensively to determine the overall extent or stage of disease, prior to the institution of therapy. Stage defines whether a tumor is localized to its site of origin or whether it has visibly spread to nearby tissues or to more distant organs by the bloodstream or lymphatic channels.

The stage of the disease has important implications for therapy, since cancers that have visibly spread widely require more intensive and longer duration treatment than localized cancers. Even for localized cancers, the risk for micrometastasis is so great that most children will require treatments that can travel to different parts of the body (such as chemotherapy) in order to eradicate these cancer cell deposits and prevent them from becoming sites of recurrence or relapse. Imaging studies, biological and chemical markers, and cytological and histological diagnostic techniques are useful staging methods.

IMAGING STUDIES

Imaging studies include the use of plain x-rays, sound waves, magnetism, or radioisotopes to provide an image of a tumor in relationship to the surrounding normal structures. The workhorse in this diagnostic repertoire is the diagnostic radiograph or x-ray. Radiographs provide a two-dimensional view of a body part or structure and provide light and dark contrasts according to the degree of penetration of the x-ray through the body tissue. A chest or a head x-ray is an example of this technique. Although helpful in screening, plain films can miss small tumor deposits. Considerable effort has gone into developing more sophisticated technologies with greater sensitivity and specificity, such as the resolution that results from developing a multidimensional view of a body part. A chest tomogram, for example, provides serial "slices" or images of the lungs and thoracic structures at different levels or depths. This provides a better opportunity to examine the chest cavity as a three-dimensional structure and permits a better localization of a tissue or tumor. Contrast materials, which can enhance or "light up" a tumor or surrounding tissues, can be injected into a blood vessel or a body cavity. When combined with a radiographic procedure, it becomes possible to visualize internal structures that would otherwise be indistinct.

A major advance in the ability to visualize the three-dimensional anatomy of the body was the development of CT imaging during the early 1970s. This technique has revolutionized the staging evaluation of children with cancer. Computed tomography combines x-rays produced from a tube that rotates around the body parts being examined with crystal detectors that convert the x-ray energy into electrical signals. These signals are then analyzed by sophisticated computer programs to construct an intricately detailed image. This detail can be enhanced by the use of contrast material to further highlight specific body parts. The use of CT scanning has allowed the detection of small tumors that might otherwise be invisible. CT imaging can now be done of virtually every body part including the head and brain, sinuses, spinal column, chest, abdomen, pelvis, and extremities. The disadvantages of CT scanning include exposure to x-rays and the need for the child to lie still for an extended period of time. This can be a problem for small children and sedation is often necessary in order to allow the study to be completed. Recently, so-called fast CT scanners have been developed, which may eliminate the latter problem and provide a new technology with specific application to the imaging of children. The procedure is painless, but the scanning apparatus can be intimidating and frightening to a young child. Adequate explanations and reassurance are intrinsic to the successful completion of these important studies.

During the 1980s, MRI was introduced into clinical use. This technology uses a powerful magnet that stimulates certain atomic nuclei in the body, resulting in the emission of a radio frequency that can be picked up by a receiver. This radio frequency is converted into an electrical signal, which is then processed by sophisticated computer software to create a three-dimensional image of a specific body part. MRI can produce near life-like representations of internal organs and structures, providing the physician with an extraordinary view of body tissues. This is particularly true for images of the brain and spinal cord, but other tissues including muscle can be examined in unparalleled detail. Because tumor tissue produces radiofrequency signals that can differ from those of normal tissue, MRI makes it possible to differentiate between normal and abnormal tissues. Thus, MRI is useful in evaluating localized tumors and assessing potential sites of tumor metastases. An important advantage of MRI is that it provides a means for staging without exposing a patient to additional x-rays. This technology represents an important addition to the diagnostic armamentarium in pediatric oncology.

Ultrasonography is a technique that uses sound waves to develop images of internal organs or body structures. Like MRI, ultrasound (US) is a low-risk, noninvasive procedure. Ultrasound, which is particularly useful for examination of the abdomen and pelvis, is commonly used to evaluate the liver, spleen, kidneys, and retroperitoneum. The disadvantages of US are that the image is not as detailed as that created by CT or MRI and it requires interpretation by trained evaluators.

Radioisotopes can also be used to evaluate the extent of disease. A specific radioisotope is usually injected into a vein, which distributes it throughout the body, and a special detecting camera is used to record the areas where the isotope concentrates. This creates a dotted image of the body or the specific structure that is being examined. Depending upon the isotope and carrier that is used, different body parts can be scanned. For example, technetium permits bone scanning to be accomplished; gallium binds to certain tumors including lymphomas; and the metaiodobenzylguanidine (MIBG) radioisotope marker is specific for cells that contain neurosecretory granules, such as in neuroblastoma or pheochromocytoma. Isotopes can also be used to measure the energy metabolism of organs or tumors, a technique referred to as positron emission tomography or PET scanning.

Although each of these techniques can visualize body parts and potential areas of tumor and tumor spread, they do not have the ability to identify actual tumor types. Determining a specific tumor type requires either a specific marker of the tumor or a direct examination of it. Imaging techniques do have a role in this process, however. Biopsies can be performed using fine needles under CT scan guidance, allowing tissue to be obtained without the need for surgery. This technique is being used increasingly in the evaluation of pediatric malignancies.

BIOLOGICAL AND CHEMICAL MARKERS

Certain malignancies secrete biological or chemical substances into the bloodstream or other body fluids (such as urine). These "markers"provide suggestive or inferential evidence of a tumor's presence. For example, neuroblastoma, a tumor of the adrenal glands, may produce elevated levels of catecholamines (e.g., vanillyimandelic acid and homovanillic acid) that are detectable in urine. The presence of these chemicals in conjunction with a clinical picture and imaging analysis suggestive of neuroblastoma further refine the probable diagnosis. The presence of a biological or chemical marker also provides a clue to the burden of disease. Measurements can be taken to determine whether the level of the chemical marker declines when treatment is begun.

Unfortunately, relatively few pediatric tumors produce reliable biological or chemical markers that can be used to stage or follow the course of the malignancy. However, advances in molecular biology permit the detection of very small amounts of tumor-related materials. Techniques such as the polymerase chain reaction can greatly amplify the presence of a minute quantity of a specific tumor DNA. The future will likely bring techniques that will permit the ability to diagnose and monitor tumor activity based upon the presence of specific chemical or genetic markers in blood, urine, or other body fluids.

Pathology

The gold standard for diagnosis of a malignancy is cytologic or histologic examination. In the former, cells are aspirated from a tumor through a needle or obtained from a body fluid (e.g., spinal fluid or urine). The cells are mounted on glass slides and stained with dyes that provide a contrast of the cellular structure. The specimens are examined under a microscope in order to define a specific tumor type. Histological examination involves the sectioning of a tumor tissue that was obtained either by biopsy or during a surgical procedure followed by staining and microscopic examination as in cytology. Electron microscopy magnifies structures by many thousands and permits detailed examination of cells and their components. Cytology and histology are the basis for most specific tumor diagnoses in pediatrics.

Bone marrow aspiration is commonly used in the evaluation of many pediatric malignancies, including acute lymphoblastic leukemia (ALL). This procedure involves the insertion of a needle into the inner cavity of a bone, usually of the back or the pelvis, and the aspiration or drawing-up of some of its contents. It is also important in the evaluation of solid tumors that may have spread to the bone marrow.

A bone marrow biopsy involves the use of a special needle to obtain a core of bone and bone marrow. This provides tissue other than just cells that, when sectioned and stained, provide the pathologist with the opportunity to examine the actual architecture of the bone marrow structure. Bone marrow biopsy is also done in the evaluation of acute leukemias, but is especially important in monitoring children with solid tumors. This is because small tumor metastases can become localized and difficult to aspirate and may be detectable only on careful examination of a bone marrow biopsy. Bone marrow biopsies and aspirates can be done safely and easily, but they can be painful. Appropriate education of the child along with local, and sometimes general, sedation are generally necessary.

Histological examination of tumor tissue obtained by surgical or needle biopsy is the major diagnostic procedure for pediatric solid tumors, many of which are commonly referred to as "small blue round cell tumors." Ewing's sarcoma, neuroblastoma, rhabdomyosarcoma, and lymphoma are among this group. Because the histological evaluation can be complicated, a number of sophisticated stains and procedures can be performed on biopsy material. The repertoire of techniques includes electron microscopy, immunocytochemistry (use of antibodies to highlight certain substances in the cells), cytogenetics (evaluation of the chromosomes in the cell), and a wide variety of biochemical and molecular biological techniques. Pediatric pathology has become an extraordinarily complex and complicated specialty, but refined diagnoses are increasingly possible.

Tumor Board and Staging Conference

Following the evaluation of the child with suspected cancer, it is imperative that the diagnostic and clinical care specialists meet to review the information that has been collected. This meeting usually takes the form of a tumor board or staging conference in which the pediatric oncologists, surgeons, and radiation therapists meet with the diagnostic radiologists, nuclear medicine specialists, pathologists, and other consultants to review all of the materials and test results that have been obtained. This process enables a specific treatment plan to be developed according to the diagnosis and the extent of the disease. It is also an opportunity to determine whether other procedures might be necessary in order to refine the diagnostic or therapeutic decision making. This forum also guarantees that the child with cancer will benefit from collective expertise of the group and that a plan can be formulated that will provide the greatest opportunity for cure with the lowest chance for unnecessary side effects and morbidity.

PRINCIPLES OF TREATMENT

Once the diagnosis of cancer has been established, the therapeutic plan can be formulated. Although treatment may vary according to the specific nature of the malignancy, a number of principles of therapy are shared among virtually all of the pediatric malignancies. Central to the therapeutic rationale is the fact that pediatric malignancies often grow rapidly, generally spread to various body parts even when such spread is undetectable by current diagnostic techniques, and are often sensitive (at least initially) to currently available therapeutic modalities. For patients with solid lesions, such as bone or soft tissue tumors or abdominal masses, local treatment must be determined in addition to the systemic therapy. Local treatment refers to those techniques, primarily surgery and radiation therapy, that will eliminate, eradicate, or attempt to control the primary tumor mass. A child with cancer is also at risk for having systemic disease in addition to a localized tumor mass, so therapy must be administered that can travel to virtually all of the body parts and eradicate undetectable tumor cells. Chemotherapy, or the administration of drugs, is the major modality for providing systemic therapy.

In recent years, biological substances, in some cases materials produced by the body, have been used to enhance or amplify tumor treatment. It is frequently necessary to use two or more modalities together, an approach referred to as multimodal therapy. This concept has revolutionized the treatment of childhood cancer and is largely responsible for the improvements in survival that have been witnessed during recent decades. Although each of the components of multimodal therapy can be used individually and each has specific advantages and disadvantages, they provide a powerful means for tumor control when combined.

Cancer treatment modalities are effective against cancer cells, but they are toxic to normal tissue as well. The prospect for both acute and delayed side effects that can carry serious and incapacitating consequences for the child make it imperative that the treatment be carried out by experienced clinicians who are fully knowledgeable of the benefits and liabilities of each of these powerful modalities. These individuals must be capable of working together as a team to ensure that multimodal therapy is carefully integrated into an overall plan that will maximize the child's chances for survival.

Surgery

Excision or removal of a solid tumor mass is often the first step taken to control a malignancy. For many pediatric malignancies, however, even amputation of a limb can still fail to effect a cure because of the presence of micrometastasis. This not only underscores the importance of adjuvant chemotherapy, but also has lead to a new view of the extent of surgery that should be performed on a growing child. Today, surgical management is guided by two principles. The first is that no child should be considered to have such advanced disease that an attempt at treatment is ruled out. Second, although extensive surgical procedures may sometimes be necessary to control a pediatric malignancy, every attempt should be made to minimize those that have deforming or disabling consequences.

In recent years, a number of revolutionary procedures have been introduced. These include the use of limb-sparing procedures and "neoadjuvant chemotherapy," the latter being the use of anti-cancer drugs to shrink the size of a tumor in order to make it more easily resectable.

Limb-sparing procedures have had a major impact upon the management of bone or soft tissue malignancies. Whereas in the past amputation might have been the only means for tumor removal, limb sparing allows the surgeon to excise tumor-containing bone and tissues and replace it with an artificial prosthesis that allows continued (albeit limited) function of the affected limb. Limb sparing procedures are sophisticated and complicated and must be performed by experienced surgeons. Candidates for limb-sparing must be carefully evaluated. When this procedure is feasible, it can be highly effective in preserving limb function while still providing the opportunity to remove the tumor.

Some large tumors can only be removed by extensive surgical procedures. In some cases the administration of chemotherapy prior to surgery can reduce the size of the tumor to the point where it can be more safely and easily resected. This use of neoadjuvant chemotherapy can, in certain circumstances, allow surgery to be both more successful and more tolerable for children with cancer.

Surgery has another role in cancer treatment. During the past 15 years, it has become increasingly common for children receiving cancer chemotherapy to have intravenous access devices implanted surgically. These catheters are composed of a soft rubber substance called silastic and, when implanted by a surgeon, permit access to veins for blood sampling and the delivery of chemotherapy. The most frequently used device of this type is the Hickman-Broviac catheter, which is tunneled under the skin of the chest wall, usually exiting around the sternum. Generally, four to eight inches of the catheter extend beyond the skin surface and this extension is usually capped and taped to the chest wall. These catheters are painless to wear and to operate, but they have an impact on the patient's awareness of his or her illness and can cause self-image problems for teenagers who may wish to wear bathing suits. Another type of device is the subcutaneous port, which can be surgically implanted under the skin to serve as a reservoir. Although these devices have the advantage of not being visible from the skin, access to them requires the use of a needle. Both of these surgically implanted devices have significantly improved the quality of life for children undergoing cancer therapy by reducing the number of painful procedures they must endure to receive their treatments.

Radiation Therapy

Like surgery, radiation therapy has been a cornerstone of the anti-cancer armamentarium because of its usefulness in local tumor control and in combination regimens. Radiation therapy is a sophisticated science requiring careful planning and simulation to assure that the treatment is delivered to the tumor in effective doses, while at the same time sparing surrounding normal tissue. This is particularly important in the pediatric age group in whom radiation therapy can have long-term effects on growth, development, and organ function. It is imperative that children receiving radiation be evaluated in centers where expertise in pediatric radiation therapy is available. As with imaging studies, children undergoing radiation treatments must remain still, to prevent ineffective delivery to the tumor and unnecessary damage to healthy organ tissues. For younger children, generally those younger than 5 years of age, immobilization and sedation are essential components of radiation treatment planning.

Although radiation treatments themselves are painless to receive, higher dose levels can produce uncomfortable skin irritation. The sensitivity of normal tissues to the damaging effects of radiation therapy varies greatly; some organs are relatively resistant and others are exquisitely sensitive. To some degree, sensitivity to radiation depends upon the degree of cell turnover in a specific organ. For example, cells of the skin, mucous membranes, gonads, and the hematopoietic (blood forming) system are very sensitive to the effects of radiation therapy because of their high multiplication rates.

A general goal of radiation treatment is to encompass the entire tumor within the radiation field while sparing as much normal tissue as possible. In some cases, radiation therapy is delivered to the entire body as part of a preparative regimen for bone marrow transplantation, a procedure referred to as total body irradiation (TBI). This form of radiation therapy has a significant impact upon the hematopoietic and immunological systems, and this effect can be fatal if reconstitution is not accomplished by bone marrow or peripheral blood stem cell transplantation. Like chemotherapy, total body irradiation is a form of systemic therapy because radiation is administered to virtually all areas of the body.

Chemotherapy

More than any other anti-cancer treatment modality, chemotherapy has had a pivotal role in improving survival. Chemotherapy drugs are referred to as cytotoxic agents because they result in cell death. These compounds may act on a cell during a particular phase of the cell cycle, or may be effective regardless of the stage of a tumor cell's reproduction and development. Some of these drugs act by interfering with the cell's genes or DNA, others with its RNA, while others interrupt protein synthesis. Regardless of the exact mechanism of action, the common thread is that the tumor cell is rendered unable to carry on its functions of growth and reproduction.

Chemotherapeutic agents may favor the destruction of tumor cells that are multiplying, but they are also capable of causing similar damage to normal body tissues that are also multiplying and dividing. This is the main reason that the administration of chemotherapy is associated with so many side effects and sequelae. Normal tissues with high cell turnover rates (e.g., hair follicles, the lining of the mouth and digestive tract, and the blood-forming cells of the bone marrow) are most susceptible to the adverse affects of chemotherapy. Thus, common side effects associated with chemotherapy include hair loss, nausea and vomiting, sores in the mouth and gastrointestinal tract, and suppression of the bone marrow. Each of these side effects has an impact upon the pediatric cancer patient and family. Hair loss can be devastating to adolescents because it will make them feel and look different from their peers at a time in their life when appearance is so important to self-esteem. Mouth sores can be painful and can affect the child's ability to eat and maintain proper nutrition. Suppression of the bone marrow can be life-threatening. In light of potential side effects, chemotherapy schedules must be carefully designed and monitored. Accordingly, children receiving chemotherapy should be cared for in centers that have expertise in pediatric oncology. It is also important for the child and family to understand both the beneficial effects and side effects of chemotherapy and to become partners in the care and support necessary to sustain the treatment program.

Most schedules include combinations of agents. This approach maximizes the activity of the regimen by using agents that work in different manners, thereby taking advantage of their additive effects in the destruction of tumor cells. Combination regimens also minimize the ability of cancer cells to escape destruction by having developed resistance to a particular drug. Usually, chemotherapy regimens are administered in cycles, often on a monthly basis, to give the patient adequate time to recover from treatment effects and lessen the buildup of toxicity.

The immediate goal of chemotherapy is to produce a remission of the cancer; that is, all measurable components of the cancer have been eliminated. Remission does not mean that all the cancer has been eradicated, because many tumor cells can be present in the body and yet escape detection by even the most sophisticated technologies. Chemotherapy is often administered over many months, and in some diseases over years, to maintain control of the malignancy. During this period of maintenance therapy, the goal is to continue reducing the body's tumor burden with the ultimate goal of eradicating it and thus producing a cure.

INVESTIGATIONAL PRINCIPLES

Tumors vary in their sensitivities to various cytotoxic drugs, and it is by trial-and-error that physicians have ascertained which agents are most active against a particular malignancy. The evaluation of investigational agents is critical to future success in the treatment of children with cancer. If preclinical (laboratory) testing suggests a new drug may be useful, further testing in clinical trials will be undertaken. Three phases of clinical trials are followed in the evaluation of chemotherapeutic agents. Phase I testing involves the assessment of safety and tolerance of a new agent and is basically designed to determine the dose that can be tolerated. In general, Phase I testing does not begin in children until testing has proceeded in adults. The development of therapeutic agents for children with HIV infection, however has forced a reconsideration of this policy. It is anticipated that the pace of drug development for children with cancer might also he accelerated as a consequence of these insights. Once a dosage of a chemotherapeutic agent has been found to be safe and tolerable, the agent then undergoes Phase II testing, in which its activity against different tumor types is determined. The tumors that might be most likely to respond to a new chemotherapeutic agent can be discerned in part from the results of testing in experimental in vitro systems as well as in animal experiments. If a drug appears to be active in Phase II testing against a specific tumor, it is then ready for Phase III trials in which its activity is compared to known agents. In general, Phase I testing requires only a small number of patients to ascertain safety, tolerance, and dose findings. Phase II testing might require 25 to 100 or more patients. Phase III comparative studies generally involve hundreds or thousands of patients.

Comparative assessment using randomized clinical trials is an essential component of drug development. It is the only way to avoid bias and assure the activity of a new agent. A new drug or a combination of drugs is assessed within the context of a protocol that spells out the exact details of the regimen to be studied and allows the data to be accrued in a way that accurate interpretation is assured. Because pediatric malignancies are uncommon, many of the protocols conducted in the United States are done as part of multi-institutional studies, in which centers around the country collaborate and cooperate to evaluate new treatment concepts or to fine-tune those that have already become established. Most of these cooperative trials have been performed under the auspices of the Pediatric Oncology Group and the Children's Cancer Study Group. These groups, which are now being combined into a single national group, are supported by the NCI, and have been successfully enrolling more than 50% of children with cancer into clinical protocols (Weiner, 2000). By assuring that as many children as possible are being enrolled in state-of-the-art treatment protocols, the prospect exists for improving the outcome for future children with cancer.

CHEMOTHERAPY ADMINISTRATION PRINCIPLES

Chemotherapeutic agents are generally administered orally or intravenously. In some protocols, agents are administered into the artery (intra-arterial chemotherapy) to deliver therapy to a specific tumor site. Certain chemotherapeutic agents, including vincristine, daunorubicin, and doxorubicin, can cause considerable damage if they infiltrate or extravasate out of the vein. This problem is largely avoided by the use of Hickman-Broviac catheters.

Because cancer cells can survive in areas of the body in which chemotherapy has limited access (e.g., the central nervous system [CNS]), it is sometimes necessary to deliver the agents into the spinal fluids. This approach, called intrathecal therapy, is integral to the treatment of several childhood cancers, most notably leukemias and lymphomas, and is a component of CNS prophylaxis.

It is an important aspect of pediatric cancer care that all members of the patient's health care team be aware of the range of potential side effects so that appropriate support for the patient can be given. Some of these treatment modalities carry delayed or chronic toxic effects in addition to acute side effects. For example, during or shortly after administration of chemotherapeutic agents, patients may experience nausea and vomiting because of the drug's impact on the trigger zones in the areas of the brain that control the vomiting reflex. Antiemetic medications can suppress this reaction. Nausea and vomiting represent an uncomfortable treatment side effect, but the occurrence of hair loss and mouth sores represent both the stigmata of cancer treatment as well as sources of pain and discomfort. Depending upon the child's preferences, the hair loss can be creatively masked by scarves, wigs, or caps, and the mouth sores aided by good oral hygiene. Chemotherapy-related bone marrow suppression, however, represents a true limitation of treatment because all three cell components of the blood (white blood cells, red blood cells, and platelets) can be suppressed as a consequence of cancer treatment. Depleted red blood cells and platelets are treatable with either packed red blood cells or platelet transfusions, thereby allowing therapy to continue. Also, modifying the dosage and frequency of the chemotherapy can attenuate some of these marrow-related side effects. Suppression of the white blood cells, however, constitutes a major problem for both the child and the medical care staff. A white blood count that falls to low levels, particularly when it remains low for days to weeks at a time, increases the risk for developing a life-threatening infection. Most of the organisms that contribute to these infections are endogenous, arising from the body's own microbiological flora. In the absence of the body's defending cells, these organisms can result in serious infections. In a child undergoing cancer therapy, any sign of infection, particularly when the white blood cell count is low, should be immediately brought to the attention of the child's physician. Any fever in conjunction with a low white blood cell count is reason for immediate evaluation and almost certainly will result in the child's admission to the hospital for intravenous antibiotic therapy. This approach of quick response to signs of infection has largely overcome the life-threatening sequelae associated with low blood counts and infection. This points out the need to include the parents and the child, when appropriate, as part of the health care team so that they are well educated about the adverse effects of therapy and, in particular, when to call for help.

Many of the therapeutic effects and side effects of chemotherapy are directly related to the intensity or the amount of therapy that is being administered. Intensity is either a high dose of a drug or combination of drugs administered at any point in time, or the very frequent administration of chemotherapeutic agents. Generally, more intensive chemotherapy regimens are associated with a greater degree of therapeutic effects and side effects. Situations occur in which high-dose chemotherapy regimens are essential in order to provide the maximum chances for survival, as in the treatment of acute leukemias or high-risk solid tumors. In these situations, very high doses of chemotherapy may be necessary to provide the maximum degree of tumor cell eradication.

Perhaps the most extreme examples of this are the regimens used in bone marrow stem cell or peripheral blood stem cell transplantation, which in the past decade became an important component of childhood cancer treatment. Stem cell transplantation was first established for the treatment of children with leukemia, and subsequently for lymphoma, and has more recently been used in the treatment of a number of solid-tumor malignancies. Stem cell transplantation is a reconstitution or rescue regimen. The major strategy is to be able to deliver the highest possible dosage of chemotherapy and other modalities, such as radiation therapy, in order to have the greatest impact on the tumor. Because such intensive therapy can result in profound suppression of the hematopoietic (blood-forming) cells of the bone marrow for very long periods of time, the administration of hematopoietic stem cells might hasten the patient's recovery and attenuate some of these toxic side effects. The experience gained during the last decade has demonstrated that bone marrow transplantation can reconstitute the marrow in patients who have received very high dose regimens.

There are two sources of bone marrow that can be administered to patients. Autologous bone marrow is the patient's own bone marrow, harvested at a time when the disease is in remission, often treated to eradicate any residual cells, and frozen and stored until it is administered back to the patient. With allogeneic bone marrow transplantation, the source of the marrow is someone other than the patient. The best source of an allogeneic bone marrow transplantation donor is a sibling or family member of the patient. During recent years, a number of registries have been developed so that persons unrelated to the patient whose marrow might be compatible with the patient can be identified as possible donors. Increasingly, stem cells harvested from the peripheral blood are supplementing the need to obtain such cells from the bone marrow per se.

Transplantation of stem cells can be successful in the treatment of acute leukemias in particular, but it is still considered an investigational procedure for many of the other pediatric malignancies. It is essential that these transplantations be performed at centers that are equipped to deal with the medical and psychosocial needs of children who undergo these procedures.

BIOLOGICAL THERAPIES

The advances in molecular biology and recombinant DNA technology made it possible during the 1980s to generate large quantities of molecules that serve as chemical signals affecting the body's immune and hematopoietic systems. Among these agents are cytokines, a generic term for nonantibody proteins released by certain types of immune system cells on contact with a specific antigen. These act as intercellular mediators, as in generating an immune response.

Agents known as the granulocyte macrophage-colony stimulating factor (GM-CSF) or granulocyte colony stimulating factor (G-CSF) both appear to be capable of accelerating the time to bone marrow recovery following the administration of cytotoxic chemotherapy. The integration of these "biologicals" or "growth factors" into chemotherapy schedules may lessen some of the side effects, in particular reducing the duration of low white blood cell counts (neutropenia) and the associated risk for developing serious infections. Studies evaluating these biologicals in children with cancer are under way, and it is anticipated that their role in the treatment of pediatric malignancies will be discerned within the next several years. Cytokines eventually may play a pivotal role in the care of children with cancer by both decreasing toxicity and enhancing the tumoricidal activity of chemotherapy.

The interleukins and the interferons are other molecules that may play an important role in the treatment of malignancy or in the supportive care of pediatric cancer patients. These agents are being evaluated in children and their role in combination regimens should be discerned within the next several years. The ability to use the immune system as part of cancer treatment has been demonstrated in several adult malignancies, particularly renal cell cancer and melanoma. A strategy combining the administration of interleukin 2 with lymphokine-activated killer cells has been shown to exert an impressive effect in some adult malignancies. Additional strategies being explored in adults include the use of tumor infiltrating lymphocytes, which may be more specific in their destruction of a tumor. These adoptive immunotherapy regimens have only begun to be explored in children, but they may play an increasing role in the future. Studies to evaluate tumor infiltrating lymphocyte cell therapy for neuroblastoma, for example, are under way at the NCI.

Another important strategy is the blockade of new blood vessel formation necessary to feed tumor cells. This approach called "antiangiogenesis" is currently under investigation and should it prove successful, it will have an impact on a number of solid tumors of childhood, perhaps most notably brain tumors.

Future Considerations in Pediatric Cancer Treatment

The major goal in the treatment of the child with cancer is to utilize therapies that are specific for the tumor and that spare the child as much toxicity as possible. The evolving understanding of the molecular basis of cancer may well facilitate the ability to treat pediatric malignancies by novel mechanisms. In addition to the application of biologicals, it may be possible to reprogram tumors to differentiate and to stop multiplying, thus rendering them incapable of spreading locally or metastasizing to other parts of the body. Insights gained from in vitro studies suggest that a number of chemical agents and biological agents may be useful in accomplishing this cellular reprogramming, and further work is expected. If successful, these strategies could further improve the impact of cancer treatment as well as enhance the quality of life of the children who receive treatment for the disease.

PRINCIPLES OF THE MULTIDISCIPLINARY APPROACH TO CARING FOR CHILDREN WITH CANCER

When malignancy is suspected in a child, many resources and technologies must be integrated in order to determine whether a cancer exists, the nature of a primary cancer that is diagnosed, and the extent to which the disease may have spread prior to the initiation of therapy. This comprehensive assessment requires the expertise of pediatric oncologists, surgeons, radiation therapists and radiologists, nuclear medicine specialists, pathologists, and cytologists. All play intricate roles in the overall evaluation of the child with probable or proven cancer. Once the diagnosis is established, cancer treatment requires the integration of many resources and skills to maximize the child's chance of survival and minimize the toxic effects of treatment that might ensue. Skilled physicians and nurses form the base of the medical therapeutic alliance. However, treatment without the psychosocial support and care of the child and his or her family would be incomplete. Thus, essential members of the multidisciplinary team also include social workers, psychologists, physical and occupational therapists, recreational therapists, teachers, and members of the clergy. Each contributes insight, care, and understanding to the child with cancer. Many therapies must be administered in a hospital or outpatient clinic, so interruption of family life cannot be avoided. As much attention as possible must be given to helping the pediatric cancer patients and their families lead as normal lives as are possible. Part of this supportive approach is to help the child remain in school and look forward to the prospect of successful treatment and even cure. Contact with schools and community services represents an arm of the cancer treatment program that requires the assistance of the multidisciplinary team.

Survival rates for most childhood cancers have steadily improved over the past 25 years. Although a number of young people have been cured of their underlying disease, they will also have experienced side effects related to treatment. Whether these include impaired growth, sterility, heart problems, or physical limitations, it is important to learn from the experiences of children who have survived cancer treatment, and thus to develop even better treatment strategies in the future.

REFERENCES

Malkin, D. (1997). Molecular biology of childhood cancers. In V. T. DeVita, S. Hellman, & S. A. Rosenberg (Eds.), Cancer: Principles and practice of oncology (5th ed., pp. 2083-2091). Philadelphia: Lippincott, Williams, & Wilkins.

Pizzo, P. A., Horowitz, M. E., Poplack, D. G., Hays, D. M., & Kun, L. E. (1993). Solid tumors of childhood. In V. T. DeVita, S. Hellman, & S. A. Rosenberg (Eds.), Cancer: Principles and practice of oncology (4th ed., pp. 1738-1791). Philadelphia: Lippincott, Williams, & Wilkins.

Pizzo, P. A., & Poplack, D. G. (1996). Principles and practice of pediatric oncology (3rd ed). Philadelphia: Lippincott, Williams, & Wilkins.

Weiner, M. A. (2000). Principles and practice of pediatric oncology. In R. Bast, D. Kufe, R. Pollock, R. Weichselbaum, J. Holland, & E. Frei (Eds.), Cancer medicine (5th ed., pp. 2125-2127). Hamilton, Ontario, Canada: B. C. Decker.

CHAPTER 6

COMMON ISSUES AND CHALLENGES FOR FAMILIES DEALING WITH CHILDHOOD CANCER

Marie M. Lauria, MSW, LCSW

The diagnosis of cancer in an infant, child, or adolescent creates an immediate and frightening crisis in the lives of patients and all family members. The prospect of the pain and suffering that is widely perceived as an inevitable part of the disease and its treatment adds greatly to parents' fear and anxiety. The persistent association of cancer with death further intensifies these feelings.

As core members of multidisciplinary teams, pediatric oncology social workers collaborate with other team members, young people, and families to understand and help them address the socioeconomic and emotional aspects of childhood cancer. All team members find the work fast-paced, intense, and emotionally difficult.

> The diagnosis exposes the vulnerability of children and adults; magnifies the already awesome responsibility of the medical professionals; and heralds enormous, irreversible, and often unforeseeable changes in the family. Health professionals become intimate partners with individuals, heretofore strangers, whose lives become greatly influenced by these relationships and by actions undertaken on their behalf. Staff, in turn, are profoundly affected by patients and family members, by the

extent of their responsibility, and by the meaning and importance of their mission. (Ross, 1993, p. 214)

Childhood cancer moves from the crisis stage of diagnosis through subsequent stages of chronicity and recurrent crises. For the fortunate majority of young people, treatments end, normality returns, and lifetime monitoring becomes a way of life. For the less fortunate, death, sadness, grief, and mourning result. In the beginning, there is no certainty about what will happen. This makes it reasonable to treat each child as a potential survivor, to foster normal growth and development, and to promote adaptive family functioning, despite the difficulties and uncertainties of treatment outcomes.

All children and families require some assistance in handling the multiple issues confronting them at each illness stage. Most have never had any direct experience with cancer or other serious illness, or with the complex system of current health care. They quickly learn that the standard of quality care in pediatric oncology is a comprehensive, coordinated approach attentive to both the medical and psychosocial aspects of care. It offers all family members the diverse services of a multidisciplinary team to help them manage this demanding and extended experience. Oncology social workers cannot spare families the profound social, emotional, spiritual, and economic distress of a child's diagnosis and subsequent experiences with cancer. What they can do is use knowledge of all aspects of childhood cancer, its treatment and the clinical expertise they possess to help make a difference in the quality of care patients and families receive.

This chapter discusses the *common psychosocial themes or issues of childhood cancer* faced by patients and families from the period of diagnosis, through treatment, and into long-term survivorship or bereavement. It considers them within a framework of adaptational tasks and challenges related to the different stages of the illness and its treatment.

COMMON THEMES AND ISSUES IN CHILDHOOD CANCER

Clinical Observation and Research

Many clinical observers have shared their experiential wisdom and many researchers have added to our understanding of patients' and families' very complex needs and of the common issues and themes of childhood cancer. They created a body of psychosocial research and relevant literature (Redd, 1994). They explored topics such as open communication (Foley, 1994; Claflin & Barbarin, 1991); expression and management of emotions (Nelson, Miles, Reed, Davis, & Cooper, 1994; Mulhern, Fairclough, Douglas, & Smith, 1994); coping with painful procedures (Dahlquist, Power, Cox, & Fernbach, 1994); the roles of family and extended family members (Grootenhuis & Last, 1997; Kupst, Natta, Richardson, Shulman, Lavigne, & Das, 1995); changes in self-esteem and body-image (Arnholt, Fritz, & Keener, 1993; Sanger, Copeland, & Davidson, 1991); school reintegration (Deasy-Spinetta, 1993); cognitive functioning (Stehbens, et al., 1994; Katz & Varni, 1993); survivorship (Speechley & Noh, 1992; Christ, Lane, & Marcove, 1995; Weigers, Chesler, Zebrack, & Goldman, 1998); and end-of-life care (Whittam, 1993).

Researchers have also captured concerns about sexuality and fertility (Weigers, et al., 1998). They studied the effectiveness of behavioral and other interventions to reduce anxiety, fear, and discomfort and to manage pain and other treatment side effects (Zeltzer, LeBaron, & Zeltzer, 1984). They have examined family quality of life issues, such as adjustment to diagnosis, treatment, and survival (Varni, Katz, Colegrove, & Dolgin, 1994); marital relationships (Dahlquist, et al., 1993); sibling needs (Bendor, 1990; Chesler, Allswede, & Barbarin, 1991); peer relationships (Noll, Bukowski, Davies, Koontz, & Kulkarni, 1993); the indirect costs of treatment and family finances (Eaton, 1993); employment and insurance issues (Hays, 1993); and overall family coping and adaptation (Hersh & Weiner, 1993; Overholser & Fritz, 1990).

Oncology social workers incorporate many of these findings into clinical practice. For example, they create patient and family-friendly environments, treat each new patient as a potential survivor, provide detailed information, and communicate more effectively. They understand the importance of helping all family members with coping and adaptation during active treatment or bereavement, and recognize the need to continue learning more about the growing body of long-term survivors.

Common Issues

What the literature teaches and what experienced social workers know from their practice is that although each child and family is unique, there are issues common to all in the experience of childhood cancer. They include:

- KNOWLEDGE AND INFORMATION NEEDED TO DEAL WITH ALL ASPECTS OF CANCER

    Acquiring and processing information on childhood cancer is essential if families are to be informed participants throughout the course of the disease and its care. Patients also are part of this process and receive information tailored to age and development. Parents often must not only absorb the information they are given, but also relay it to other children or family members. Information needs change over the course of treatment and into survivorship. The team must address any impediments to understanding, such as language or cognitive ability and recognize that high levels of anxiety often prevent parents from hearing and processing information well. Information-seeking behavior can be a good antidote to anxiety and a strategy for regaining control over a situation in which parents and patients feel powerless. Oncology social workers and others can facilitate these activities by providing written and audiovisual materials and guiding families to use the Internet (Sharp, 1999).

- THE PHYSICAL IMPACT OF THE CANCER ON AN INFANT, CHILD, OR ADOLESCENT

    The physical effects of cancer and its treatment on the body distress both patients and parents. They are difficult for the patient to endure and for the family to watch and try to assist. Diagnostic tests, surgery, monitoring procedures, and treatment bring discomfort, pain, nausea, vomiting, fevers and infections, fatigue, changes in appetite, and sleep disturbances. Infants sometimes must have their mobility limited and their feeding and sleeping routines disrupted. Toddlers also find constraints on their movements distressing and are fearful of treatment procedures and separations from parents for surgery or radiation treatments. Older children and adolescents are upset by hair loss and changes in appearance, by interruption of their school, social lives, and usual activities, and by renewed dependence on parents for physical care.

Parents quickly realize that the major share of helping their children comply with the treatment plan and cope with the effects of treatment will fall to them. They will be responsible for care of right atrial catheters, for monitoring temperatures, and for worrying about nutrition. Some are more at ease and comfortable with these tasks. Others are unsure of their own competence and find it challenging to urge compliance with painful or invasive procedures or persuade their children to take unpleasant medicines. Parents of pre-verbal children are anxious about having to interpret the meaning of their children's crying or lethargy. Some parents, often fathers, are uncomfortable with providing physical care. When the patient is an adolescent, the parent of the same sex is usually the best caregiver around some physical needs. All parents have concerns about their ability to care for their child's physical needs and about how to incorporate these responsibilities into daily life. End-of-life care presents special difficulty as physical functioning deteriorates and pain management becomes an issue. Parents and patients require education and active support from various team members to help them handle these many issues comfortably.

- EMOTIONAL REACTIONS OF ALL FAMILY MEMBERS

Parents often describe being on an emotional rollercoaster. The feelings they report seem to be normal ones all parents commonly experience. What they actually say or do to express these feelings differs. How they handle their emotions usually reflects variations in life situations, cultural norms, and their individual coping styles in responding to major distress. The feelings common to all parents include:

Shock. Parents report feeling numb or having received an almost physical blow. They report feeling confused, or being unable to hear, remember or think clearly when given information about their child's diagnosis or treatment plan. Such numbness may serve to deaden the very painful feelings the diagnosis brings and to give parents time to face gradually those difficult emotions.

Disbelief/Denial. Disbelief or denial of the accuracy of the diagnosis, progressive disease, or the likelihood of death often serves to buffer very painful feelings. It is an adaptive way for parents and patients to gain time for adjusting to disturbing realities. Only when denial delays timely treatment, results in futile pursuit of questionable alternative therapies, or interferes with decision-making about ending aggressive treatment is it maladaptive. Team members should not confuse denial with reluctance or unwillingness to talk about what is happening.

Fear/Anxiety. Anxiety and fearfulness when events and their outcome are unfamiliar and beyond our control is a normal human reaction. Fear of cancer is universal. A family's only first-hand experience may be with cancer treated in an older family member. Fear of the intensive treatment, an uncertain future, the unknown, and death is very understandable.

Guilt. Questions of guilt arise soon after parents accept that their child or adolescent really does have cancer. Parents have major responsibility for protecting their child from danger and harm. Initially, they question what behavior or action of theirs may have contributed to their child's life-threatening disease. Addressing the questions parents have can relieve feelings of guilt. It is important not to let guilty feelings distract parents from the many tasks they face when their child has cancer.

Sadness/Feelings of Depression. Sadness and feelings of depression are normal and understandable reactions of parents to their child's cancer diagnosis. Every parent hopes and dreams that life for their child will be healthy, happy, and carefree. Cancer and its treatment defer that dream. Parents must grieve the loss of their hopes. Young people also need to express their sadness and grief over the changes and losses the disease brings.

Anger. The fact that cancer threatens the life of an innocent and blameless child makes parents feel angry at the cruel and random injustice of life. When someone we love is seriously ill it seems natural and normal to fight back and to look for someone to blame. Family members can direct anger at God, at physicians who didn't recognize or misdiagnosed the cancer, at one another for past behaviors that they think contributed to the diagnosis, or even at themselves for being in some way responsible. Some parents conceal their anger or even deny that they feel angry since they consider expression of such feelings as "not nice" or destructive. Others express their anger in explosive and hostile ways. Anger may also serve as a mask for feelings of depression and powerlessness. Young people of every age become angry at the unfairness of fate, at the loss of control they experience and at the indignities they suffer as cancer patients. Since parents, patients, and care providers must collaborate it is important to identify anger and help find appropriate ways to express anger and resolve legitimate complaints.

Most parents and patients require education and suggested strategies from oncology social workers and other team members to help them identify, express, and master the powerful feelings evoked by the difficult events of childhood cancer. Some need only validation that they are managing their feelings appropriately. Seasoned oncology social workers realize that with such education, validation, and support, families and children generally are able to cope effectively and adjust well to cancer and its treatment. A recent Australian study found "...in the longer term, the number of psychological problems experienced by children treated for cancer and their parents does not differ from that in the general community" (Sawyer, Antoniou, Toogood, Rice, & Baghurst, 2000, p. 219). Occasionally, of course, there are parents or young people experiencing special difficulty in coping who need referral for therapy that is more intensive or for medication.

- INFLUENCE OF CANCER ON CHILDREN AND ADOLESCENTS' NORMAL GROWTH AND DEVELOPMENT
The rapid pace of children and adolescents' growth and development will not await completion of treatment. Young people are "works in progress" and it is essential for oncology social workers and other team members to assist parents in promoting and supporting normal developmental activities and behaviors. Cancer treatment does not always make this an easy task. Furthermore, the young person's natural tendency to "regress" in the face of the disease's assault, coupled with parents' natural inclination to guard and protect children present additional obstacles. Over the many years of treatment and for those who move into long-term survivorship, there will be shifts in the developmental needs of young people and a corresponding need for team members to change the approach to care.

Each developmental period brings its particular challenges:
- *Infancy* (0–2). Infants need uninterrupted nurturing, predictable routines, and emotional stability. This is difficult to achieve during treatment.
- *Early childhood* (2–5). Toddlers require parental guidance and opportunities to learn self-care and exert some control. Their concrete thinking may cause confusion when patients and others try to explain illness events to them. They can be very anxious about separation from parents and about being hurt physically. Play offers an important means of reassurance and

mastery of experiences.

- *Mid-childhood (5–11)*. Young people in this period are developing abilities to comprehend what they are experiencing. They are beginning to understand cause and effect and may search privately for information about their cancer. They vary in their capacity for integrating information and explanations when they are overwhelmed emotionally. They are interested in clear rules and expectations. Involvement in school, sports, and other activities may be a problem because of treatment interruptions, fatigue, or concern about appearance. At these ages, children have a beginning awareness of the permanence of death and see it as an external, frightening force.

- *Adolescence (12–18)*. Adolescents have an appreciation of the relatedness of disease and death. They want complete information, but have difficulty asking direct questions. Self-esteem, independence, socialization, sexuality, and body image are important concerns in this period of developing a personal identity. Parents are often the "safe" targets of their anger and hostility. They may have trouble verbalizing or admitting to feelings of sadness and depression. They may actively search for the meaning in having and battling cancer, and can turn to faith in God for support.

Parents sometimes require education by social workers and others about their children's developmental needs and help in understanding how the experiences of childhood cancer affect them.

- EFFECTS OF THE CANCER EXPERIENCE ON FAMILY LIFE AND ON INDIVIDUAL FAMILY MEMBERS

Childhood cancer is widely acknowledged as a family disease. The life of the family and the lives of each family member are affected by the events of diagnosis and treatment, by the paradoxical joy and uncertainty of survivorship, and for some, by death, grief, and mourning. Families provide the context in which childrens' and adolescents' cancers occur and are managed. Young people need their families to nurture and love them, to protect them, to provide for basic needs, to foster growth and development, to teach about communicating with and relating to others, and to communicate values, culture, and spiritual beliefs. Carrying out these family functions is very difficult in the face of cancer and its demands. Parents are sometimes emotionally and physically exhausted. They must try to juggle attention to their ill child with their personal needs and those of other children, careers and jobs, financial concerns, or the needs of aging parents. There may be existing problems in the marital relationship or they may be single parents struggling to handle the tasks of two parents. Parents may be divorced, in second marriages, have blended families, or have conflictual relationships with former spouses. They may have their own problems with alcoholism, physical illness, abuse, or mental illness. Differences in temperament, styles of coping, communication, and decision making may be sources of tension. They may have difficulty disciplining, or lack other parenting skills necessary to assist their child.

Siblings sometimes suffer in the separation from parents occasioned by treatment in centers distant from home. The attention and time given to an ill brother or sister may be distressing and a cause of resentment and jealousy. They may have fears about their own health or their chances of getting cancer. Parents must find the energy to attend to the siblings' growth and development, to listen to their worries and to provide the love and support they require.

Social supports are critical to the coping of families with the pressures of daily life, especially during illness crisis periods and when disease progresses or death occurs. Some families have natural support systems, but others may need encouragement to develop, seek or use support available through neighbors, churches, or communities.

- PATIENT AND FAMILY INTERACTIONS WITH HEALTH CARE SYSTEMS
A cancer diagnosis brings patients and families into the complex and sometimes frightening world of modern medicine. Hospitals and major medical centers usually are vast and confusing places with endless corridors, many buildings, and impersonal inpatient rooms. Bone marrow transplant units are both isolating and intimidating. Professionals ask numerous and repetitive questions, perform endless tests, and give extensive information. The language can seem almost foreign and the technical terms used bewildering. There are forms and more forms to be completed. Contact with insurance or managed care providers increases and is frequently a source of frustration as families check coverage arrangements, seek approval for tests and procedures, or question payment for care. Families are unsure who is in charge of decision-making for their children. The schedules and routines of daily family life alter to incorporate an often-complicated treatment regimen and trips between home, doctors' offices, and medical center multiply. Parents find they must yield some control of their child and place their trust in team members. Families' interactions with community medical and other health care providers also increase as pediatricians, family practice physicians, and home health nurses assist with treatment.

With time and experience, patients and families become familiar with the medical centers and other places where treatment is given. They find the spots that offer privacy. They bring blankets and pictures from home to brighten inpatient rooms. They learn to pack snacks, toys, and books for clinic visits. They master the way to the cafeteria. They learn to navigate around the miles of hallways. They memorize the route and all the shortcuts from home to the hospital. They find ways of communicating with personnel in insurance, managed care, and government agencies. They learn to advocate for their children and themselves. Team members become real people and important sources of support. Families learn to distinguish the differing roles of professionals they encounter and trust their skills. Patients and parents adjust and become reluctant experts in childhood cancer. Oncology social workers and other team members often are central to families' advocacy efforts.

- UNCERTAINTY REGARDING TREATMENT RESPONSE AND SURVIVAL
One of the most challenging issues confronting young people with cancer and their families is the need to live each day with heightened awareness of the fragility of life. No one has a guarantee of life beyond the present moment, but that is not a thought on which most people care to dwell. Cancer and its treatment, however, bring constant reminders of mortality. Families' personal experiences with cancer and observation of the lives of other patients make them value and appreciate the gifts of good health and life. Some individuals find it particularly difficult to tolerate uncertainty. They are comfortable only when they know what will happen and feel assured that the plans they make for the future have a good chance of working. Others are more naturally pessimistic, always expecting that the worst will happen. However, the majority of patients and families cope with uncertainty about the future by investing in hope.

The hope or optimism that things will turn out all right and that tomorrow will be brighter is very strong in most human beings, no matter how difficult the adversity they face. Young people and their families begin feeling hopeful about future survival when they hear about available treatment and the remarkable progress made in curing childhood cancers. At the time of diagnosis, each individual patient, whatever the relevant statistics, has every reason to believe that he or she will respond well to treatment and achieve eventual cure. Such belief sustains many through the demanding months and years of treatment. If the cancer progresses and death appears the likely outcome, patients and families moderate their hopefulness to wish for things other than life, such as moments of pleasure or pain-free hours. When treatment ends and a lifetime of survivorship begins, uncertainty persists but is diminished since cancer is no longer the central fact of daily life.

- THE SEARCH FOR MEANING

  Hope, for some, is bolstered by faith that there is a reason for what has happened, even if they do not understand what that reason is. Some consider cancer a test from God to see how they will respond. For others, it is a summons to return to faith in God or to church attendance. Still others consider the bad things that happen as random events, but believe that they will receive whatever strength they need from God to handle the experience. Occasionally, there are some who see the diagnosis as a punishment from God for current or past behaviors, and others who are angry, believing that God has allowed their child to develop cancer. There are people who do not believe in a Supreme Being or God or Creator. They try to interpret the diagnosis or the suffering and trauma of their child in light of whatever beliefs and cultural attitudes they have about the nature and meaning of illness, life, and death. Although parents vary in their ability to convey such thoughts, beliefs, and attitudes to their children, it is common for young people to reflect their views. When death is likely, there usually is renewed interest in and discussion of religious and spiritual issues and traditions as family members try to help young people deal with the ending of life. Ministers, priests, rabbis, hospital chaplains, and other spiritual leaders assist with exploration of questions and concerns throughout the cancer experience, but especially at the time of death. Conversations begun at the time of diagnosis with oncology social workers about faith and beliefs generally continue through all phases of treatment.

ILLNESS STAGES AND USE OF A FRAMEWORK OF ADAPTATIONAL TASKS

The many common issues in the experience of cancer occur and recur, requiring attention at different phases of the illness experience. Oncology social workers and their colleagues benefit from having a strategy for organizing both assessments and clinical interventions to help patients and families anticipate what they can expect. A stage of illness framework that incorporates issues and related tasks can serve that purpose.

There have been several efforts to identify a framework of illness-related coping tasks, one a classic in the social work literature (Mailick, 1979); another specific to adult cancer patients (Christ, 1993). One framework, tailored to pediatric oncology, builds on work by several others interested in adjustment to illness (Lauria, Hockenberry-Eaton, Pawletko, & Mauer, 1996). It is a framework of family adaptational tasks, compatible with an approach based on coping and adaptation and specific to the different phases of the cancer experience. Division of cancer-related events into stages or phases is arbitrary, of course, but one possible division is the following:

- Diagnosis and initial treatment
- Treatment when remission is sustained
- Treatment when disease recurs
- Progressive disease and death
- Treatment completion and survival.

What follows are descriptions of each stage and a listing of the adaptational tasks or challenges relevant to them (see Table 1).

Treatment Stages and Adaptational Tasks

STAGE I: DIAGNOSIS AND INITIAL TREATMENT

The first stage begins with evaluation of a child or adolescent's symptoms because of concern about a possible malignancy, and continues into diagnosis and the early weeks of treatment. Parents often describe this as a period of turmoil and emotional upheaval for all family members. As they struggle to absorb the fact that their child is seriously ill with a life-threatening disease, the cancer and its treatment sweep them into a complex and unfamiliar health care system. Parents and patients try to process detailed information about the diagnosis and about available treatment options. Parents must give permission for numerous tests and procedures, learn about

TABLE 1

Family Adaptational Tasks in Stages of Childhood Cancer

Stage I. Diagnosis and Initial Treatment
- Acquiring and processing knowledge and information
- Providing emotional support to infant, child, or adolescent
- Assisting patients with the physical aspects of disease
- Expressing and managing emotional reactions to diagnosis and treatment
- Adapting family life to balance the needs of all members
- Attending to relationships within and outside the family
- Mobilizing essential social supports and other resources
- Learning to function in the health care system
- Facing uncertainty and loss of control
- Searching for meaning

Stage II. Treatment when Remission is Sustained
- Addressing changing informational needs
- Sustaining hopefulness through chronicity and crisis periods
- Assisting the patient with side-effects, body image, self-esteem, schooling, and changes in personal aspirations
- Mastering feelings regarding child or adolescent's disease and treatment experiences
- Fostering patient's normal growth and development
- Maintaining satisfactory family functioning
- Dealing with reimbursement issues, government program regulations, or legal rights
- Securing and using social and emotional support
- Anticipating the completion of treatment

Stage III. Treatment when Disease Recurs
- Coping with emotional responses evoked by disease recurrence
- Processing information and participating in decision-making about possible new treatments
- Assisting child or adolescent to understand and accept recurrence and cooperate with new plan for treatment
- Regulating hopefulness about outcome

Stage IV. Progressive Disease and Death
- Coping with emotional responses to disease progression and eventual death
- Assisting the patient with physical deterioration, discomfort, and pain
- Maintaining adequate family functioning
- Preparing the child, siblings, and other family members for impending death
- Reshaping hope to focus on the good events of each day
- Helping the child or adolescent live until death occurs
- Making arrangements for funeral or memorial services
- Ending formal relationships with team members
- Grieving and mourning the loss of child or adolescent
- Finding meaning and purpose in life without the child's presence

Stage V. Treatment Completion and Survival
- Managing the conflicting emotions of completing treatment
- Adjusting to any long-term effects of treatment
- Acquiring information about issues and resources relevant to survivorship
- Resuming "normal" individual and family life
- Arranging and maintaining appropriate lifetime follow-up for the patient

Note. Adapted from Lauria, et al. (1996). Psychosocial protocol for childhood cancer: A conceptual model. *Cancer, 78(6)*, 1349-1352.

clinical trials or other treatment options, sign consent forms, and participate in making important decisions about their child's care. The necessity for moving quickly to bone marrow transplantation confronts a few families and presents a different set of treatment and management issues. Parents or other caregivers must assist their child's adjustment to all that is happening, while managing their own emotions and communicating to siblings and other family members about the diagnosis and treatment. The crisis of the diagnosis either can expose weaknesses and problems in individual family members and in the family system, or can demonstrate the strength and resilience of the family.

The cancer and its treatment disrupt ordinary daily life. Divorced parents come together to help their child or resume old struggles with one another. Previously uninvolved parents appear on the scene. Parents require time away from work to be with their child. One parent may take a leave of absence or quit a job. Financial concerns and insurance or managed care coverage issues emerge. Travel to distant medical centers may present problems. Relatives, friends, or neighbors help with siblings left at home. Some families find they lack the familial, social, and community resources they need to provide support.

The ill child becomes the major focus of family time and attention, temporarily setting aside other individual or family problems. Many families have immediate concerns about limited or inadequate finances; insurance or managed care coverage and the potential cost to them of extensive treatment. Some parents find that the diagnosis causes a questioning of religious, philosophical, or spiritual beliefs.

Family adaptational tasks of the diagnostic stage are:

- Acquiring and processing knowledge and information
- Providing emotional support to infant, child, or adolescent
- Assisting patients with the physical aspects of disease
- Expressing and managing emotional reactions to diagnosis and treatment
- Adapting family life to balance the needs of all members
- Attending to relationships within and outside the family
- Mobilizing essential social supports and other resources

- Learning to function in the health care system
- Facing uncertainty and loss of control
- Searching for meaning.

STAGE II: TREATMENT WHEN REMISSION IS SUSTAINED

There is no clear point in time when the first stage ends and the next begins. Stage II is that period of time when treatment patterns become established and the cancer appears to be under control. Patients and families move from the crisis time of diagnosis and the newness of treatment toward greater familiarity with childhood cancer and its regimens. They now are knowledgeable about childhood cancer and better able to formulate questions. They have their emotions in check and are able to offer their children the comfort, support, and encouragement they need. Families adapt to a chronic situation in which family life returns to a more normal state, although altered to fit the new reality of treatment protocols.

In the early days of this stage, families have heightened anxiety as they, and perhaps community physicians and nurses, assume more responsibility for care. Clinic visits, scheduled tests, and re-admissions join other planned events on families' calendars. Team members become familiar and trusted. Families learn to tolerate the inevitable small setbacks and treatment delays occasioned by their child's particular response to therapy. They struggle to deal with government program regulations or insurance and managed care reimbursement issues. They turn their attention to the needs of their other children and to family matters. They count on support from friends and family and begin to make connections with patients and families in situations similar to theirs.

This is the stage in which families permit themselves to hope that cure will be the outcome, even while remaining aware of the uncertainty of the future. For some fortunate families, the majority of those whose children have cancer, there is steady progress toward the end of the treatment plan and the beginning of long-term monitoring.

Family adaptional tasks of the stage of sustained remission are:

- Addressing changing informational needs
- Sustaining hopefulness through chronicity and crisis periods

- Assisting the patient with side effects, body image, self-esteem, schooling, and changes in personal aspirations
- Mastering feelings regarding child or adolescent's disease and treatment experiences
- Fostering patient's normal growth and development
- Maintaining satisfactory family functioning
- Dealing with reimbursement issues, government program regulations, or legal rights
- Securing and using social and emotional support
- Anticipating the completion of treatment.

STAGE III: TREATMENT WHEN DISEASE RECURS

A child's recurrent disease stuns the family anew, bringing a resurgence of fear and dread. This stage may occur in the early months of treatment or months after treatment has ended. Families must learn about new treatment strategies, make new decisions, offer their child or adolescent fresh encouragement, and regulate their own and the family's hope and optimism. They now are knowledgeable about cancer and the health care system, but there is new information to digest. For a few, transplantation becomes a final option and a search for "matches" or unrelated donors begins. Transplantation, when it occurs, moves patients and families into a new crisis situation. Siblings or parents may become bone marrow donors, opening new issues and concerns. Moving forward with normal family life is difficult in this stage. Cancer becomes again the factor that dominates everyday events and family energy shifts to the needs of the patient. Some young people respond well to transplantation or new medications and eventually complete this second round of treatment. Others experience repeated cycles of remission and relapse until achieving remission is no longer a possibility.

Family adaptational tasks of the stage when disease recurs are:

- Coping with emotional responses evoked by disease recurrence
- Processing information and participating in decision-making about possible new treatments
- Assisting the child or adolescent in understanding and accepting recurrence and cooperating with the new treatment

- Regulating hopefulness about outcome.

STAGE IV: PROGRESSIVE DISEASE AND DEATH

The death of a child or adolescent can occur precipitously because of rapid disease progression or because of an unforeseen consequence of treatment. When that happens this is a very brief stage in the illness experience. Most, however, come to a moment, different for each patient and family, when there is realization that potential life-saving treatments are exhausted and that death is inevitable. During the weeks and months of this phase, while parents may go to work and siblings to school, the anticipation of death is an ever-present preoccupation. Family members generally want information that will help them understand what is likely to occur. They still have decisions to make about their preferences about end-of-life care. It is often difficult for many to move from a belief in aggressive treatment to an acceptance that palliative care is best. Teams generally support the wishes of patients and families, but sometimes must mediate the disagreements that occur about what to do.

Parents and other family members mobilize to help their child live every day. Surprisingly, it is not a period devoid of hope or happiness. It can, if time and circumstances allow, be a rich and treasured episode in the life of a family. Family members reshape hope to focus on providing immediate comfort, marking small milestones, and arranging simple pleasures. They remember the good times in family life. Some young people find enjoyment in life until very close to death. Others have a more difficult and uncomfortable course. Parents have the anguishing task of helping their child to prepare for death. Infants need comforting and cuddling, and toddlers the verbal reassurance that parents will be there. Older children and adolescents require information about what is happening to them. They also need an opportunity to discuss fears and parents' beliefs about what happens after death. Oncology social workers, and other team members, remain involved to counsel, educate, and assist in practical ways.

Family members also try to prepare themselves intellectually, emotionally, spiritually, and practically as they watch the child's physical deterioration. Death often is a welcome relief from suffering. Families make funeral and burial arrangements and end their active involvement with most team members. Oncology social workers often maintain telephone contact in the year following death. Some offer bereavement counseling or bereavement groups; others refer to community bereavement programs. All family members face lifetimes of mourning and grieving. Even when they reinvest in the future, the death of a child remains a chronic sorrow.

Family adaptational tasks of the stage of progressive disease and death are:

- Coping with emotional responses to disease progression and eventual death
- Assisting the patient with physical deterioration, discomfort, and pain
- Maintaining adequate family functioning
- Preparing the child, siblings, and other family members for impending death
- Reshaping hope to focus on the good events of each day
- Helping the child or adolescent live until death occurs
- Making arrangements for funeral or memorial services
- Ending formal relationships with team members
- Grieving and mourning the loss of child or adolescent
- Finding meaning and purpose in life without the child's presence.

STAGE V: COMPLETION OF TREATMENT AND SURVIVAL

This stage is the one longed for by all patients and families. Treatment ends and plans are made for the coming months and years of follow-up care. Many effects of the experience and the treatment persist, as do many unanswered or unanswerable questions. This is a period, however, that will last for a lifetime. There is much reason to celebrate reaching the desired goal of surviving cancer and having the prospect of a long life. Young people move on with growing and developing. Families, although forever changed, return to a normal life. The experience damages some; but the majority of families gain strength from what they endure. Anxiety about cancer and its possible recurrence persists for most parents and adolescents, but generally diminishes as time passes. Ideally, teams monitor the health of these young people in long-term survivor clinics, where oncology social workers are available to assess continuing or new psychosocial concerns. The strong ties to team members loosen. Care eventually is transferred to adult care providers armed with knowledge about the patient's relevant medical history.

Family adaptational tasks of the stage of treatment completion and survival are:

- Managing the conflicting emotions of completing treatment
- Adjusting to any long-term effects of treatment
- Acquiring information about issues and resources relevant to survivorship
- Resuming "normal" individual and family life
- Acquiring information and resources relevant to survivorship
- Arranging and maintaining appropriate lifetime follow-up for the patient.

SUMMARY

This chapter, in exploring families' common experiences with childhood cancer, suggests use of a framework of family adaptational tasks to guide social workers' assessments and clinical interventions throughout the stages of cancer and its aftermath. Social workers in pediatric oncology are important members of the care team. They must be well prepared for the difficult work they do. Their special knowledge and skills position them to work with young people, families, and team members to achieve the best possible social and emotional outcomes, whatever the demands of the disease and its treatment.

The increasing number of surviving and cured children and adolescents, if given adequate support and assistance during the periods of active treatment, are able to move forward more confidently into productive futures. Social workers can continue to assist these fortunate young people as they return to medical centers for periodic monitoring.

Families, of course, always survive childhood cancer, even when children die. The attention and care they receive from dedicated and competent social workers can have lifetime impact, doing much to avoid adverse psychosocial effects and strengthen family functioning. Families and young people demonstrate daily an admirable ability to use the help available to them to rise to the many challenges of childhood cancer. Oncology social workers feel privileged to work with these special young people and their families. They are daily witnesses to small and large acts of courage, to human resilience, to the struggle to preserve life, and to the triumph of the human spirit over adversity.

REFERENCES

Arnholt, U.V., Fritz, G. K., & Keener, M. (1993). Self-concept in survivors of childhood and adolescent cancer. *Journal of Psychosocial Oncology*, *11(1)*, 1-16.

Bendor, S. (1990). Anxiety and isolation in siblings of pediatric cancer patients: The need for prevention. *Social Work in Health Care*, *14(3)*, 17-35.

Chesler, M. A., Allswede, J., & Barbarin, O. O. (1991). Voices from the margins of the family: Siblings of children with cancer. *Journal of Psychosocial Oncology*, *9(4)*, 19-42.

Christ, G. H. (1993). Psychosocial tasks throughout the cancer experience. In N. M. Stearns, M. M. Lauria, J. F. Hermann, & P. R. Fogelberg (Eds.). *Oncology social work: A clinician's guide* (pp. 75-99). Atlanta, GA: American Cancer Society.

Christ, G. H., Lane, J. M., & Marcove, R. (1995). Psychosocial adaptation of long-term survivors of bone sarcoma. *Journal of Psychosocial Oncology*, *13(4)*, 1-22.

Claflin, C. J., & Barbarin, O. A. (1991). Does "telling" less protect more? Relationships among age, information disclosure, and what children with cancer see and feel. *Journal of Pediatric Psychology*, *16(2)*, 169-191.

Dahlquist, L . M., Czyzewski, D. I., Copeland, K. G., Jones, C. J., Taub, E., & Vaughan, J. K. (1993). Parents of children newly diagnosed with cancer: Anxiety, coping and marital distress. *Journal of Pediatric Psychology, 18,* 365-376.

Dahlquist, L. M., Power, T. G., Cox, C. N., & Fernbach, D. J. (1994). Parenting and child distress during cancer procedures: A multidimensional assessment. *Children's Health Care, 23(3),* 149-166.

Deasy-Spinetta, P. (1993). School issues and the child with cancer. *Cancer Supplement, 71(10),* 3261-3264.

Eaton, A. P. (1993). Financing care for children with cancer. *Cancer, 71(10),* 3265-3268.

Foley, G. V. (1993). Enhancing child-family-health team communication. *Cancer, 71(10),* 3281-3289.

Grootenhuis, M. A., & Last, B. F. (1997). Parents' emotional reactions related to different prospects for the survival of their children with cancer. *Journal of Psychosocial Oncology, 15(1),* 43-62.

Hays, D. M. (1993). Employment and insurance issues. *Cancer, 71,* 3306-3309.

Hersh, S. P., & Weiner, L. S. (1993). Psychosocial support for the family of the child with cancer. In P. A. Pizzo & D. G. Poplack (Eds.). *Principles and practice of pediatric oncology* (pp. 353-382). Philadelphia, PA: Lippincott, Williams, & Wilkins.

Katz, E. R., & Varni, J. W. (1993). Social support and social cognitive problem solving in children with newly diagnosed cancer. *Cancer, 71(10),* 3314-3319.

Kupst, M. J., Natta, M. B., Richardson, C. C., Shulman, J. L., Lavigne, J. V., & Das, L. (1995). Family coping with pediatric leukemia: Ten years after treatment. *Journal of Pediatric Psychology, 20(5),* 601-617.

Lauria, M. M., Hockenberry-Eaton, M., Pawletko, T. M., & Mauer, A. M. (1996). Psychosocial protocol for childhood cancer: A conceptual model. *Cancer, 78(6),* 1345-1356.

Mailick, M. (1979). The impact of severe illness on the individual and family: An overview. *Social Work in Health Care, 5(2),* 117-124.

Mulhern, R. K., Fairclough, D., Douglas, S. M., & Smith, B. (1994). Physical distress and depressive symptomatology among children with cancer. *Children's Health Care, 23(3),* 167-179.

Nelson, A. E., Miles, M. S., Reed, S. P., Davis, C.P., & Cooper, H. (1994). Depressive symptomatology in parents of children with chronic oncologic or hematologic disease. *Journal of Psychosocial Oncology, 12(4)*, 61-77.

Noll, R. B., Bukowski, W. M., Davies, W. H., Koontz, K., & Kulkarni, R. (1993). Adjustment in the peer system of adolescents with cancer: a two-year study. *Journal of Pediatric Psychology, 18(3)*, 351-364.

Overholser, J. C., & Fritz, G. K. (1990). The impact of childhood cancer on the family. *Journal of Psychosocial Oncology, 8(4)*, 71-85.

Redd, W. H. (1994). Advances in psychosocial oncology in pediatrics. *Cancer, 74(4)*, 1496-1502.

Ross, J. W., (1993). Understanding the family experience with childhood cancer. In N. M. Stearns, M. M. Lauria, J. F. Hermann, & P. R. Fogelberg (Eds.), *Oncology social work: A clinician's guide* (pp. 199-236). Atlanta, GA: American Cancer Society.

Sanger, M. S., Copeland, D. R., & Davidson, E. R. (1991). Psychosocial adjustment among pediatric cancer patients: A multidisciplinary assessment. *Journal of Pediatric Psychology; 16(4)*, 463-474.

Sawyer, M., Antoniou, G., Toogood, I., Rice, M., & Baghurst, P. (2000). Childhood cancer: A 4-year prospective study of the psychological adjustment of children and parents. *Journal of Pediatric Hematology/Oncology, 22(3)*, 214-220.

Sharp, J. W. (1999). The Internet: Changing the way cancer survivors obtain information. *Cancer Practice, 7(5)*, 266-269.

Speechley, K. N., & Noh, S. (1992). Surviving childhood cancer, social support, and parents' psychological adjustment. *Journal of Pediatric Psychology, 17(1)*, 15-31.

Stehbens, J. A., MacLean, W. E., Kaleita, T. A., Noll, R. B., Schwartz, E., Cantor, N. L., Woodard, A., Whitt, J. K., Waskerwitz, M. J., Ruymann, F. B., & Hammond, G. D. (1994). Effects of CNS prophylaxis on the neuropsychological performance of children with acute lymphocytic leukemia: Nine months post-diagnosis. *Children's Health Care, 23(4)*, 231-250.

Varni, J. W., Katz, E. R., Colegrove, R., & Dolgin, M. (1994). Perceived social support and adjustment of children with newly diagnosed cancer. *Journal of Developmental Behavioral Pediatrics, 15(1)*, 20-26.

Weigers, M. E., Chesler, M. A., Zebrack, B. J., & Goldman, S. (1998). Self-reported worries among long-term survivors of childhood cancer and their peers. *Journal of Psychosocial Oncology, 16(2)*, 1-23.

Whittam, E. H. (1993). Terminal care of the dying child: Psychosocial implications of care. *Cancer, 71 (10)*, 3450-3462.

Zeltzer, L., LeBaron, S., & Zeltzer, P. M. (1984). The effectiveness of behavioral intervention for reduction of nausea and vomiting in children and adolescents receiving chemotherapy. *Journal of Clinical Oncology, 2*, 683-690.

CHAPTER 7

SOCIAL WORK INTERVENTIONS WITH CHILDREN AND ADOLESCENTS

Michelle Fillios Cox, MSW, LMSW
Allison Stovall, MSW, LMSW

The diagnosis of cancer in childhood quickly involves the child or adolescent, parents, and all family members in the complex world of present-day cancer treatment. This world acknowledges the importance of treating the child with a disease, not just the disease itself. The child brings not only a biological reality to this world, but also a social and psychological one. The nature of the disease and the intensity of the treatment it requires produce physical, social, and emotional effects that demand attention for the child, family, and society.

Medical and psychosocial team members share common and interrelated goals for patient and family. They commit themselves to preserving or extending the life of the child and minimizing suffering, while interfering as little as possible with normal growth and development. Health care professionals attempt to assist families to function in ways that enable individual family members to realize their needs. This chapter notes the usual elements in psychosocial care programs, discusses social work issues in providing services, and examines the varied services and interventions social workers in pediatric oncology use to assist young people and families with the social and emotional impact of cancer and its treatment.

PSYCHOSOCIAL CARE PROGRAMS

Oncology social workers in pediatrics provide services as part of an overall program of psychosocial care generally offered in pediatric oncology centers. There is consensus that such psychosocial care should be part of quality care for all cancer patients (Arceci, Reamon, Cohen, & Lampkin, 1998). Currently, each pediatric oncology center team determines what staff, programs, and clinical services to offer. Recently, oncology social workers and other clinicians have recognized the value of working toward establishment of a psychosocial protocol. This protocol would help clinicians respond to the challenge of articulating clearly what they do, standardizing their approaches, and researching the efficacy of their clinical efforts (Lauria, Hockenberry-Eaton, Pawletko, & Mauer, 1996). Despite a lack of overt consensus about the specifics of psychosocial care, however, there are some usual components found in the programs available in almost all centers. These components include:

- Incorporating psychosocial services into coordinated, comprehensive care programs
- Offering continuity of psychosocial care to all patients and families from diagnosis through treatment and into extended survivorship or bereavement
- Sharing responsibility for psychosocial care among multidisciplinary team members
- Offering a wide range of clinical services, such as advocacy, supportive counseling, and other therapies, behavioral interventions, stress management, education, and resource provision and referral
- Providing varied support programs, such as parent, sibling, or other support groups, school re-entry programs, summer camps, buddy programs, recreational activities, bereavement groups, and survivor programs
- Using medical center volunteers in special programs to supplement the work of psychosocial professionals
- Collaborating with community and national voluntary health

and other organizations to expand psychosocial care through shared programs and initiatives.

Providing such a broad array of services and programs is a challenging task for all team members involved in psychosocial care. Social workers new to pediatric oncology will need time to learn about what is possible in their particular work setting, but they also need awareness of what is "standard" in well-respected institutions. They also may wish to refer to the Standards of Practice developed by the Association of Pediatric Oncology Social Workers (see the Appendix or their Web site at www.aposw.org). They may find that staffing, funding, and resource allocations often are not sufficient to support delivery of quality psychosocial care. Psychosocial clinicians everywhere report pressure to "do more with less." In this era of concern about costs in health care, they also face challenges to provide data to support the efficacy of services and programs they deliver. Fortunately, there is usually a strong commitment by those in the field and an exchange of mutual support among team members that make the tasks easier.

ISSUES IN THE DELIVERY OF SOCIAL WORK SERVICES

To provide effective services and programs in pediatric oncology, social workers must understand several issues that influence and shape the services they offer. These include:

* THE MULTIDISCIPLINARY TEAM
  The complexity of providing comprehensive care for children and adolescents with cancer led to the creation of multidisciplinary teams in most major medical centers. In addition to social workers, teams include professionals of several disciplines who have responsibility for or shared interest in these issues: physicians, nurses, psychologists, psychiatrists, child life workers or recreation therapists, school teachers, chaplains, and

others. Despite respect for differing contributions, differences in professional training, mission, goals, and attitudes can create divisions among team members. Teams often struggle with issues of authority, roles, boundaries, leadership, responsibilities, and decision-making. Members must be alert to the potential these differences have for adversely affecting patients and families.

Teams meet regularly, often during daily inpatient rounds, to devise a comprehensive approach to caring for each child or adolescent followed in their center. Teams usually work more effectively when there are mechanisms in place to facilitate regular communication about patient care. Development and use of multidisciplinary care plans also improve team communication and collaboration. Good teamwork enhances patient care and is essential to quality care.

- ## ROLE CLARITY AND LIMITS

The social worker assumes many roles with patients and families: evaluator, counselor, educator, advocate, case manager, group worker, discharge planner, and liaison to hospital and community resources. In addition, professional concern for the needs of all the patients and families being served may lead to other roles including case manager, program planner, teacher, resource developer, and researcher. It is important for social workers to articulate clearly to team members and families the various roles they can play and the areas in which they can offer patients and families assistance. They also may need to speak to the limits of what they can do. Families coming to a medical center do not expect to receive the many services that are part of a comprehensive care approach. Sometimes, families' misperceptions about social workers or previous negative experiences with social work pose problems. Most families welcome the help available, but each family must be free to accept or reject assistance and services. Well-functioning families may need only a minimum of clinical services and validation that they are responding normally to this new experience. Families with many problems may require intensive help. Almost all families appreciate the education, support, and special programs available to their children and to them. Social workers new to pediatric oncology may need to learn that some problems and situations will not be resolved. Social workers understand that they only can offer help and support, not impose it. If families reject services initially, continuing interest on the part of the social worker sometimes results in a request for help at a later phase in the illness experience. Physician support for psychosocial assessment and supportive interventions as a basic and essential part of team care usually elicits cooperation from even reluctant parents.

At times, physicians and other team members also require help in understanding what social workers can and cannot do. For example, they may need reminding that social workers are not able to "fix" patients and families whose attitudes or behaviors cause problems or interfere with adherence to the treatment plan. In such situations, social workers often can make a positive difference. They can serve as mediators, raise issues that others find uncomfortable to discuss, or help identify and solve an underlying problem that is the real issue.

- ## PROFESSIONAL BOUNDARIES

The intimacy of the work sometimes makes it difficult for team members to maintain appropriate professional boundaries with patients and families during the many intense months of treatment. Young people have enormous appeal and the plight of particular patients and their parents will touch the heart of any caring individual. Most oncology social workers will at some time in their careers struggle with boundary issues. Becoming a personal rather than a professional friend threatens one's ability to retain objectivity and provide services in a professional manner. It also makes it difficult to give each patient and parent the equal attention they deserve. Experienced oncology social workers know that it is possible to show compassion and caring while preserving the emotional distance necessary to helping effectively. Consulting with a supervisor or a peer who has had similar experiences can make a difference in understanding and managing one's own reactions.

- EMOTIONAL STRESS

  The intensity of social workers' involvement with children and families coupled with awareness of the enormity of the problems they face can create cumulative stress. Such stress may interfere with the ability of an individual to sustain the energy demanded by this work. At times, a worker's life situation will pose problems in handling a pediatric oncology assignment. Social workers who are in their childbearing years may have particular difficulty watching the anguish of children and parents with whom they can identify. Others may be experiencing serious loss in their personal lives. Additionally, when social workers are responsible for diverse services to very large numbers of patients and families during multiple crises and periods of chronicity, they can expect to feel very stressed. Some find they are temperamentally unsuited to work in pediatric oncology. Most social workers, however, can handle the day-to-day pressure they experience if they are attentive to its effects and use the same time and stress management strategies they recommend to patients and families.

- ETHICAL CONCERNS

  Social workers in pediatric oncology also must be attentive to the many value issues that are an integral part of work in this area.

  > Ethical issues arise from many factors: The uncertainty of outcome; the manipulation of children who cannot make decisions for themselves; the difficulty of obtaining informed consent because of the complex nature of the disease and treatment; the intense long-term involvement of patients and families with medical staffs and treatment centers; the sometimes conflicting interests or researcher, healer, parent and patient, and the varying roles and expectations of many caregivers. (Ross, 1993, p. 233)

  At different times and in different situations, social workers represent themselves, the profession, the team, and the institution to patients and families. At other times they act or speak on behalf of patients and families to the team, the institution, and other agencies and organizations. They must be vigilant in respecting confidentiality and maintaining the trust placed in them by all these parties as they confront ethical dilemmas regarding their own actions and counsel parents about the difficult ethical decisions they face. Many facilities offer opportunities for formal consultation on ethical issues through clinical ethics committees. Social workers also can turn for guidance on ethical matters to the National Association of Social Workers "Code of Ethics" (NASW, 2000; www.nasw.org).

- KNOWLEDGE AND SKILLS
  Pediatric oncology social workers must possess excellent clinical skills in order to offer the array of social work services which children and families require for coping with childhood cancer. Along with those skills, they must have knowledge about particular cancer diagnoses and about the common issues pediatric patients and families generally confront in dealing with a cancer diagnosis. They must also be familiar with theories underlying a variety of interventions and with the results of published psychosocial research findings and clinical observations (see Chapter 6). With this knowledge, the social worker can then move to the critical tasks of assessing the uniqueness of each child or adolescent and planning appropriate interventions.

ASSESSMENT OF PATIENTS AND FAMILIES

High-Risk Screening

In some cancer centers, social workers assess all patients and families who present for consultation and treatment. While this is ideal in working with individuals facing a frightening diagnosis, social work staffing patterns may not make it possible to see all patients. In these instances, social workers usually develop high-risk screening methods, often a checklist, to determine which patients and families are most in need of services, such as those at risk for problems with adaptation or basic social needs. Social workers assist at times in finding financial and other resources to facilitate bringing a new patient for diagnostic evaluation. Community professionals may alert social workers to problems with or concerns about a child, adolescent, or family.

Purpose of the Psychosocial Assessment

The initial assessment process sets the stage for the development of a therapeutic relationship between the social worker and the family. It serves as the essential basis for the delivery of effective services and demonstrates to the child and family the importance the multidisciplinary team gives to understanding the impact of the cancer diagnosis on all family members. Assessment information is important because it provides the team of caregivers with an individualized picture of the child or adolescent, a unique individual with personal attributes who is developing socially within the context of a family, a school environment, and a home community. Assessment of the family's understanding about a social work referral may help team members know when clarification is necessary regarding the social worker's role.

Assessment Data

While social workers can observe each family's ways of managing during the crisis of the diagnostic phase, as Last and Grootenhuis (1998) have emphasized, it is important to learn from parents about the "emotional and behavioral reactions and coping strategies" that existed in the family prior to the diagnosis. Social workers need to know the strengths possessed by the child or adolescent, the siblings, the parents, and other significant members of the family. At the time of diagnosis, there may be a tendency for family members to protect each other because of the fears often attached to the idea of cancer. Family members may need help in understanding the value of openness and honesty in providing information on their history and life situations, formulating questions, and communicating with team members. They also need to hear how the social worker will use the information provided.

Information on the composition of the family and the nature of family relationships is essential. It also is important to identify which family members are central in the life of the child or adolescent. The social worker should obtain information on the family's socioeconomic status and on the employment situations of each parent. Exploration of economic resources on hand for covering the costs of treatment and out-of-pocket expenses helps identify families needing referral to financial assistance agencies. It is helpful to learn about the degree of closeness or tension within the family and about the friendship networks of the patient. This information helps in predicting the tangible and emotional supports available to patients and families struggling to achieve stability or alerts the team to potential problem areas. Information on other problems of family members, such as alcoholism, severe cognitive limitations or illiteracy, or serious mental illness is also important. Exploration of formal and informal spiritual resources assists the social worker in understanding the family's values and beliefs as well as the meanings the family assigns to the occurrence of a serious, life-threatening illness in their child. A complete assessment also takes into consideration the ethnic group to which the child and family belong and their primary language. Membership in ethnic minorities may bring special viewpoints regarding illness that the health care team should understand.

Format of the Assessment

The first section of the assessment reports the data gathered in the initial interviews, with careful delineation of information reported by family members about their personal situations. This includes:

- Initial reactions to diagnosis, proposed treatment, and possible outcomes
- Observations of prevalent communication, coping, and decision-making styles and affect of family members
- Child's or adolescent's emotional, cognitive, and developmental status
- The child's level of academic performance, both long-term and prior to diagnosis

- Attitudes toward informing the school of the child's medical situation
- Issues of particular concern to the child and family
- Information on the composition of the nuclear and extended families
- Descriptions of support networks in neighborhood, community, church, or school
- Sources of family income and insurance, public assistance, or managed care coverage
- Distance family lives from treatment center and home setting (urban/rural)
- Information on the suitability of the home for home health care
- Information on spiritual, religious, and cultural values, beliefs, and philosophy of life.

The social worker should follow this descriptive data by a section that highlights the strengths of the patient and family members and indicates how those strengths can help in developing positive ways of coping with the stresses imposed by the child's cancer. It is important also to include the patient's and parents' perspectives on how they are managing at this point. Any problems or high-risk factors should be noted in this section. Finally, the assessment should include a list of the social worker and team's plans for any specific problems cited. Since assessments and psychosocial care plans should identify the strengths families bring to the experience, social workers should consider sharing the contents verbally with most families. Parents are often reassured that the team thinks that they will be able to cope effectively with the experience.

There are several ways to document assessment data. When there is a high volume of parents, or when an institution mandates brief chart entries, social workers may use a checklist with room for a few comments. Some departments of social work adopt a format that combines descriptive narrative with a list of problems, strengths, and resources. When time allows, a concise narrative format may be used to communicate with the team about the functioning of a new patient and family. In some settings, social workers may document their assessment and proposed interventions in a multidisciplinary care plan developed with other team members. Good clinical practice also requires periodic updating of assessment information to capture changes in the patient or family situation.

CLINICAL INTERVENTIONS WITH PATIENTS AND FAMILIES

Crisis Intervention

When parents learn that their child has cancer, they experience loss of stability both individually and within the family system. This loss of balance constitutes the crisis situation characteristic of the diagnostic phase of the illness. Parents and other adults in the family become anxious about the possible loss of the child and the suffering that treatment may bring. The child's siblings worry about the sick brother or sister, develop fears about their own health, or resent the absence of their parents, even when they can understand the reasons for that absence. The anxieties of the patient vary with age, but concerns about painful medical procedures, physical discomfort induced by treatment, and changes in appearance are common. The social worker and other team members can help children and families recognize that the diagnosis of a severe, chronic illness can bring about upsetting feelings. Further intervention is directed at exploring and clarifying the feelings of each family member. Expression of fear, anger, and other common emotional responses can relieve the child or adolescent and family members of some anxiety and feelings of helplessness. As Clarke-Steffen (1997) reported in a review of studies of family coping with childhood cancer, "...parents tended to use their usual coping strategies, and marriages remained stable over the course of the illness and survival." The social worker can help family members to understand how to manage feelings, how familiar coping mechanisms can be valuable in this new situation, and how to learn new ways of coping. When the patient's initial discharge from the hospital or clinic is imminent, the social worker can help the family members contemplate the activities and emotions connected with the return home. This is a good time to provide the parents with information on agencies in their home community that offer emotional, social, and financial support. When the child returns for the first time to the treatment center, the crisis work can move to completion with a review of how child and family members handled encounters with friends and relatives at home.

The process of crisis intervention is limited, but the social worker may employ it on a recurring basis when working with families. Even when the initial crisis of the diagnosis is substantially resolved, other crises may arise throughout the course of treatment. During ongoing therapy a crisis may ensue if a child requires surgery, especially if the need arises from an emergency. A significant crisis can develop when the disease recurs, once a remission has been attained. When treatment has been successful and families face the termination of therapy, the patient and family may experience a crisis as they learn to function with much less dependency on the treatment center staff.

The most demanding crises arise when staff must make the family aware that the child's cancer has progressed despite the use of proven therapeutic agents. After addressing this disturbing news together, the child, the family, and the multidisciplinary team must put their energies into attaining another remission. The health care team may suggest the option of a bone marrow transplant to the child and family. This becomes a viable treatment choice based on the child's clinical status and emotional health. If bone marrow transplant is neither advisable nor possible, then the medical team generally recommends maintenance therapy.

When it is not possible to bring about a second remission, or if the disease recurs following new treatment or post-transplant, physicians discuss the gravity of the child's or adolescent's prognosis with the family. Although many pediatric oncologists are skilled and experienced in communicating such difficult news, team members may also be involved, suggesting age-appropriate ways to communicate with the child or adolescent. The team may present the option of treating with Phase I or II protocols in an effort to gain some temporary control of the disease. Most patients and parents continue to find some reason to hope that something will happen to prove the team wrong about the outcome for their child. When there are no further treatment options, the team begins preparing patient and family for the likely death of the child or adolescent. It usually begins with a discussion of shifting from active treatment to end of life supportive care. The issue of considering a referral to home hospice may be raised. Strategies similar to those employed during the crisis of diagnosis are used throughout the phases of the illness to help young people and their families cope with these difficult periods.

Supportive Counseling

Throughout the course of treatment, the social worker may engage in supportive counseling to maintain functional behaviors in all family members. Based on the team's psychosocial assessment of the child's and family's functioning, the social worker will employ interventions grounded in theories of normal family functioning, communication, stress management, cognitive/behavioral techniques, brief problem-focused therapy, and insight-oriented psychotherapy (Lauria et al., 1996).

Families may experience increased anxiety in anticipation of clinic visits, particularly in the early months of therapy. As part of ongoing work with child or adolescent and family, the social worker may need to review current issues periodically and assist with problem solving. It can be useful to help families anticipate problems arising from normal life changes or predictable illness events. Parents may ask for help in dealing with normal growth and development issues of their ill child or other children. At times, parents may need to hear a simple "vote of confidence" in how they are managing daily life. By maintaining an active interest in the successful adaptation of the child and family, the social worker demonstrates positive regard for them and their welfare. This enhances the individual's feelings of worth and strengthens the therapeutic relationship.

Family Counseling

The social worker must keep the family context in mind when working with the child and available family members since all members of the family system are affected by the changes resulting from the cancer diagnosis and treatment. It is important to help parents anticipate common changes in family functioning. They may need help in evaluating how to balance the needs of all of the family members. This is particularly crucial to keep in mind as shifts occur in the roles assumed by family members as a consequence of the demands of the child's treatment (Lauria et al., 1996). When conducting the initial assessment, it is wise to address the needs and reactions of the patient's siblings. If they are not present because of the distance from home, it is still important to attend to their concerns in discussions with family members. When hospital staff pay attention to the family as a unit, they give a sense of importance to the siblings and the parent who usually remains at home with them (Bendor, 1990). Typically, the family therapy practiced by a pediatric oncology social worker has as the underlying framework the impact of the child's cancer on family life

Collaboration with the Multidisciplinary Team

Social workers may turn to other mental health professionals in the treatment center to assist in working with the family when families present with long-standing problems in the marital relationship or with serious problems in individual or family functioning. These may include other social workers or psychologists and child psychiatrists who specialize in behavior therapy, individual psychotherapy, group work, or family therapy. The social worker may undertake the significant therapeutic task of preparing a child or family member for psychological counseling or neuro-psychological assessment. Psychologists may be team members, employed in pediatrics, or affiliated with the center's psychiatry department. In most centers, child psychiatrists are available, on a referral basis, to assess the need for medications to facilitate coping and adaptation.

Many pediatric oncology social workers practice in university teaching hospitals and work with child life specialists or recreation therapists in attending to the mental health needs of children and family members. Social workers and child life specialists often act as mutual referral agents. The social worker focuses on the patient and family but may work most actively with the parents, especially if the patient is a preadolescent child. The child life specialist or recreation therapist may be aware of family issues but will use the media of play and activity to focus on work with the child. Child life specialists, social workers, and psychologists often work closely with parent consultants (i.e., parents hired to work with multidisciplinary teams). Occasionally, parents may refuse the social worker's attempts to offer support and other kinds of intervention. In those instances, the social worker may offer consultation to other members of the team. They may also choose to stay in touch with the family on a superficial level and find that the family becomes receptive to their involvement later.

Social workers are aware that patients and families often face spiritual and ethical concerns, so they work closely with or refer to hospital chaplains. Religious belief systems can be central to individual and family coping with illness. Sometimes patients and families begin to question their religious beliefs. Often parents try to find meaning in the occurrence of illness and struggle to come up with explanations of why their child has become ill. They may question their faith by wondering if the child's illness represents punishment for previous or current behaviors. Throughout the course of the child's treatment, parents and other family members are likely to express hope for a miracle or some form of divine healing. Adolescent patients may present additional challenges to the team if they hold religious views that differ from those of their parents.

Collaboration with Volunteers

Volunteers in health care settings often choose to spend time with children with cancer to create opportunities for the children and their families to enjoy themselves despite the difficulties of treatment. When the resources of the volunteer department of the hospital allow for it, volunteers can join with the child life specialists or recreation therapists in offering regularly scheduled parties and holiday observances. They may sponsor buddy programs with volunteers befriending patients and their siblings. Volunteers serve as counselors in camp programs for patients and their brothers and sisters. They organize fund raising activities to support the educational and recreational programs that promote the cognitive, social, and emotional adjustment of children with cancer and their family members. Members of voluntary health organizations supplement the work of hospital volunteers with a variety of beneficial programs. The American Cancer Society (ACS) has adapted the "Look Good, Feel Better®" program for teenagers in order to help them with their concerns about appearance. In addition, they have information on childhood cancer posted on their Web site (www.cancer.org). The Patient Aid program of the Leukemia and Lymphoma Society (LLS; www.leukemia-lymphoma.org) helps families with the expenses of travelling to treatment centers when their children have leukemia, lymphoma, or related diseases. Its "Back to School" program helps with school re-entry. Informational resources and support are available from many organizations, such as the Pediatric Brain Tumor Foundation of the United States (PBTF; www.pbtfus.org). Social workers can provide families with information on accessing these programs and others that may have a regional scope of service.

Child Management Interventions

The social worker's repertoire of interventions needs to include techniques for modifying behaviors within the family. For some parents, positive nurturing skills that reinforce adaptive behavior come easily. Others use practices that are ineffective or have negative repercussions. In working with parents, social workers need to remember how devastated parents are by the cancer diagnosis of their child and by the helplessness they feel in watching the pain and trauma their child experiences. Even parents who are aware of the importance of a consistent approach to discipline are tempted to overindulge or overprotect a child with a serious illness. The social worker can assist parents in dealing with any ambivalence they have by acknowledging that it is normal and understandable to want to indulge the whims of a child with cancer. Temporary periods of extra attention and indulgence may even be beneficial, offering important comfort and consolation to patients and satisfaction to parents who feel they are providing the additional time and extra love their ill child needs. Parents eventually may need support and encouragement to resume their usual disciplining and limit setting. While young people like increased attention, they also want reassurance that their illness is not so terrible that they must be the focus of family life. Parents also may find that singling out a child or adolescent with cancer for prolonged special treatment is likely to disrupt normal development of each child in the family and adversely affect patient sibling relationships. Studies of siblings of children with cancer have noted the pain and isolation which they report feeling when an ill sibling receives excessive parental attention (Bendor, 1990). The challenge facing parents is one of striking a balance. Parents must move between exercising reasonable caution and encouraging the child or adolescent to participate in normal, age-appropriate activities, and social interactions. Social workers can assist families with these issues by noting the successful approaches and strategies reported by other families in similar situations.

Behavioral Techniques

Behavioral techniques serve to reduce anxiety, to distract from the perceived source of pain, to provide physical comfort, and to give the child greater feelings of control (Redd, 1994). Social workers who are trained and experienced in the behavioral techniques of desensitization, relaxation, visual imagery, and hypnosis use them to help patients who experience anticipatory nausea and vomiting related to treatment, heightened anxiety over invasive medical procedures, or mild pain. In many centers, however, psychologists and child life workers are more likely to be the team members using these interventions with young patients. Physicians and nurses are attentive to pain management strategies, often combining medication with behavioral interventions by other team members. Social workers often are more involved in assisting parents by teaching them behavioral strategies to reduce anxiety and help with the management of stress.

Education

Family members who are educated about cancer and its treatment and helped to anticipate common issues the family will experience will feel more competent as they participate in treatment. Provision of medical information to the sisters and brothers of patients helps them also reduce their anxiety and sense of vulnerability about the patients and themselves (Bendor, 1990). The educational activity of information seeking and sharing can enhance the sense of control needed by both patients and family members. The social worker often works closely with team nurses and doctor to reinforce some of their education of the family. It also is important for families to learn about the structure and function of the hospital and the system of health care, so that they will feel more comfortable and knowledgeable about this new environment. Families who receive information about hospital and community resources as well as techniques for coping tend to adapt more positively (Lauria et al., 1996; Sloper, 1996).

Patient and Family Advocacy

Families may need the case advocacy skills of a social worker to secure access to special or limited services in the hospital or from community agencies when particular services have been denied. Linking families or patients with available resources is not advocacy, although the two sometimes are confused. Social workers also teach parents to advocate for their children, coaching them in appropriate ways to convey information about changes in family income or insurance status to the hospital business office or to community agencies that offer financial assistance. Social workers may need to advocate with insurers, managed care companies, or public and private agencies when their guidelines for reimbursement or service do not address patients' needs. They also may need to advocate for parents and young people to assure that they receive the protections offered by current laws to all cancer patients (Hoffman, 1996).

Social workers in pediatric oncology engage in other advocacy activities. They serve as liaisons between family members and staff when they have communication problems or conflicting views on the value of treatment. The social worker may assist parents in influencing treatment decisions involving their child by assisting them with preparation for conferences with the team and by creating opportunities for parents to ask questions and express views during these conferences.

Group Work

Social workers may organize and provide groups for children, adolescents, and families to assist them in adapting to the cancer experience (American Cancer Society, 2001). Professionally led groups based at the treatment center need to be support groups not therapy groups. These groups help individuals strengthen their coping skills and benefit from the experience of mutual support. They may feature an educational component with a program on a topic of interest or an activity followed by a discussion period in which personal experiences are shared and mutual support given. There are various models for structuring groups. They may include patients and their siblings or there may be separate groups for each. Patient groups are often age-related. Bendor's (1990) findings indicate the value of having programs specifically directed at the needs of siblings. In two groups for siblings, they discussed many of the concerns that distressed them about having an ill sister or brother. Group interventions vary according to ages and developmental levels of the members. Activity groups may enable children to lose themselves in art or a game and talk together about their experiences. Parents' support groups offer opportunities to educate and address parenting issues that are relevant to maintaining effective communication and discipline. Recreational activities designed for parents encourage mutual sharing and can reduce families' sense of social isolation. Some treatment centers offer groups for bereaved family members, creating a separate forum for addressing their special needs.

Parents of children with cancer may embrace a self-help group model. While parents may want to set the agendas for such groups, they often welcome assistance from the social worker in locating sites and speakers for program meetings. Social workers also serve as consultants to parents' groups regarding group formation and process. Affiliation with a hospital social worker may legitimize the self-help group in the eyes of the hospital staff.

For families who are motivated to use it, the Internet is a valuable resource for identifying sources of support and information (Sharp, 1999). There is great variation in the quality and breadth of the information available due to the dynamic nature of the Internet (see Chapter 14).

SOCIAL WORK ACTIVITIES THROUGHOUT TREATMENT PHASES

Case Management

Information obtained during the initial assessment assists the health care team in anticipating and planning with the family for discharge needs. From the outset, pediatric oncology social workers assess the family's ability to comply with prescribed home care regimens. They identify the adaptations that family members and the new cancer patient must make when they return to the home community

In the role of case manager, social workers coordinate referrals to social support systems and to agencies that offer material and practical assistance. These referral activities aid families in managing successfully following discharge. During hospital or outpatient treatment the child and family establish ties with other families and form relationships with staff members. Affiliation with support groups in the home community reinforces the benefits of mutual sharing learned in the treatment center. The social worker can assist the family in locating available community organizations.

When indicated, the social worker may help the family access a community medical facility near home. Third-party payers often require the use of local medical providers to augment the services available in the oncology treatment center. Families benefit when they know that the staff at the cancer center has good communication with the hometown team of caregivers who will take responsibility for monitoring the child's health, and often, for administering some of the therapy. The social worker can help community care-givers respond to the family's needs by communicating with them, with permission from the family, information about the responses, and adaptation of the family to the initial phase of treatment at the cancer center. When adjustment problems are severe, the hospital social worker may work with community caregivers to help access local mental health or support resources.

Social workers also provide help to families who consult other centers for second opinions or experimental therapy or for special-ized treatment such as bone marrow transplant. When parents desire a second opinion regarding treatment for their child, the social worker can explore with the family their rationale for this and work with other team members to make necessary arrangements. Social workers must assure families that they support their right to seek other treatment options.

When the family takes the child to another center, the referring social worker, with the parents' sanction, can establish contact with the social worker in the new setting. Such social work intervention is important when the patient may undergo a bone marrow trans-plant or investigational treatment. The social worker at the receiv-ing clinic or hospital can be informative about living arrangements and institutional procedures. A child and family who trust the pedi-atric oncology team attending to them from the time of diagnosis may find it hard to transfer that trust to a new set of health care providers. The work of pediatric oncology social work colleagues on behalf of the family can enhance the parents' ability to make a suc-cessful transition at a critical stage in the treatment. This same kind of cooperative work is desirable when a family needs to transfer a child's care to another hospital due to a geographic move.

School Interventions

Some medical centers include hospital teachers on the psychosocial team. They offer bedside instruction, teach in a hospital-based schoolroom, and serve as liaisons to personnel in the students' home school districts. In consultation with the medical team, they determine the child's current level of school activity so that they can help the child continue working toward their educational goals. Varni, Katz, Colegrove, & Dolgin (1994) point out that schools provide the opportunity for ongoing socialization and social support. The social worker and family members can discuss options for preparing school personnel and classmates for the child's return to school. Some children are comfortable helping teachers explain the illness to classmates, while others prefer that classmates be informed before they return. Social work intervention should focus on the development of open lines of communication among family members, school personnel, and the cancer center (Deasy-Spinetta, 1993).

Pediatric oncology nurses can serve as effective liaisons with school nurses in helping children resume normal school activity, educating school nurses and students about treatment and anticipated side effects. The nurse's interpretation of medical information can complement the social worker's communication with school personnel regarding adjustment issues. Hospital teachers take responsibility for discussing academic issues with personnel from the child's school. In some centers, a school coordinator is the team member who takes the lead in communication with the school using others on the team as resource people. School personnel in the home school have the benefit of knowing the quality of the child's school performance prior to the diagnosis of cancer. They can assist in the process of planning for the child's return to the school by sharing this information with involved hospital staff (Deasy-Spinetta, 1993). In some centers, team members have worked together to develop information packets and workshops for school personnel. When medical information is given to patients' schools, or decisions are made about the timing of patients' re-entry into school, it is important that the pediatric oncologist serve as a consultant. The multidisciplinary team must also consider the needs of the patients' siblings when communicating with school personnel. Healthy siblings of children with cancer are at high risk for having emotional and social distress unless preventive mental health measures are undertaken (Bendor, 1990).

INTERVENTIONS BEYOND ACTIVE TREATMENT

Long-term Survivors

After the completion of active treatment, children return to cancer centers for follow-up examinations at lengthening intervals. Some institutions hold separate clinic sessions for the long-term survivors and, in others, the child continues to be followed by a primary pediatric oncologist. Social workers focus on helping long-term survivors with resumption of normal childhood activities. Social workers need to be aware of vocational and emotional rehabilitation resources to assist survivors in dealing with the psychosocial outcomes of treatment. Cancer survivors still face discrimination from some employers and insurance providers. Social workers, as noted previously, need to be prepared to serve as patient advocates in these instances, as well as educators about the rights and legal protections available to young people and their parents.

Bereaved Families

Unfortunately, a significant although decreasing number of pediatric cancer patients die of the disease or of causes related to treatment each year (Greenlee, Murray, Bolden, & Wingo, 2000). Parents need to know that the professionals who cared for their child have not forgotten them and are still interested in assisting them as they grieve the loss of their child. If families are willing to continue in counseling following a child's death, parents and siblings may be seen individually or in groups in some centers. When counseling is not feasible because of logistics or reluctance to enter into scheduled counseling sessions, the social worker can set up a routine for follow-up telephone contacts. When desired by families, social workers may refer parents or siblings for bereavement counseling to chapters of Compassionate Friends (www.compassionatefriends.org) or to special hospice programs in their communities. Some social workers supplement their contacts with families by providing books or articles written to address bereavement issues. In some centers, members of the multidisciplinary team collaborate to offer a memorial service in honor of patients who have died. This provides a good opportunity for families and staff to have closure.

SUMMARY

Oncology social workers face the challenge of providing optimum psychosocial interventions and resource referrals in a time when the health care system continues to implement cutbacks in staffing in response to institutional needs to stabilize revenue and expenses. In these circumstances, social workers encounter many barriers to provision of comprehensive services including decentralization of social work departments and assignment to other clinical services in addition to pediatric oncology. The pressures of managed care may make it necessary for them to assume responsibility for tasks pertaining to utilization management and discharge planning to a greater extent than in the past. Despite this situation, as pediatric oncology social workers come to know families in crisis, they draw from the knowledge base that is the foundation of their profession to help these families cope with the impact of having seriously ill children. Pediatric oncology social workers direct their efforts at helping families successfully integrate the experience of childhood cancer into their lives with minimal disruption. This time of disruption can make it difficult for families to achieve the goal of coping successfully with the cancer experience. Social workers in pediatric oncology continue to enhance work toward that goal by offering their knowledge of family functioning, their experience with appropriate helping techniques, and their compassion.

REFERENCES

American Cancer Society (2001). *Cancer support groups: A guide for facilitators*. Atlanta, GA: American Cancer Society.

Arceci, R. J., Reamon, G. H., Cohen, A. R., & Lampkin, B. J. (1998). Position statement for the need to define pediatric/oncology programs: A model of subspeciality care for chronic childhood diseases. *Journal of Pediatric Hematology/Oncology*, 20 (2), 98-103.

Bendor, S. J. (1990). Anxiety and isolation in siblings of pediatric cancer patients: The need for prevention. *Social Work in Health Care, 14 (3)*, 17-35.

Clarke-Steffen, L. (1997). Reconstructing reality: Family strategies for managing childhood cancer. *Journal of Pediatric Nursing, 12 (5)*, 278-287.

Deasy-Spinetta, P. (1993). School issues and the child with cancer. *Cancer, 71*, 3261-3264.

Greenlee, R. T., Murray, T., Bolden, S., & Wingo, P. A. (2000). Cancer statistics, 2000. *CA: A Cancer Journal for Clinicians, 50 (1)*, 7-33.

Hoffman, B. (1996). *A cancer survivor's almanac: Charting your journey.* Washington, DC: National Coalition of Cancer Survivorship.

Last, B. F., & Grootenhuis, M. A. (1998). Emotions, coping and the need for support in families of children with cancer: A model for psychosocial care. *Patient Education & Counseling, 33 (2)*, 169-179.

Lauria, M. M., Hockenberry-Eaton, M., Pawletko, T. M., & Mauer, A. M. (1996). Psychosocial protocol for childhood cancer: A conceptual model. *Cancer, 78 (6)*, 1345-1350.

National Association of Social Workers. (2000). *Code of Ethics of the National Association of Social Workers.* Washington, DC: NASW.

Redd, W. H. (1994). Advances in psychosocial oncology in pediatrics. *Cancer, 74*, 1496-1502.

Ross, J. W. (1993). Understanding the family experience with childhood cancer. In N. M. Stearns, M. M. Lauria, J. F. Hermann, & P. R. Fogelberg (Eds.), *Oncology social work: A clinician's guide* (pp. 199-236). Atlanta, GA: American Cancer Society.

Sharp, J. W. (1999). The Internet: Changing the way cancer survivors obtain information. *Cancer Practice, 7(5)*, 266-269.

Sloper, P. (1996). Needs and responses of parents following the diagnosis of childhood cancer. *Child Care, Health & Development, 22 (3)*, 187-202.

Varni, J. W., Katz, E. R., Colegrove, R. Jr., & Dolgin, M. (1994). Perceived social support and adjustment of children with newly diagnosed cancer. *Journal of Development & Behavioral Pediatrics, 15 (1)*, 20-26.

CHAPTER 8

SPECIAL PROGRAMS FOR CHILDREN WITH CANCER AND THEIR FAMILIES

Nancy F. Cincotta, CSW, ACSW, CCLS

SPECIAL PROGRAMS

Childhood cancer is emotionally, physically, and financially demanding on the entire family. The range of responses to the disease can affect coping in multiple domains such as school performance for the child, work productivity for parents, and emotional functioning for all family members. Children and families have a variety of adverse responses to cancer and its treatment protocols. Parental well-being is crucial to a child's ability to adjust to the diagnosis of the disease and its varied implications. Depression, anxiety, loneliness, helplessness, and uncertainty are all anticipated responses of parents to a diagnosis of cancer in their child (Grootenhuis & Last, 1997).

The negative impact of the illness can often be minimized through programmatic interventions designed to meet the unique psychosocial needs of the patient and family. These programs, which originate primarily under the auspices of hospitals and the community of cancer organizations, offer services to address emotional sequelae or other consequences inherent in the course of childhood cancer. At critical stages during a child's medical care, a respite program, a "wish" for the child and family, an individualized activity for the child, or arrangements for a family member to stay at a Ronald McDonald House can alleviate stress and lessen the burden of the disease.

The social worker has varied roles in specialized programming. Most often it is the social worker's role to accurately assess a family's needs throughout the course of treatment and to make referrals to appropriate programs. In certain settings, the social worker's charge may be to establish a program to meet an identified need. The decisions about whether a particular center will develop a program (e.g., an afternoon for siblings, a back-to-school program, a children's group, or a bereavement program) will depend on a number of factors including, but not limited to, the level of staffing and volunteer support available, skill and interest of the particular staff member, the funding required for the program, the size of the patient population, and the type of program.

Networking with other social workers locally and nationally, through groups such as the Association of Pediatric Oncology Social Workers (APOSW) or the Association of Oncology Social Work (AOSW) is vital to learning about existing resources and creative programming. Community organizations that serve cancer patients, such as the American Cancer Society (ACS), the Leukemia and Lymphoma Society (LLS), or Cancer Care are invaluable in providing information regarding local and national resources. Cancer-related publications provide another avenue for the social worker to obtain information (e.g., *Coping* magazine contains practical information for patients and families). *Cancer Practice* and the *Journal of Psychosocial Oncology* provide program descriptions, program evaluation and outcome data, and other significant research findings.

Even when maximized to make it the most positive experience possible, utilizing a child-friendly environment, sensitive medical staff, and the provision of supportive services, including child life programming and hypnotherapy/pain management interventions, the routine of chemotherapy, radiotherapy, hospitalizations, and clinic visits can be an onerous experience. Life routines are altered; normal experiences with one's peer group (e.g., school, class trips) may be changed or averted. The whole process of cancer treatment infringes on a child's and family's own rhythm.

Whether a special program is designed to provide respite, education, socialization, psychotherapy, diversion from the illness, or some combination of these, its positive impact should not be minimized. Certain opportunities, (e.g., a referral to a wish program, applying for camp) may seem incidental to treatment. To the contrary, they are integral to many families' experiences. They stand out from the regular clinic visit, the planned and unplanned hospitalizations, and the "drudgery" that comes with treatment. It is often the memories resulting from these programs that families cherish long after their child is off treatment or deceased.

Since childhood cancers affect the entire family, special programs have been created to address the concerns of siblings, parents, grandparents, or the family as a whole. Whether assessing needs, establishing a program or making referrals, the social worker must consider the child's age, strengths, and limitations, the stage of illness, and the family's emotional and financial status. Programs separate from the child's medical care offer families and patients opportunities to share information, thoughts, and experiences which further enable them to cope with feelings of depression, anxiety, isolation, and immobilization.

PROGRAMMING FOR CHILDREN

There are multiple services available to help children deal with the impact of the illness in ways consistent with their stage of development. Many centers employ child life specialists, pediatric social workers, child psychologists, and creative arts therapists who have developed skills in play therapy, hypnotherapy, art and music therapy, and other creative enterprises to help children understand, express and adapt to their illness and its treatment. Information on therapeutic activities specifically designed to meet children's needs can be accessed through members APOSW and AOSW who have developed expertise in this area. A particularly useful book, *101 Play Therapy Techniques*, can be helpful to the clinician in developing and implementing such activities (Kaduson & Schaefer, 1997).

Children who attend clinic exclusively for chemotherapy may

resist coming and frequently will not enjoy the visits. Children who come to a clinic where chemotherapy is only a part of their experience, where art work, game playing, and other therapeutic activities are commonplace, will feel that they are more active participants in their care and are more likely to take pleasure from their visits.

Therapeutic activities designed to help the child with the overwhelming nature of the cancer experience are invaluable. For children who are apprehensive about procedures, the opportunity to rehearse them through doll play will enhance their coping ability and minimize negative effects during and after the procedure. Innovative programming, such as that provided by the Starbright Foundation, has allowed children to connect in cyberspace, adding yet another dimension to social support (Holden, Bearison, Rode, Rosenberg, & Fishman, 1999).

Rooming In

Pediatric inpatient hospital programs allow for rooming in of parents or caregivers when a child is admitted, but there are variations on who can stay, when, and how. Some centers actually provide a comfortable bed for one parent, whereas others may provide a lounge chair. While many institutions offer special sibling visiting programs, others are still reluctant to allow young children to visit. Bone marrow transplant and intensive care units have their own visiting arrangements and often require off-site accommodations. Some programs have hotel-like, hospital-affiliated accommodations for parents, and many different organizations have begun to develop alternative housing possibilities (e.g., programs which have volunteers who provide housing for parents more than 25 miles from home, volunteers who find hotels willing to accept cancer patients or family members for a free night's stay before, during, or after treatment.)

Ronald McDonald Houses

Ronald McDonald Houses began when the original house in Philadelphia opened its doors in 1974. There are now more than 200 Ronald McDonald Houses in 19 countries with more than 3,000 bedrooms available each night. Families of children with cancer can stay at a Ronald McDonald house during the course of inpatient and outpatient treatment. This is particularly helpful if the family's home is a considerable distance from the treatment center or if the child is critically ill.

At times when the child is hospitalized and only one person can stay in the hospital, the other parent (and a sibling) may stay at a Ronald McDonald House. In certain situations such as bone marrow transplantation during which a parent may not be permitted to remain in the hospital, the family's stay at Ronald McDonald House can facilitate daily visiting. A Ronald McDonald House stay may allow an earlier discharge of the patient, affording the ability to stay in close proximity to the hospital, facilitating a quick return if a crisis should occur. Some Ronald McDonald Houses have affiliated professional psychosocial staff to provide support services. The oncology social worker serves as liaison to the House, referring families, assessing the family's ability to pay a minimal amount for their lodging, and making recommendations regarding the family's emotional and financial needs to the house managers. For those from other countries, it may be at the Ronald McDonald House that family members begin to learn crucial information about this country.

Ronald McDonald Houses are run as communities in which living, dining, kitchen, and sometimes bathroom space is shared. Parents cook for themselves and are assigned cleaning tasks. At times, House staff members orchestrate special events such as helicopter rides and holiday activities. However, this model may not be right for everyone. There are some parents who may prefer more anonymity that a Ronald McDonald House might offer.

Groups for Patients and Families

Historically, group work has been an avenue used by social workers for offering assistance to persons faced with similar, difficult situations. Groups can offer children with cancer and their family members the opportunity to share their own illness-related experiences and learn from the experiences of others. The social worker, alone or with other team members, can play various roles in relation to groups offered in a particular institution or community. The social worker can:

- Assess the need for a particular hospital-based group, design it,

and provide leadership for it (e.g., monthly sibling group)
- Help facilitate the development of a self-help group (e.g., a Candlelighters group)
- Design and serve as facilitator for a group that addresses a specific need (i.e., coming off treatment, limited session group)
- Serve as planner, leader, or facilitator for community-based groups that often are under the auspices of local units of the ACS or chapters of the LLS, Cancer Care, or other cancer-related agencies
- Refer to existing groups in the community.

Groups can target populations of patients, parents, siblings, or families. They can be designed for particular age groups, to address the changing issues of different treatment phases, to provide a forum to share information or to teach skills.
Examples of age-related groups:
- Play or activity groups for preschoolers or younger children to help them deal with surgery or painful procedures
- Adolescent rap groups to encourage peer discussion of treatment experiences
- Grandparent groups to help deal with the emotional issues of helping their child (parent) and their grandchild (patient).

Examples of groups designed to address the issues of different treatment phases:
- Groups for parents of newly diagnosed children
- Groups dealing with post-treatment concerns (long-term survivors' group)
- Bereavement groups.

Examples of groups for imparting information:
- Groups about medical information "understanding your child's protocol"
- Groups about nutritional issues for the child with cancer
- Groups about resources (e.g., camp programs for children with cancer).
Examples of groups for teaching a skill:

- Groups for learning stress management techniques
- Groups for learning hypnotherapy skills
- Groups for learning effective ways to communicate with the physician.

Groups can be time-limited (for a fixed number of sessions), open-ended (for an indefinite number of sessions), or one-time events. They can take the form of generalized support or educational groups without any predetermined agenda. They may meet in inpatient, outpatient, or community settings during the day or in the evenings. The time of day at which a group is offered will automatically make it accessible to some while excluding others (e.g., daytime groups may eliminate working parents).

While groups can supplement more individually tailored interventions with children and families, participation should be by invitation rather than expectation. Interest in group involvement on the part of children, parents, or siblings is not universal. The value that groups can offer must not obscure the fact that individual needs and preferences should be respected. Families may he more open to group work services at certain stages than at others. For children and family members who are amenable to group work services, such programs can afford them immeasurable support and strength. For additional, in-depth information about support groups, readers can contact their local ACS office to order the publication entitled *Cancer Support Groups: A Guide for Facilitators* (ACS, 2001; Code #4660).

Self-Help Groups

Parents' self-help groups arise in many forms. Some groups begin with professional leadership (e.g., a group for parents of children who are newly diagnosed) and at the completion of the group, parents decide that they want to continue to meet. In other cases parents may attend retreats, or groups established under other auspices and decide upon return to their center that they want to have a group with other parents. In oncology centers parents often come together in the interest of a project (a fundraiser, a picnic, a holiday party), and then remain connected in the interest of mutual aid.

The Candlelighters Childhood Cancer Foundation (CCCF; www.candlelighters.org), a national organization established in 1970 by parents of cancer patients to advocate for the needs of their children and to foster communication among affected families, has fostered many parent self-help groups. The aim of parents helping parents is empowerment through mutual support and dissemination of information and resources. The national office of Candlelighters can refer a parent to a local group, if one exists, or to a contact person in the area. Each Candlelighters group is different, as membership and activities vary from community to community. In some areas, a hospital social worker may serve as co-leader or consultant to the Candlelighters group. Parents who must travel great distances from the treatment center, who are interested in peer support, or who are uncomfortable taking part in a hospital-based group, might benefit from participation in a community self-help Candlelighters group.

Candlelighters publishes three newsletters: *Candlelighters*, for parents and professionals, *The CCCF Youth Newsletter*, for young patients, survivors, and siblings, and *The Phoenix*, for adult survivors of childhood cancer. These newsletters provide parents and children with helpful ideas about coping, communicating, and living with cancer during and after treatment. Children who are reluctant to talk about their treatment may benefit from reading about someone else's feelings or experiences. Seeing in writing that others share your experience offers immeasurable support on the cancer journey.

It is possible for a child to find a pen pal through the Candlelighters newsletter. This may be particularly significant for a child who is inactive or temporarily bedridden due to the illness. There are many pen pal programs for children with cancer and children with a chronic illness, such as the Children's Hopes & Dreams Wish Fulfillment Foundation. The various parameters (i.e., who is screening applications and monitoring communication) of these and other programs need to be understood before making a referral.

School Programs
School is the "workplace" of the child and provides an environment for learning and socializing. It is a societal expectation that all children will

attend school. Whether a child likes or performs well in school or not, most children recognize that school is something that they and their peers must participate in. Integrating school into the child's life when the child is in the middle of a medical crisis can challenge all involved. School absence can impede intellectual and emotional growth and development and deny a child age-appropriate opportunities for further development of positive self-esteem.

The family's and child's feelings about school will play a role in their responses to school attendance after diagnosis. A child who never liked or fared well in school is unlikely to be excited about reentering the classroom and may see the illness as an opportunity to avoid it. A child who enjoyed school and misses the experience may have an easier period of reintegration.

Returning to school after diagnosis and treatment can be traumatic for a child. Feelings of anxiety about seeing peers or teachers and feelings of confusion about who and what to tell about their illness, are common, as are anxieties about school performance. Parents as well as children may need help as they prepare for a child's return to school. Many medical centers and local organizations have helpful videotapes about school re-entry that they sell, lend, or rent.

There is recognized educational, developmental, and social value of the school experience for the child on treatment. Teachers, peers, and the routine and structure of the school day can provide support, encouragement, and diversion for children occupied with the details of their diseases. Whenever possible, returning to school is the best alternative for the young patient. Knowing how important it is in our society, if school attendance isn't emphasized, the child may conclude that he or she is gravely ill.

Most children who have undergone chemotherapy fear that they will be teased in school because of their appearance. Many feel apprehensive about the academic and social activities they have missed. If they are not feeling well, they may worry about keeping up with the demands of their schoolwork. Periodic absences, while necessary, may be stressful and may also impede learning. When indicated and available, adjunctive tutoring can be helpful.

Certain types of cancer require rigorous protocols that may

involve prolonged hospitalization, during which time children may be so ill that they are unable to attend school. In these cases, local school districts will provide in-home tutoring after receiving documentation from the treatment center specifying the child's particular physical strengths and limitations. Many treatment centers have on-site academic tutors for pediatric patients; some have a schoolroom within the medical unit. Some children are never able to emotionally or physically negotiate the illness, its treatment, and the responsibilities of school. Whether a child survives or dies, parents rarely regret the choices that they make about school. However, activities, which are connected to school, the prom, graduation, and special events, are those most often highlighted by parents. In the end, families and staff must agree upon an educational plan for the child that seems in the best interest of the child in the context of his or her family.

For children who are unable to physically return to school, ongoing contact with the class, including cards, visits, and evens homework assignments, will enable the child to remain optimistic about reentry at a later time. Peer relationships are critical to a child's well-being. Efforts to maintain these connections are important (Bluebond-Langner, Perkel, Goertzel, Nelson, & McGeary, 1990). A child who is kept informed about school activities will feel less anxiety about the gaps in attendance. Encouraging visits from a school counselor or teacher can be helpful.

Understanding and dealing with cancer or other severe illness in the classroom can be difficult. Many pediatric oncology centers offer training sessions for school staff to learn about the physical and emotional aspects of childhood cancer. Health care personnel are in a unique position to offer vital information and can help school staff maximize their ability to help their students with cancer. In this milieu, informed professionals can also explore and deal with anxiety that the school staff have about an ill child's return to school. Some treatment centers have school visiting programs in which members of the child's treatment team go to the school and meet with the teacher, the nurse, the class, or an assembly of children, depending on the needs and wishes of the school and family. Other centers offer one-day programs at the medical center for school and community agency staff that provide similar information (Ross, 1984). School reentry programs are all focused on the same goals of helping the child have a favorable experience with school, to further a sense of normalcy for the child and overcome psychological, physical, environmental, and family issues related to school reentry (Worchel-Prevatt et al., 1998). Different stages of illness may dictate differential approaches to school reentry (Madan-Swain, Fredrick, & Wallander, 1999).

The LLS has developed a Back To School Program which is available through local chapters to help professionals in their efforts to acclimate the child to the classroom. The ACS has published comprehensive educational materials aimed at parents and schoolteachers; contact your local ACS for more information. Other materials can be found on the Internet (see Chapter 14 for information on how to access oncology resources).

Camp Programs

Children with cancer have fewer opportunities to experience routine activities of childhood. In recognition of these limitations, a variety of camp programs for children with cancer have been established. These programs offer positive experiences that allow children to engage in age-appropriate activities, as well as the opportunity to interact with other children with cancer who have shared common experiences. These attributes of camp can help foster self-esteem and normal development.

The side effects of rigorous treatment protocols may limit a child's regular opportunities for socialization with peers or independence from parents. Friendships made at cancer camps become important to children and can be helpful to them long after the camping season is over. Peer relationships both with healthy friends and others with the same or similar diseases are of utmost importance to children (Bluebond-Langner, Perkel, & Goertzel, 1991).

Camps for children with cancer provide environments in which they can engage in physical and recreational activities, for many for the first time since diagnosis. Children with cancer have the opportunity to master skills (e.g., boating, swimming) seemingly incongruent with their roles as cancer patients.

Children, as well as their parents, may approach the idea of camp with a mixture of enthusiasm and apprehension. Most parents experience a great deal of fear at the thought of turning their child with cancer over to strangers in a camp setting. Until parents get to know the environment and the staff, it can be an overwhelming prospect. Through discussion of concerns, the social worker can help initially reluctant parents and prospective campers recognize that camp can be a safe setting, especially since there are on-site medical and other support services. Some camps offer separate weekend programs for parents to attend during their child's stay. With support and encouragement, camp can be a therapeutic experience for all.

While certain camp programs offer sessions exclusively for children with cancer, others provide experiences for children and their siblings, and still others involve the entire family. The choice of which type of camp program or retreat to recommend to parents depends on the needs of an individual child or family and the availability of specific programs. For example, a young adolescent, struggling with an increasingly dependent role because of her illness may benefit from the autonomy inherent in a children's camp setting. The family of a dying child may find tremendous relief in a camp environment filled with opportunities for support and therapeutic activities for the whole family.

Camp programs give parents a respite from their daily routines and help them to understand that their child can function independently (in the company of responsible adults). Whether it is a children's camp or a family camp, such programs provide parents with time to attend to their own needs. A camp experience serves as a reminder of a world that exists beyond cancer. It can be the perfect escape from the intensity of treatment. This time away from the medical setting can help families refocus and replenish their energies, or can simply be a well-deserved vacation for everyone.

There are many different formats for camps, retreats, and weekend getaways. A unique example of a family camp, Camp Sunshine, in Casco, Maine accepts referrals from anywhere in the world. It is a five-day program designed for the entire family. Children have camp activities to fill their daytime hours, with family programming in the evenings. Parents have both recreational and psychosocial activities, including a five-session group program to deal with the emotional sequelae of having a child with cancer. The groups focus on various aspects of coping with critical illness, including the impact of the diagnosis, communicating with medical staff, sibling issues, gender issues, and dealing with grandparents.

A comprehensive listing of summer camps for children with cancer can be found at the Pediatric Oncology Resource Center of the Association of Cancer Online Resources (ACOR; www.acor.org/diseases/ped-onc/cfissues/camps.html) or by calling the ACS at 1-800-ACS-2345. Camp programs are sponsored by a variety of organizations, usually without cost to the family. However, the cost of transportation to and from camp may impede the ability of some to participate. Hospital social work departments or community agencies may have special funds to assist with meeting these costs. Camp is an enriching experience that should be accessible to all children with cancer and their families.

Retreat Programs

Retreats emerged in the 1980s as novel ways to help families, providing an environment secluded from everyday distractions such as telephones, television, and the demands of daily routines and responsibilities. Part of the effect of this concept is to create an intense and intimate experience for adults and children. A combination of diverting activities, as well as intensely emotional times achieve a cathartic effect, allowing parents to communicate openly about the emotional impact of the disease on the family. Some retreats are focused on the stage of the illness (e.g., a weekend programs for newly diagnosed children and their families; Ruffin, Creed, & Jarvis, 1997), while others mix children and families at different stages of illness, relying on more experienced group members to provide mentoring to newer families. Other retreats may focus on skill building (Walsh-Burke, 1992) or spiritual issues.

Outward Bound, ropes courses, and similar programs for cancer patients are designed at varying skill levels to challenge physical competence and emotional endurance. In so doing, these programs help individuals understand their strengths and their limitations. Fighting for survival in the woods parallels the journey cancer patients take, and success in this arena promotes confidence in the other.

Mentor Programs

Many institutions have programs that provide special attention to children with cancer. These can be in the form of Big Brother/Big Sister programs, in which a volunteer takes a child out for an activity, or visits during chemotherapy, radiotherapy treatments, or hospitalizations. Childhood cancer survivors (adolescents or adults) can be invaluable in this role, providing support, encouragement, and reflection of their past experience as children go through their cancer journey. An interesting example of one type of program is the Carolina Pediatric Attention, Love, and Support (PALS) group, which utilizes students at the University of North Carolina and volunteers to provide one-to-one contact and support to patients during hospital and clinic visits. In addition to patient contact this cohort is active in raising money for special programs at both annual and ad hoc events. Another program, Kidmusicmed matches musicians (music mentors) with children with cancer. The musician, with input from the child writes a song for the child. Regardless of the guise of the "buddy" program, there are many creative ways to afford children additional attention and support during the course of their illness.

Entertainment and Socialization

Programs literally focused on fun can help patients, families, and staff temporarily move away from the demanding and stressful reality of treatment. "Clown care units" have emerged as regional resources in which trained clowns utilize humor to lighten children's hospital experiences. Holiday parties, picnics, and other special events may be sponsored by wish or cancer organizations. These events give families the sense that they are not alone, that they are part of a larger community of those affected by cancer. Other activities include street fairs, outings to sporting events, masquerades, and parties of any kind.

During cancer treatment it is sometimes difficult for patients and family members to plan for the future because of the uncertainty of the outcome. Preparation for an event, although potentially stressful, can also be therapeutic. The enjoyment of planning an event, followed by the anticipation and the memories of it are worthy of note. For example, an adolescent planned and worked diligently with staff to plan a teen party. It was great fun and required a fair amount of concentration and preparation. This child died (as did the majority of children at the party). When she was quite ill and aware that she was about to die, it was her feeling that the reason she was brought together with the other teens was so that she would know other people when she got to heaven.

End-of-treatment parties are both common and controversial. Some families feel that they want to acknowledge this time as a rite of passage, a major transition for the family. Other families and some staff members may feel superstitious about this type of event, cognizant of the possibility that the journey may not be over, and that relapse is possible. Each family must make these decisions based on what is comfortable for them.

Children have special events in their lives that are not related to their illness. It is important to work with families to help children maintain a role in the activities that are important to them such as birthday parties, community, religious, and school events.

Dream/Wish Programs

Having a wish granted, something a child would like to have or do, can be a very special event in the child's life, especially in the context of illness. Numerous organizations throughout the United States grant wishes. The criteria for eligibility vary greatly. Some offer their services only to children who are "terminally ill," while others serve children at any stage of chronic illness. The criterion of terminal illness does not mean that death must be imminent, but rather that relapse or recurrence signals that the prognosis has worsened.

Wish program staff accept referrals from professionals and families directly. There is generally paperwork, often including some medical information and liability exclusions for the family and staff to prepare. These programs are not determined by financial necessity, but rather by diagnosis. All children with cancer are eligible for these programs.

Even the most withdrawn child can become excited at the prospect of choosing and planning a wished-for experience or item. Some wish programs operate nationally with local chapters, while others are community-based. A referral to a wish organization can be a very rewarding experience for the social worker. In this task, the social worker becomes the conduit to the wish, the person who enables the family to have a positive experience that is not focused on the illness. Before a social worker refers a family to a wish organization, it is important to determine whether the child fits that group's criteria, as unnecessary disappointment for the child, family, and staff should be avoided.

Generally, wish organizations stipulate that a child cannot receive a wish from more than one program. Some treatment centers have their own funds to provide an item or trip that a child desires, but these programs are not considered "formal" wish organizations and may not make a child ineligible for another program. Often, financial restrictions are placed on the total cost of the wish. This limit, and restrictions on the number of people, who can be involved in the child's wish, varies from organization to organization. Such stipulations need to be discussed with and understood by the family from the outset.

During a time of illness-related limitation in options and control, the experience of receiving a present or trip can boost morale. The value of giving a child with cancer the freedom to choose something special, ranging from a videocassette recorder to a grand piano, or a trip to Disney World, cannot be underestimated. The social worker should be aware of strategic times during the course of treatment to consider referral to a wish program. The wish can be seen as an adjunct to treatment, revitalizing the family and helping them to endure negative aspects of the illness.

When a child is terminally ill, however, the considerations are different. The family, and perhaps the child, may see the wish as a last request. Careful consideration of the child's capabilities and limitations are crucial. Under these circumstances, the wish may provide the family with something to plan and look forward to at a time when they feel hopeless. Frequently, the wish will be among the last pleasant memories a family can create together and therefore becomes precious. In addition to the benefit of the actual experience, the child and family also have the opportunity to enjoy the excitement of planning and then the joy of reliving the experience.

Some organizations do not provide individual gifts during the year but may solicit children's wishes for "things" and then provide them at holiday time in December. Staff at the ACS, at Ronald McDonald Houses, or other social workers in the community can inform new social workers of such programs.

Hospice Programs

The impending death of a child is always a difficult period. The choice of whether a child will die at home, in the hospital, or in an inpatient hospice unit is a very personal one, made by the family in collaboration with members of the health care team. The decision may be influenced by the availability of services in a particular community.

A family's choice may depend on the amount of support that is available at home, the ages and the needs of other children, their religious perspective, or the child's wishes. Feelings about this choice may fluctuate and other options should remain available even after a decision is made. If there is a prolonged period from the time that death seems imminent and when it actually occurs, other assistance to provide additional support for families may be required. In-home support services can facilitate this difficult period for families. All family members need help when a child is dying. When a child dies at home, addressing the needs of the siblings in the house becomes an imperative. The actual experience and the memories of it (particularly the visual ones) stay with the surviving children and other family members and can be unsettling. Efforts to make the experience as comfortable and as peaceful as possible are very important while the child is dying and in the hours, days, weeks, months, and years after.

Memorial Services

Memorial services, often held at the hospital, can serve as a means to assist in the grieving process. After a child dies, family members, friends, and professional staff may feel the need for some type of closure in the form of a ceremony, beyond the funeral service. A family may wish to have a memorial event, some time after the actual funeral, to share memories and feelings with others in a way they were unable to do immediately after the death. For families such ceremonies can be a way to celebrate their child's life and are often scheduled at significant times such as the child's birthday.

There are many different ways for professionals to mourn the death of a child. Medical staff members may desire to acknowledge the lives and deaths of particular children in a formal memorial service, while privately dealing with the deaths of others. In certain situations, they may choose to invite families, in others they may not, depending on their own needs, and the particular circumstances around the death. A remembrance service at the hospital chapel or a conference or team meeting concerning the child can meet this need. Some institutions hold monthly chapel services to acknowledge the children who died during the preceding month.

Several centers have periodic memorial or remembrance programs. Parents and other family members are invited back annually, or biannually, for an event such as a luncheon or dinner program of speakers. The purposes of these programs are to offer continued support for bereaved families, to recognize the communal sense of loss for family members and staff, and to offer an opportunity for families to gain support from one another. These programs can be difficult to plan, given the intensity of feelings evoked by bringing together a large number of families of children who have died. The memorial service provides families and staff with a healing ritual, a source for closure after the death, and recognition of the relationships established between families and staff (Heiney, Wells, & Ruffin, 1996).

It is not uncommon to release balloons after a remembrance service or on a special occasion, as a token of the spiritual journey children have made. As with birthdays and other special events, balloons have come to epitomize a celebration of life in our culture and continue to do so at the time of death. Biodegradable balloons can be purchased to make these activities environmentally safe.

Bereavement Programs

As family members and professional staff struggle to cope with the death of a child, bereavement programs offer them the opportunity to share and legitimize their thoughts and feelings. Bereavement services can be offered on an individual, group, or family basis and may be hospital- or community-based. For some parents, returning to the treatment center is so painful that they will not attend group meetings at that site, while others find comfort in returning to the familiar environment. Still others view returning to the hospital as something they must master in order to move on.

Some bereaved parents choose to stay involved with activities at the treatment center, returning as volunteers in many capacities. In the interests of both the bereaved parent and families on treatment, many hospital-based programs require a 6–12 month waiting period between the time of a child's death and the parent's eligibility to return as a volunteer. Bereaved parents need adequate time to sort out intense emotions about their experience and protection from the intensity of the pain of others struggling with a new diagnosis or the demands of active treatment.

Bereavement groups can be time-limited, or ongoing with closed or open membership. The structure will depend on the auspices under which the program is offered or on the particular goal of the group. A time-limited model generally focuses on helping a number of parents at a similar stage get through either initial emotional obstacles or later effects of the bereavement process. Ongoing groups with open membership create an environment in which parents can help one another over time to recognize and deal with the various stages and tasks associated with surviving the loss of a child. Parents whose children have died several years ago can serve as role models for those newer to the bereavement process. Social workers facilitating bereavement groups need to be cognizant of the fact that some individuals need help in terminating once they have made progress in the resolution of associated psychosocial issues.

The Compassionate Friends (www.compassionatefriends.org), a national organization with local chapters, is a self-help group for parents who have had a child die from an illness, an accident, a suicide, or a homicide. In certain locations it may be the only resource available to parents who have experienced the death of a child. These groups do not have professional facilitators, so the tenor of the group varies according to those comprising its membership at a given time. Some parents will utilize the referral to the Compassionate Friends and will benefit from the experience. Other families, however, have found that it is too complicated to deal with a mixed membership that includes parents of children whose death was not disease-related.

To facilitate a bereavement group, there must be a large number of bereaved parents who potentially would participate. Therefore, it is often fruitful to have these services provided in the community or cooperatively among several organizations. Bereavement programs may be run by staff from hospitals, cancer organizations, social service agencies, hospices, counseling centers, religious groups, wellness communities, or independent practitioners. Without such a membership base, the risk is a dwindling number or participants without an adequate number to provide the most beneficial effects for those participating. A "group" of two or three is not a group, and in fact, may compromise the outcome.

Parents are not alone in their grief. Siblings, other family members, friends, and classmates all experience grief reactions and may benefit from referral to appropriate services (Stokes & Crossley, 1995; Vargas-Irwin, 1999). There are programs whose mission is to offer a safe environment for children, adolescents, and their parents to deal with their grief, such as the Dougy Center, The National Center for Grieving Children and Families, and The Center for Grieving Children.

Oncology Social Work Organizations

Oncology social work can be quite stressful. Preventive measures focusing on the role description (and conflicts) and job satisfaction need to be part of efforts made to help maintain and sustain workers in their positions (Um & Harrison, 1998). Resources that help professionals maintain themselves in oncology social work are crucial. Membership and committee involvement in professional organizations can provide the social worker with support and opportunities to maximize skills in a demanding field through networking and education.

Although some social workers practice in hospitals or organizations that have a built-in structure for support and education, there is additional benefit that can be gained from peer involvement with these national organizations.

The Association of Pediatric Oncology Social Workers (APOSW; www.aposw.org), established in 1977, is an organization of pediatric oncology social workers throughout the United States and Canada, with significant representation from other countries. APOSW is committed to addressing the psychosocial needs of children with cancer and their families. The members of this organization can provide a wealth of information and support to social workers in pediatric oncology practice. An annual conference and a quarterly newsletter provide opportunities for professionals to interact and share ideas about common areas of social work practice, program development, and research. There is an active email listserve group available to all members which affords immediate access to colleagues and their resources, ideas, and support. APOSW works in close collaboration with other organizations committed to children affected by cancer and their families.

The AOSW (www.aosw.org), a 501C3, is a national organization with a membership primarily of social workers whose mission is to educate the public and professionals about the psychosocial aspects of cancer. It also supports its membership in their work with and advocacy for cancer patients, providing continuing education, opportunities for collaborative research, newsletters, and an annual national conference, as well as regional conferences. AOSW fosters networking within its membership and in collaboration with other recognized oncology organizations and coalitions, always advocating for the support and care of people with cancer. The Children and Cancer Special Interest Group of AOSW is committed to the unique needs of children affected by cancer.

SUMMARY

Pediatric cancer can be an all-encompassing disease in terms of the problems that occur as a result of the disease as well as from its treatment. Families must work hard to deal with the illness and to maintain a somewhat normal life during the process. They must also choose which special programs will be best for their own family (e.g., one summer a cancer camp might be the best choice whereas for another summer, a regular camp may be the better choice).

The pediatric oncology social worker must consider many aspects of program development for children with cancer and their family members. Limited resources of staff, time, money, staff, patient population, or interest may impede the ability to develop particular programs. Frequently, referral to an outside program is precisely what is indicated or is the only feasible plan. Collaborative efforts between hospital and community agencies enable maximum service provision to this unique patient population.

Many organizations such as the ACS and the LLS offer educational materials and counseling services. They also advocate for pediatric patients at local and national levels. Sharing the commitment in offering service to this special group of children and their families affords the clinician a greater capability to meet their many needs. A strategic referral to an appropriate special program can be therapeutic for the family and professionally gratifying to the social worker. Childhood cancer is a demanding illness, creating multiple needs that can best be met through diverse programs.

REFERENCES

American Cancer Society (2001). *Cancer support groups: A guide for facilitators.* Atlanta, GA: American Cancer Society.

Bluebond-Langner, M., Perkel, D., & Goertzel, T. G. (1991). Pediatric cancer patients' peer relationships: The impact of an oncology camp experience. *Journal of Psychosocial Oncology, 9*(2), 67-80.

Bluebond-Langner, M., Perkel, D., Goertzel, T., Nelson, K., & McGeary, J. (1990). Children's knowledge of cancer and its treatment: Impact of an oncology camp experience. *Journal of Pediatrics, 116(2)*, 207-213.

Grootenhuis, M. A., & Last, B. F. (1997). Predictors of parental emotional adjustment to childhood cancer. *Psychooncology, 6(2)*, 115-128.

Heiney, S. P., Wells, L., & Ruffin, J. (1996). A memorial service for families of children who died from cancer and blood disorders. *Journal of Pediatric Oncology Nursing, 13(2)*, 72-79.

Holden, G., Bearison, D. J., Rode, D. C., Rosenberg, G., & Fishman, M. (1999). Evaluating the effects of a virtual environment (STARBRIGHT World) with hospitalized children. *Research on Social Work Practice, 9(3)*, 365-382.

Kaduson, H. G., & Schaefer, C. E. (1997). *101 favorite play therapy techniques.* Northvale, NJ: Jason Aronson.

Madan-Swain, A., Fredrick, L. D., & Wallander, J. L. (1999). Returning to school after a serious illness or injury. In R. T. Brown (Ed.), *Cognitive aspects of chronic illness in children* (pp. 312-332). New York: Guilford Press.

Ross, J. W. (1984). Resolving non-medical obstacles to successful school reentry for children with cancer. *Journal of School Health, 54(2)*, 84-86.

Ruffin, J. E., Creed, J. M., & Jarvis, C. (1997). A retreat for families of children recently diagnosed with cancer. *Cancer Practice, 5(2)*, 99-104.

Stokes, J., & Crossley, D. (1995). Camp Winston: A residential intervention for bereaved children. In S. C. Smith, & M. Pennells (Eds.), *Interventions with bereaved children* (pp. 172-192). London, England: Jessica Kingsley Publishers, Ltd.

Um, M.-Y., & Harrison, D. F. (1998). Role stressors, burnout, mediators, and job satisfaction: A stress-strain-outcome model and an empirical test. *Social Work Research, 22(2)*, 100-115.

Vargas-Irwin, M. (1999). Evaluation of a bereavement group for children. *Dissertation Abstracts International*, Section B: The Sciences and Engineering. 60(2 B), 0846.

Walsh-Burke, K. (1992). Family communication and coping with cancer: Impact of the We Can Weekend. *Journal of Psychosocial Oncology, 10(1)*, 63-81.

Worchel-Prevatt, F. F., Heffer, R. W., Prevatt, B. C., Miner, J., Young-Saleme, T., Horgan, D., Lopez, M. A., Rae, W. A., & Frankel, L. (1998). A school reentry program for chronically ill children. *Journal of School Psychology, 36(3)*, 261-279.

CHAPTER 9

THE IMPORTANCE OF RESEARCH IN ONCOLOGY SOCIAL WORK

Elizabeth J. Clark, PhD, ACSW

Social workers have long recognized the importance of identifying and addressing psychosocial aspects of cancer, and research in oncology social work has a 50-year history. Today, though, social workers find themselves in a changing health care arena where psychosocial care is being devalued, where even the need for oncology social workers is being questioned. As hospital stays become shorter and shorter, more cancer care is being offered in outpatient settings which traditionally have not included social work staff. In this current era of cost containment, illness episode management, and minimal standards of care, it is difficult to maintain patient services, much less engage in research activities. Yet, research may be the key to the continuation of needed oncology services and may help to safeguard clinical positions. The focus of this chapter is to discuss why oncology social work research is an important component of the profession, and to explore various types of research and their application.

RESEARCH STUMBLING BLOCKS

The stumbling blocks to doing research in the oncology setting are many, and most of them are not specific to social work (see Table 1).

TABLE 1

Barriers to Psychosocial Oncology Research

GLOBAL BARRIERS
- Lack of perceived significance (or merit) of psychosocial research within the research community
- Lack of scientific rigor in many existing studies
- Lack of trained researchers in psychosocial research
- Limited awareness of value of psychosocial intervention
- Needs of patients/survivors after treatment not considered important by medical community
- Inadequate training for cultural issues in research

NATIONAL BARRIERS
- Lack of cooperative efforts among researchers, especially across professional disciplines
- Lack of federal policy or mandate for psychosocial research
- Lack of national and private sector funding for psychosocial research

COMMUNITY BARRIERS
- Lack of collaborative research between academic centers and communities
- Lack of institutional support for research at hospitals and cancer centers
- Difficulty in recruiting subjects, especially minority subjects, for studies

Note. Reprinted with permission from Clark, E. J., Stovall, E. L., Leigh, S., Siu, A. L., Austin, D. K., & Rowland, J. H. (1996). *Imperatives for quality cancer care: Access, advocacy, action, and accountability* (p.33). Silver Spring, MD: National Coalition for Cancer Survivorship.

There is never enough time, and delivery of service always has to take precedence. Perhaps even more limiting is the belief of practitioners that they lack adequate training or experience to conduct research, especially skills in statistics and research methodology. Many masters prepared social workers acquire only six college credits in research, and few actually had the opportunity to conduct or participate in research prior to graduation. Therefore, they feel their knowledge and skills are not sufficient for undertaking research projects, for writing grant proposals, for designing studies, for analyzing data, or for publishing research findings.

The fallacy of these arguments is that many social workers already engage in research activities. These may not be classical studies that require randomization, comparison groups, and manipulation of variables — what is referred to as Research with a capital "R." What social workers often fail to realize is that there are many different types of research including focus group conduction, case studies analysis, and outcomes measurement. This research may be thought of as research with a lower case "r," but it is still important and valid for informing our clinical practice and determining the value of our interventions. It is also an important commodity for our institutions.

For example, oncology social workers sometimes are asked to work with marketing departments of their institutions to help to "sell" oncology services. Oncology has become a competitive field, and it does not matter how good the staff and services are if the community does not know about them. Focus groups are a technique often used by marketing departments. Focus groups can tell you what your cancer program is doing right and where there may be gaps in services. The same focus group approach that is valuable to marketing can help social workers understand difficulties in their own service areas, too.

Think about how often after a support group is formed, attendance becomes sporadic or there does not seem to be enough interest to run a second group. Doing some little "r" research can help social workers understand why the support groups are not working. Holding a small focus group of previous attendees might provide answers that are surprising. Perhaps the wrong population is being targeted. Maybe persons being invited are too newly diagnosed, or are not yet ready to take advantage of a support group setting. Or perhaps the age span of the group is too broad. Persons diagnosed in their twenties may not share the same social issues as those diagnosed in their fifties. Or maybe the time of the group is not conducive to attendance. There may not be parking available at the established time, or the room chosen is too far from the parking lot for people who are physically compromised while on active treatment. The important point is to find out why a support group has failed (or succeeded brilliantly). Research can help do this.

Another area of fruitful oncology research is quality improvement studies. In a hospital setting, these studies often are excellent examples of collaborative research. They frequently bring together staff from various disciplines and are creative ways of looking at a problem or issue with the goal of improving the quality of the service. These studies may involve retrospective chart review, looking to see what was done in the past, or they may be prospective, collecting data and information as the services are offered. Due to accreditation requirements, most hospital staff have become proficient in quality improvement studies, and their results are worthy of more formal research or publication. Yet, too often, a "story board" hung on the cafeteria wall is the only outlet for the findings. The value of this research effort may be lost to the broader community and to the profession.

This type of little "r" research often can be used as a springboard for a more formal research study. The study as it exists may be extended in time to capture additional longitudinal data in which observations are made at numerous points. Or, it may be used as the underpinnings of a larger exploratory study in which an attempt is made to develop an initial understanding of some phenomenon. Or, it may take the form of an ongoing descriptive study. The study may be qualitative (observation and case studies), or quantitative (numbers and statistical analysis), or a combination of both methods.

Do not be alarmed by these terms and stop reading this chapter. While they may sound like a college research course, research is not really that difficult. In fact, it should be fun.

TYPES OF RESEARCH

Again, it is important to emphasize that there are various levels of inquiry. Social workers do not have to begin with the classic experimental design that requires control groups, advanced statistical techniques, and major funding. There are many different approaches to research that are valuable for oncology social work.

A few examples may help to make this point. First, consider an exploratory qualitative study that had a great impact on the field of oncology social work. This study, done in the mid-sixties, looked at the changing communication patterns of cancer patients. It was conducted by Ruth Abrams, one of the first oncology social workers. She worked at Massachusetts General Hospital, and she eventually wrote a book about her study entitled *Not Alone with Cancer: A Guide for Those Who Care* (Abrams, 1974). In her preface to *Not Alone with Cancer*, Abrams stated that it was her hope that her "observations will help to break through the wall of silence, uneasiness, and despair that has been traditionally, and for too long, a burden to the patient with cancer and those who care for him." This book is not filled with tables and charts of statistical analysis, but with words and descriptions of patterns. It is based on astute and careful observations of a skilled clinician. A main task of qualitative research is to determine the ways that people in particular settings come to understand, account for, and manage their day-to-day situations, and the researcher is the main "measurement device" in the study (Miles & Huberman, 1994).

Another ground-breaking study may help to make the point about the importance of qualitative research. All oncology social workers are familiar with the work of Elisabeth Kubler-Ross. Kubler-Ross began her work in thanatology by accident. She was working with theology students who had been assigned a paper on "crises in human life." The students had chosen death as the most major crisis that people face, and they asked Kubler-Ross the following questions: "How do you do research on dying when data are so impossible to get and when you cannot verify your data and set up experiments?" They concluded that observation and talking with persons who were dying and their family members would be the best that they could do.

At the conclusion of their study, they delineated five stages through which a dying patient may pass during the dying process (denial and isolation, anger, bargaining, depression, and acceptance). While they acknowledged that not all dying persons experience all stages, and that there may be some repetition of stages, there is a typical, observable sequence (Kubler-Ross, 1969). Think of the impact that this rather simple research study has had on the field of thanatology and on the way services for the terminally ill are still structured and delivered today. Social workers and other therapists are well equipped to do qualitative research. They are skillful in interviewing, in participant observation, in case recording and case analysis. Social workers often have one additional advantage: they look at the social setting and take into account the various levels of analysis from the individual to the societal. This results in particularly rich qualitative data.

EXPLORING ONCOLOGY SOCIAL WORK RESEARCH OPPORTUNITIES

Why do some social workers do research? Maybe they liked their research courses in graduate school and are simply interested in why some events occur and some interventions work while others do not. Maybe they are affiliated with a medical school or research institution that has a research tradition, and engaging in research studies will help them stay interested in their field. Perhaps, they have a desire to add to the research literature and knowledge base of the field. Maybe they need to show their administration that what they do is important and should be continued. Whatever the reasons, the opportunities for research, and for involvement in research, are many.

Social workers who have not participated previously in a formal research study may wonder what they possibly can bring to the project. They might be concerned that they will be embarrassed by not knowing, or not being able to recall, statistical terms or components of research design. Maybe they never quite understood randomization or sample selection. Or, conversely, maybe they were a whiz in their research class, but have never put what they learned to work and would welcome the opportunity to be a part of a research team.

The first thing to remember is that oncology social workers do have important specialized knowledge and clinical experience. Many researchers lack this firsthand knowledge, and many have never worked in a clinical setting. Think about all of the journal articles that simply make no sense from a clinical perspective. Furthermore, think about how many research articles seem to have no clinical application. They conclude with phrases such as "more research needs to be done." It is for reasons such as these that multidisciplinary studies are so important in psychosocial oncology, and why oncology social workers need to play a larger role in research activities.

This is easy to understand when we consider that oncology is a multidisciplinary field. Treatment decisions are made by a team of oncology specialists with input from various disciplines. It stands to reason that research studies also would benefit from this multidisciplinary perspective. Think of the gaps that might exist if only the intrapsychic factors were considered in studying the impact of cancer. Adding social and relationship factors, financial and workplace concerns, and looking at the social context of the illness experience would give a much broader understanding of the overall impact.

Skills of Oncology Social Work Researchers

What skills and experiences can oncology social workers contribute to the research team? Table 2 lists a variety of research activities in which oncology social workers can participate. A few areas should be highlighted. Social workers with clinical oncology experience should be an asset for hypothesis generation. They can help other researchers decide what questions need to be asked.

TABLE 2

Possible Areas of Research Involvement for Oncology Social Workers

- Formulating the research process
- Conceptualizing the research problem
- Generating hypotheses
- Designing the research plan
- Protecting the rights of research subjects
- Assuring cultural sensitivity
- Defining the sample
- Determining respondent burden
- Selecting subjects
- Collecting data
- Analyzing data
- Interpreting the findings
- Recognizing clinical applicability
- Disseminating the findings

Note. Adapted from Clark, E. J. (1994). An overview of psychosocial oncology research issues. In B. Rabinowitz, E. J. Clark, & J. Hayes, (Eds.), Demystifying oncology research: A handbook for psychosocial and nursing practitioners (p.3). Trenton, NJ: Joint Psychosocial and Nursing Advisory Group to the New Jersey Commission on Cancer Research.

Social workers also can play a role in the safeguarding of the ethics of the research study and the study design. Protecting clients' rights is a well-established function of social work practice, and one to which social workers have a strong commitment. Having a social worker involved from the beginning in the design of the study might alleviate future problems.

Similarly, social workers can help academics and other researchers understand why some study designs simply will not work in their clinical setting. They can describe issues such as the lack of, and need for, patient privacy for questionnaire completion or interviewing. They can discuss the tight schedules and work patterns of clinical staff, and they can help to show the value of participating in the study to those working in the clinical setting. They also can help to bring a culturally sensitive approach to the study design and can make certain that the research team recognizes the need for materials that match the literacy level of the chosen sample.

Two other important roles for the oncology social worker come at the conclusion of the data analysis. Once the statistical analysis is completed, it is up to the researchers to try to make sense of the findings, to understand the variances found in the data. The social worker brings clinical knowledge and expertise to this task. Their understanding of the broad range of oncology issues, their hands-on experience with patients and families, and their knowledge of the social system in which the research was conducted all help to explain the research results. Without a clinician on the team, the researchers might miss important explanations about the findings.

Finally, the last area where the oncology social worker can be of particular service to the research team is in clinical application. Who better to describe the impact that the findings can, and should, have on the clinical setting and for the patient population studied than the social worker who practices in such a setting. This is an area where academic researchers often fall short, and the utility of their findings go unrecognized by clinicians.

GETTING HELP WHEN GETTING STARTED

If oncology social workers are not yet at the level where they can design, obtain funding, and conduct their own research projects, how can they get started and gain research experience? First, they need to let others know about their interest in being part of a research project. If not at an institution where research is a priority, they should contact their local college or university. Talks with social work and nursing faculty may be valuable. Many academics need clinical settings and experienced clinicians for their research projects. Practitioner-researcher partnerships can lead to creative collaboration (Hess & Mullen, 1995), and many academics would welcome social workers as part of their team.

If the institution has a formal research program, social workers can explore how they might become a member of their institutional review board (IRB) that reviews and monitors research protocols with respect to the protection of human subjects. IRBs are required to have members from various disciplines, and finding a member from the behavioral sciences is not always easy.

Social workers might also want to explore ways to sit on various review panels for research and development grants. They can check to see if there are local groups that award oncology funding. For example, a local women's club or breast cancer group may give small awards to be used within the community. These awards are often described in the newspapers. There may also be some drug companies that offer some small competitive awards. Check with colleagues to see if they know of any opportunities. Sitting on review panels or boards will help social workers understand the types of research that get funded, and it will help them learn the pitfalls that result in good ideas never seeing the light of day.

Clinical Trials Research Opportunities

Another entrée into oncology research is through clinical trials. Clinical trials are experiments that are designed to determine the

potential value of therapies in human subjects. Larger medical institutions usually participate in clinical trials research. Smaller institutions that provide cancer services may also participate in cooperative groups that conduct clinical trials on a regional basis. Social
workers may already be part of the clinical trials program. They may
help provide education to patients about the benefit of clinical trials
participation, may act as advocates in helping individuals enroll in
appropriate trials, and may help patients understand their rights
regarding continuing in or withdrawing from a clinical trial.

However, clinical trials also have research roles in which social
workers might engage. Protocol design, accrual, data collection,
and data management are areas for exploration about the fit of
social work skills. Becoming better informed about clinical trial
research might open avenues to other oncology social work
research opportunities.

National Resources

Do not overlook national resources that are available to social workers. For instance, both the Association of Oncology Social Work
(AOSW) and the Association of Pediatric Oncology Social Workers
(APOSW) have special interest groups in research. This past year,
the AOSW special interest research group (called SWORG or the
Social Work Oncology Research Group) developed a kit designed
to aid oncology social work clinicians evaluate their practices. It
includes a resource guide for practical research study designs, both
quantitative and qualitative, with application to clinical case examples. The AOSW also has a special interest group in computing. For
more information on these special interest groups, consult their
Web sites: AOSW Web site: www.aosw.org; and APOSW Web site:
www.aposw.org.

Case Example: Collaborative Research Across Institutions

Collaborative research with oncology social work peers is a particularly good way to get started in oncology social work research. An
excellent case example of oncology social work collaboration is pre-

sented in an article titled "Prevalence of Psychological Distress among Cancer Patients across the Disease Continuum," written by Zabora et al. (1997). Oncology social work researchers from 12 medical centers around the country designed and implemented a research study to investigate the prevalence of psychosocial distress across the disease continuum to determine if any differences existed in a large random sample of 386 adult cancer patients ranging in age from 18 to 85 years. The study was approved by the IRB of each institution.

The study used two well-established research instruments and demographic data were collected during a brief interview. Data from the 12 institutions were sent to the first author's institution for coding and review. All analyses were completed at one of the other participating institutions. The sociodemographic findings indicated that the sample was fairly representative of the adult cancer outpatient population seen in oncology clinics across the country, and the study findings were consistent with previous studies of the prevalence of distress among cancer patients. Furthermore, they suggested that a significant number of patients who were not in counseling might benefit from social work or psychiatric intervention.

This case example shows the value of collaboration that permitted oncology social work researchers at numerous institutions to participate in a national study. Also, by combining the numbers of subjects seen at 12 institutions, the research increased its sample size and explanatory power.

Case Example: Collaboration Across Disciplines

Another example of collaborative research is an educational project called the *Cancer Survival Toolbox*®, a self-advocacy training program for persons with cancer. Three cancer organizations joined together to develop this project. The groups were the AOSW, the Oncology Nursing Society, and the National Coalition for Cancer Survivorship (NCCS). Each group selected two members to work on the project. This team wrote a grant proposal and received an unrestricted educational grant from Genentech BioOncology.

They began with a variety of research activities. They first completed needs assessment surveys of cancer survivors (n=569) and of oncology social workers and oncology nurses (n=833). They were interested in finding out what skills cancer survivors needed to develop in order to manage their cancer. Once they had the survey data, they next conducted pilot groups with cancer survivors. Based on these findings, the content of an audiotape training program was written. This content was then sent to 15 cancer organizations for review and feedback, and the training program was revised accordingly (Walsh-Burke & Marcusen, 1999).

Combining the three perspectives of social worker, nurse, and cancer survivor, and making the content data-based helped the research team feel certain that the resulting product was comprehensive and that it would meet the needs of the cancer survivor population. The collaboration across disciplines was a very important aspect of the program.

A National Study of Cancer Survivors

Another potential opportunity for collaborative research is a nationwide longitudinal retrospective and prospective study of 100,000 cancer survivors that is currently underway through the Behavioral Research Center of the American Cancer Society (ACS). Called the Study of Cancer Survivors, the study's mission is broad. It seeks to examine what long-term needs of survivors are unmet, treatment effects, possible prevention of late effects including second cancers, psychosocial factors, behavioral patterns, and support necessary for good survivorship and quality of life. A pilot study was conducted in four states (Georgia, Iowa, Minnesota, and Wisconsin) in 1996–1997. The full study will run until 2006.

This is a major research undertaking and there may be a variety of research participation opportunities for oncology social workers across the nation. Contact your local division of the ACS to see if the study is underway in your area. For more general information, check the ACS Web site at www.cancer.org.

FORMAL ONCOLOGY SOCIAL WORK TRAINING

Each year the ACS offers Clinical Oncology Social Work Training Grants to qualifying hospitals and medical centers. There are two types of grants. The first is the master's training grant that introduces social workers to the special needs of cancer patients and their families. The second type of award is for post-master's candidates. This type focuses on training individuals to conduct psychosocial oncology research. The training grant provides an excellent opportunity for starting a research initiative within an institution and gives oncology social workers some financial support while they hone their research skills. Check the ACS Web site for more information.

Acquiring Additional Academic Skills

Sometimes the easiest way for social workers to acquire research skills is to take a formal course. Social workers who have been out of school for a long time and feel their research skills are too rusty, or feel that they lack the self-confidence needed to become part of a research team, might want to check their local college, university, or community college to see if they can audit a research course. A class is often more fun if the student is not being evaluated. Social workers in an audited class might be required to write a research proposal that will receive helpful critique from their instructor. Choosing a "real" topic—one from a clinical setting—can lay the groundwork for an actual research study. Going to class also might provide some valuable contacts with others who are looking for an opportunity to collaborate on a research project.

Another possible option is to take a class in grant-writing. Finding funding is an essential part of conducting research. Most clinicians are intimidated by the grant-writing process, but it actually is a process that is easily learned. What is needed is the blueprint for the process. This includes choosing a topic carefully and making sure it fits the interests of the funding agency. Next, the audience (the grant reviewers) need to be addressed appropriately. This may mean defining terms and making the research goals and methodology clear. The timeline will need to be designed and the budget will have to be developed. These topics are all covered in a grant-writing course. The course may not totally prepare an individual for acquiring a grant, but it could be a major step forward.

Finally, a social worker with an interest in research may want to explore working on obtaining a doctoral degree. There is a great need for more trained oncology social work researchers. Social work framed the field of psychosocial oncology. Yet, the current psychosocial oncology literature indicates that the social work profession lags far behind nursing and psychology in conducting research and publishing relevant articles. Oncology, psychiatry, religion, and health education are also fairly well represented. This is quite evident on examination of the table of contents for the journal *Cancer Practice: A Multidisciplinary Journal of Cancer Care* published by the ACS. On average six full-length articles are published in each issue. Nurses comprise the majority of authors with generally only one article per issue written by a social worker. *The Journal of Psychosocial Oncology*, edited by two social workers, fares a little better, but oncology social workers still are not the dominant profession represented in the articles.

TURNING IDEAS INTO PUBLISHABLE RESEARCH

The barriers to publishing for practitioners are similar to those of conducting research. Practitioners cite lack of time, lack of publishing skills, lack of formal research participation, and lack of self-confidence as reasons they do not contribute more to the social work literature. Yet, few people are better prepared to write about intervention techniques, program planning, implementation and maintenance of social work services, or the actual application of theories and research findings (successes and failures) than those working in clinical settings.

Oncology social workers have valuable experiences that need to be documented and made available for others to use as models and for validation of their own efforts. Yet, only infrequently, do we see such articles in the literature. Publishing is not a critical part of the clinical mission. Consequently, few oncology social workers make it a priority.

Even if they are not involved in structured research activities, oncology social workers can write important pieces that expand the literature, identify issues for possible future research, and simply make others consider a topic more fully. Perhaps these articles can be described as "thought" pieces rather than research reports.

Publishing Case Example

One excellent example of this type of article is "Psychosocial Consequences of Inadequate Health Insurance for Patients with Cancer" published in *Cancer Practice* by Myra Glajchen (1994). The article explores several domains of life of persons with cancer that can be affected by a lack of health insurance. Dr. Glajchen uses brief case studies to make her points about the physical, emotional, financial, social, and employment burdens of cancer caused by inadequate insurance. The article ends with clinical recommendations for professionals to help alleviate these burdens for their patients.

As noted in the article, while several aspects of financial burden of cancer have been studied and documented (such as the costs of cancer and lost wages), the psychosocial aspects of health insurance coverage had received scant attention in the literature. Dr. Glajchen's article raised awareness about this issue for many practitioners and offered suggestions for interventions. This "thought" piece served a valuable function for other oncology social workers and for persons with cancer.

Publishing as a Process

Just as research is a process, so, too, is publishing. There are numerous hints for helping social workers and other practitioners publish. Perhaps most important is setting personal goals for publishing. For example, the writer may decide to submit one article for publication by the end of the year. Time for writing will not magically appear; time needs to be made for it. It is important to develop a timeline and stick to it. Next, the writer should choose a topic to write about (one that the writer knows well makes the writing much easier), and decide when the literature search will be completed. It helps to keep a file on related articles and any thoughts or notes about the topic. It is surprising how quickly random thoughts add up to paragraphs and pages. Another hint is to jot down checklists or brief case examples as they come to mind. If a computer is used regularly, items should be stored in a separate computer file for the article. As a relevant reference is found, it should be added to the reference list.

It is important to study carefully the format of the articles that have previously been published in the journal of choice. The writer should also become familiar with the journal's guidelines for authors and the bibliographic style, and these should be followed exactly.

Except in eighth grade English class, no one ever insisted that an article be written "in order" from opening sentence to the last. Sometimes it helps to begin writing the sections that are easiest. Eventually there will be a number of sections that can be knitted into a whole. It may be useful to complete the case studies (if case studies are being used), and work back to the introduction. Many people write their abstracts last, and the final title may not be evident until the article is completed.

Once the article is written, it should be given to a few friends to read. The writer should listen carefully to the suggestions, but not feel compelled to include them all. It is essential that writers stay true to their own work. Only they know what they are trying to convey.

Also, it is important to note that almost all journals will require revisions. It is a rarity to submit an article and have it published without changing some aspects of it. Do not be discouraged if revisions are requested. Almost all journals ask for revisions, and that is a very good sign that the article is publishable.

If the article is rejected by the journal of choice, it should not be assumed that it is unpublishable. If possible, get comments from the editor. Make changes and submit the revised manuscript to another journal. Most importantly, the writer should not give up. Instead, they should be flexible and persistent. The publication of oncology social work articles is critical to the profession, and oncology social workers have an obligation to help develop the literature.

TOPICS FOR FUTURE RESEARCH

What are important research topics for oncology social workers? How should future efforts be structured? Topics will vary considerably from institution to institution. Selection may depend upon available patient populations, the structure of the oncology practice, and even upon funding opportunities. However, some general guidelines for needed future psychosocial oncology research can be provided.

In 1995, the NCCS convened the First National Congress for Cancer Survivorship. In preparation for the Congress, surveys were sent to health providers, government officials, professional and advocacy organizations, scientists, and others regarding critical issues facing the eight million cancer survivors in this country. Over 300 persons responded. The survey data were used as the basis for discussion at the Congress, and the results were published in a report called *Imperatives for Quality Cancer Care* (Clark, Stovall, Leigh, Austin, & Rowland, 1996).

The areas deemed most important for psychosocial oncology research in the next decade are listed in Table 3. It is a broad list that emphasizes the importance of, and the need for, oncology social work research. While research efforts for many of these topics are currently underway, there is still much work to be done. Research efforts need to be increased so that the knowledge base of oncology social work is documented and expanded, and so that we continue to honor the tradition of oncology social work research that began half a century ago. It is a challenging time for oncology social work, but it is also an exciting time, and oncology social workers are up to the challenge.

TABLE 3

The Most Important Areas for Psychosocial Oncology Research that Should be Undertaken in the Next Decade

OUTCOMES RESEARCH
- Health-related quality of life studies of outcomes of medical care should be linked with clinical trials
- Impact of psychosocial services on financial and health outcomes
- Differential effectiveness of different types of psychotherapeutic interventions in influencing survival and improving adjustment to cancer
- Psychosocial and behavioral links that may be predictive of cancer outcomes
- Psychosocial impact of involvement in clinical trials on quality of life
- Psychosocial impact of reduction of medical services and professional support
- Evaluation of outreach efforts to the underserved (what works and why)

EXPLORATORY STUDIES
- Impact and burden of cancer care on family caregivers
- The meaning of survivorship across cultures
- Examination of critical factors that contribute to or inhibit patient decision-making
- Psychosocial issues related to childbearing and impact of infertility secondary to cancer
- Long-term psychosocial sequelae of cancer survivorship
- Identification of resiliency factors of cancer survivors
- Ways that cancer changes spiritual/existential meaning for the individual

COMPARATIVE/INTERVENTION STUDIES
- Testing of case management models for effectiveness and appropriateness for populations served
- Effect of participation in a psychotherapy group versus a support or self-help group with comparison of facilitators from various professional disciplines and peer groups
- Identification and investigation of psychosocial and educational interventions that enhance patient satisfaction, quality of life, adherence to medical regimens, optimal coping, and high functioning
- Testing of life extension hypothesis of psychosocial intervention
- Evaluation of cancer-related self-advocacy training on quality of life
- Effect of cancer diagnosis on persons with a history of psychiatric diagnosis
- Systematic comparison of in-home and residential hospice care to in-hospital care with regard to cost and family adjustment
- Clinical trials for reducing symptom distress

DEVELOPMENT OF PSYCHOSOCIAL ONCOLOGY TOOLS
- Need for reliable and valid assessment tools for understudied populations such as the poor and elderly
- Need for culturally and ethically sensitive measures
- Need for standardization of quality of life measures

Note. Reprinted with permission from Clark, E. J., Stovall, E. L., Leigh, S., Siu, A. L., Austin, D. K., & Rowland, J. R. (1996). *Imperatives for quality cancer care: Access, advocacy, action, and accountability* (pp. 32-33). Silver Spring, MD: National Coalition for Cancer Survivorship.

REFERENCES

Abrams, R. (1974). *Not alone with cancer: A guide for those who care.* Springfield, IL: Charles C. Thomas.

Clark, E. J. (1994). An overview of psychosocial oncology research issues. In B. Rabinowitz, E. J. Clark, & J. Hayes (Eds.), *Demystifying oncology research: A handbook for psychosocial and nursing practitioners* (pp. 1-4). Trenton, NJ: Joint Psychosocial and Nursing Advisory Group to the New Jersey Commission on Cancer Research.

Clark, E. J., Stovall, E. L., Leigh, S., Siu, A. L., Austin, D. K., & Rowland, J. H. (1996). *Imperatives for quality cancer care: Access, advocacy, action, and accountability.* Silver Spring, MD: National Coalition for Cancer Survivorship.

Glajchen, M. (1994). Psychosocial consequences of inadequate health insurance for patients with cancer. *Cancer Practice, 2(2),* 115-120.

Hess, P. M., & Mullen, E. J. (1995). *Practitioner-Researcher partnerships: Building knowledge from, in, and for practice.* Washington, DC: NASW Press.

Kubler-Ross, E. (1969). *On death and dying.* New York: Macmillan.

Miles, M. B., & Huberman, A. M. (1994). *Qualitative data analysis* (2nd ed.). Thousand Oaks, CA: Sage.

Walsh-Burke, K., & Marcusen, C. (1999). Self-advocacy training for cancer survivors. The Cancer Survival Toolbox. *Cancer Practice, 7(6),* 297-301.

Zabora, J. R., Blanchard, C. G., Smith, E. D., Roberts, C. S., Glajchen, M., Sharp, J. W., BrintzenhofeSzoc, K. M., Locher, J. W., Carr, E. W., Best-Castner, S., Smith, P. M., Dozier-Hall, D., Polinsky, M. L., & Hedlund, S. C. (1997). Prevalence of psychological distress among cancer patients across the disease continuum. *Journal of Psychosocial Oncology, 15(2),* 73-87.

CHAPTER 10

PROFESSIONAL ISSUES IN ONCOLOGY SOCIAL WORK

Naomi M. Stearns, MSW, ACSW

Working with cancer patients and their families can be one of the most professionally stimulating and rewarding experiences of a social worker's career. As patients and families confront the daily challenges posed by a chronic, life-threatening illness, they are generally receptive to social work involvement. This is particularly true at the various crisis points that arise during the course of treatment. The preponderance of social workers that provide services to cancer patients do not practice in cancer centers or in major teaching hospitals; in fact, most do not work exclusively with cancer patients. However, it is safe to suggest that most social workers, regardless of the setting in which they practice, will at some time during their careers have the opportunity and challenge of dealing with either cancer patients or their families. For this reason social workers should become familiar with the variety of professional issues that have an impact on oncology practice.

Treatment options continue to expand at a rapid pace and the survival rates for many cancer patients have increased. In addition, economic factors that influence funding, staffing, and reimbursement continually change the way health care is delivered. Each of these changes has a major impact on oncology social work practice. Oncology social workers have been redefining their role to meet the increased demands imposed by more complex treatment modalities and shrinking resources. In many settings, their role has been re-defined by administrators whose understanding of social work practice, especially in oncology, may be limited. The implications for oncology social workers and their patients are significant and at times ambiguous.

While medical social work originated at Massachusetts General Hospital in 1919, oncology social work has been a recognized specialty for over 25 years. The incumbent professional issues have not necessarily changed but, rather, have expanded as the nature of practice has shifted to a case management model. Some professional issues might appear to relate more directly to social workers practicing in larger medical settings or cancer research centers. However, all social workers are affected by these changes, which demand flexibility and creativity as well as a large measure of forbearance. Oncology social workers must be sensitive to the impact of all this change on the entire health care team. The more one understands the larger picture, the greater the chance one will develop new and effective ways to increase social work visibility and value to the team.

In addition to the core knowledge about the impact of medical illness, oncology has its own vocabulary and unique qualities. There are many ways to develop clinical expertise in oncology, with experience being the best teacher. Social workers can also read numerous professional texts, as well as a plethora of first-person accounts of the cancer experience. Several cancer centers offer clinical skills courses in oncology social work that range in length from several days to a week.

TEAMWORK

The team delivery of health care is never more crucial than in oncology, and the concept raises numerous professional issues regarding collaboration. Twenty-five years ago, cancer researchers who treated patients may or may not have included a social worker on their relatively small team. Oncology social workers have proven the wisdom and appropriateness of their participation on the team, although the social work role may differ among institutions. In 1992, the Association of Community Cancer Centers (ACCC; www.accc-cancer.org) first articulated a standard for social work services, stating that qualified individuals provide social work services to meet the psychosocial needs of patient/families. The most recent statement regarding standards was completed in 2000. More recently, the Association of Oncology Social Workers (AOSW; www.aosw.org) developed its own standards of practice in 1997 that are applicable to social work practice within cancer centers, teaching and community hospitals, and agencies serving cancer patients and their families. Even in hospitals where the role of the social worker has been restructured, cancer patients and their families are expected to receive social work services. This places the social worker in a unique position on the team, but it also raises questions regarding role differentiation and expectations about who should provide what to patients and families. The social worker frequently is the pivotal person in facilitating continuity of care in a system where so many professionals provide that care. Social workers who are cognizant of the potential for fragmentation are in a unique position to use their skills to increase communication among team members.

Educating others on the team about the diversity of the social work role can be challenging and at times frustrating. The perceptions of others on the health care team generally define their expectations of social work and influence their understanding of what it offers patients and families. Social workers whose major function is discharge planning may feel that their clinical assessment and therapeutic skills are not fully appreciated. It would be wise to consider the clinical expertise involved in helping a patient and family deal with a nursing home placement for instance, which is often perceived as abandonment and the end of life. Social workers who are considered part of the mental health team are often perceived as lacking adequate understanding of the patient's practical needs.

While social workers might feel the need to explain to others what professional education and skills they possess, the most effective way to demonstrate those abilities is by example. By demonstrating knowledge of and respect for the integration of the biological, psychological, social, and practical needs of cancer patients and their families, the social worker is able to provide a model for patient care. Tensions within the team are bound to surface, especially in times of shrinking resources and growing demands on staff energies.

Turf issues present yet another arena for professional conflict. In any multidisciplinary setting there are bound to be some conflicts. While a certain amount of team tension can be stimulating and healthy, it is important to separate the administrative issues from those related to the emotional intensity of the work itself. A work environment that respects the emotional drain on its staff and that encourages professional development among its team members certainly enhances everyone's ability to continue to function effectively.

"Teamwork involves a fully functioning group, characterized by a common mission, defined leadership, and systems of operation that capitalize on the best of the professional disciplines represented" (Hermann & Hilderly, 1993, p. 329). In most settings, social work plays a vital role on the case management team. While it may be difficult to accept, the social worker should understand that not all patients require social work intervention. However, all patients require information and that is often the entrée one has to the patient and family. Within the framework of case management, the patient will often choose a support person from the team. The patient's choice might well be someone other than the social worker. This is not generally an indictment of the social worker or a reflection of the social worker's competence. Rather, it is human nature to gravitate to the person with whom we feel a strong connection. Also, patients can be depleted of energy trying to sustain close relationships with multiple team members. It can also be helpful to remember that there are plenty of patients to go around. Competition among team members is often a waste of energy considering the plethora of unmet needs found in any population of people with cancer.

ETHICAL ISSUES

Oncology social workers often articulate concerns regarding the ethics involved in cancer care. They are involved on a daily basis with issues of truth telling, patient autonomy, self-determination, informed consent, and quality of life. Cancer diagnosis and treatment have spawned ongoing debates around disclosure; randomized clinical trials, curative vs. palliative care (treatment oriented to symptom management), appropriate limits of treatment, and orders not to resuscitate (DNR orders). New workers, in particular, are forced to define and confront on a daily basis the concept of a "burdensome" life. In oncology practice, professional staff often finds themselves grappling with competing values. Certain patient care decisions may threaten to force the caregivers to compromise their integrity. Social workers are particularly vulnerable in situations where treatment choices appear to undermine patient autonomy. Self-determination has been the foundation of social work training; as technology advances, the burden of choice increases. Patients are forced to consider the tradeoff between high-tech medical treatments, such as bone marrow transplantation and biological therapies, and what they and their families consider an acceptable quality of life or death. "Ethical decision making has often been described as a choice between two rights. Without clear-cut answers, practitioners often have to choose between alternatives" (Ferrell & Rivera, 1995, p. 94).

The social worker frequently is asked to assist patients in sorting out the treatment options presented to them by the physician. One soon learns just how difficult the choices can be. Adjuvant treatment for breast cancer is but one example of this type of dilemma for patients for whom the options may seem confusing. Adjuvant treatment for cancer usually refers to additional therapy such as chemotherapy given after surgery and radiation to decrease the likelihood of a recurrence. In general, there is an ongoing debate within the medical community regarding the "best treatment" for a number of types of cancer. How does the patient choose? A dilemma arises for social workers when they feel pressure to support a specific treatment, especially when its benefit for the patient is unclear.

Maintaining a neutral stance can be difficult and, at times, inappropriate. The more the social worker is able to learn about the available options, the greater the ability to respond to the patient's questions and concerns in an appropriate manner.

Communication between the physician and social worker is essential. The social worker's role in the patient-physician relationship must be clarified and the physician should keep the social worker apprised of what information the patient has been given. Having a social worker present during physician-patient discussions allows all participants to hear what the physician tells the patient about proposed treatments and possible side effects, both medical and psychosocial. It also helps social workers identify areas that need further explanation by the physician in order to facilitate the patient's decision-making process. The social worker's presence also allows observation of the interaction between the patient and physician and the patient and family, which helps in understanding how information is being given and received. Including social workers in such meetings enhances their credibility as vital members of the team.

Other ethical conflicts relate to the social worker's expectations regarding the goal of treatment. While one might prefer to think in terms of cure, it is helpful to understand that, at times, cure is not the objective, despite the aggressiveness and difficulty of the treatment. Frequently, treatment is an attempt to both manage the symptoms and maximize the quality of the patient's life within the constraints imposed by the disease, or perhaps, to think in terms of slowing down a terminal process when that is consistent with the patient's goals. An untreated cancer can cause serious disruptions of bodily functions and for that reason alone, palliative treatment is often recommended.

The issue of self-determination, a basic principle in the generic practice of social work, is highlighted in every discussion of ordinary vs. extraordinary means. Do-not-resuscitate orders, living wills, and artificial feeding are among the most commonly debated issues of self-determination in cancer care. Self-determination is a professional issue that social workers are well-equipped to debate, but one that often creates anxiety for the staff as they try to interpret patients' and families' wishes and concerns to the other members of the team. This is especially true when the patient's desires conflict with those of the family or those of the physician.

Certain legislative action should encourage earlier discussions about patients' wishes and provide direction to family members and staff. The Patient Self-Determination Act became effective nationwide in December 1991. The Act mandates that all hospitals, HMOs, and nursing homes that receive Medicare and Medicaid reimbursements provide written information to patients regarding their rights to refuse care, to create Advance Care Directives, and to appoint agents (proxies) to make decisions for them should they become unable to do so. It is important to know the way this policy is being carried out in one's work setting, where applicable, and how the social workers are involved.

When considering these ethical issues, a frequent concern is whether medicine has the right to create a "burdensome" life with its interventions. How does one define " burdensome?" What may seem to the medical team to be rather ordinary medical intervention may seem to certain patients radical or extraordinary and, indeed, burdensome in their own circumstances. The terminology used in discussing professional ethical issues is often vague. The term " heroic measures," for example, is wide open to interpretation. It is necessary to find out the patient's interpretation of these words. The physician's interpretation is equally important. While one physician might consider admission to an intensive care unit a heroic step, another might interpret cardiopulmonary resuscitation as routine, rather than heroic. Discussions about prognosis can be extremely misleading, as even the most considered medical prognostication is cloaked in uncertainty and bias. Social workers and others on the health care team must understand the impracticality of absolute prognoses.

In most medical settings there is a tendency to generalize and at times decisions reflect what is more convenient or less disruptive for the hospital than for the patient and family. Ethical practice dictates that care be individualized. While this is conceptually sound, it may be difficult to implement institutionally. One of social work's goals is to return to patients some of the control they relinquish upon entering a medical setting. This particular issue should be of utmost concern to oncology social workers.

It is important for social workers to be in basic agreement with the philosophy of the institution in which they work. For example, social workers in cancer research centers soon learn that they work in an environment where there is generally always another treatment to be tried when one treatment fails to elicit a favorable response. That kind of aggressive approach may raise significant quality-of-life issues for social workers, especially those new to the field. It is important that social workers allow enough time to fully understand an institution's orientation so that they can make informed judgments about their ability to fit in. Each of us brings to our work a set of beliefs and values that influence our handling of ethical dilemmas. It is important to understand that all medical decisions ultimately are made by two or more persons, each with his or her own moral and ethical traditions; sometimes they match, and at other times they are in sharp contrast. At some time, each of us is convinced that there is only one way to decide—my way! If social workers are unclear about or misunderstand the goal of a particular medical treatment and the social work role, then the conflicts will most certainly be exacerbated. In order to help patients understand their options social workers need to clarify their own values and learn to respect the values of their colleagues, even when they differ. It is the development of the relationships between the patient, physician, social worker, nurse, and other members of the team that encourages a respect for a variety of beliefs, thus helping everyone to negotiate the difficult ethical issues.

PEER SUPPORT

Another component in professional development is the importance of peer support. Having colleagues who immediately understand the work one does, without having to explain, contributes to a sense of professional satisfaction. Social workers who work in teaching hospitals or cancer centers may have easier access to such support, but there are options for those with less built-in support.

In many parts of the country, local or regional groups of oncology social workers meet regularly to provide ongoing education and support. These groups are open to any social worker with an interest in oncology. The AOSW is an international organization whose mission includes advocating sound public and professional programs and policies for cancer patients, creating professional standards for oncology social work practice, and providing valuable services to its members. AOSW sponsors a yearly educational conference, publishes a quarterly newsletter; and offers consultation through its extensive network of members. Involvement with a local social work oncology group, as well as the international organization, guarantees access to a variety of learning experiences and other resources that are crucial to developing a sense of competence in this specialized area. Cancer Care, Inc. is a national non-profit social service organization that provides a wide range of free professional services to cancer patients, families, caregivers, and health care professionals. It can be reached through its 800 number and Web site. Cancer Care also sponsors regular teleconferences about medical and psychosocial topics and is a wonderful resource to learn about cancer. For professionals acting as the sole oncology social worker in a particular setting, the peer support offered through these organizations can dramatically reduce the sense of isolation, in addition to providing excellent educational benefits.

Mailing lists and list servs are another way to access information. One of these is the Social Work Oncology Network (SWON), which is available to AOSW members. It provides on-line support including resource sharing, clinical expertise and clinical consultation. Each subscriber receives a separate copy through email of each item that is posted. Mailing lists are a free resource for oncology social workers to speak with one another about particular topics of interest. This service is particularly valuable to those social workers in rural settings or overseas who might feel particularly disconnected from their oncology social work peers.

PROFESSIONAL DEVELOPMENT

Rapidly changing treatment developments and the increased longevity of patients mandate the need for oncology social workers to continually expand their knowledge and their repertoire of interventions, many of which have been discussed in other chapters of this book. While many programs and materials exist to meet the oncology social worker's professional development needs, it can be difficult, if not impossible in the current economic climate for many social workers to be given time away from the workplace as well as the financial assistance to attend seminars and courses. A number of avenues are worth exploring to obtain money for travel and conference registration, for example, the oncologists in your setting, community agencies, or drug companies. Some institutions have restricted staff from soliciting funds from pharmaceutical firms. Consider asking for smaller amounts from several sources rather than just one. On the job, oncology social workers ought to expect adequate and thorough orientation to their jobs. It is particularly helpful when your supervisor has specific oncology experience. Some new oncology social workers have been successful in obtaining outside specialized supervision when it is not available on site. While not a substitute for clinical supervision, the AOSW listserv encourages clinical discussion of difficult cases and an opportunity for creative problem solving. The institution has a responsibility to provide support to staff and the social worker has the right to request supervision. This is an investment that pays off for the institution since it means not having to constantly replace inadequately trained, overwhelmed staff members who have been insufficiently prepared for their jobs. The AOSW Standards of Practice (1997) and their document *Managed Care: A Survival Kit for the Oncology Social Worker* (1995) may be useful in helping institutions appreciate the broad range of skills necessary for comprehensive psychosocial care.

The Journal of Psychosocial Oncology, published by The Haworth Medical Press, is the official journal of the Association of Oncology Social Work. A subscription to the journal is one of the benefits included in AOSW membership. It offers a wide range of articles of research and clinical interest. Oncology social workers are encouraged to submit practice and research papers for possible publication. Likewise, *Cancer Practice*, a journal of the American Cancer Society, is interested in oncology social workers as potential sources of practice-related articles.

The American Cancer Society, through its Divisions and Units, provides a variety of educational programs at little or no cost to attendees. Many of the programs are scheduled at the end of the workday or on Saturdays in order to accommodate health professionals who cannot attend at other times.

The annual educational conferences held by the AOSW and APOSW are excellent ways to build skills and network with colleagues from around the world.

PROFESSIONAL GRIEF OR MANAGING THE INTENSITY OF THE WORK

Oncology social workers frequently are asked to explain how they manage the intensity of their work over time. This query is generally followed by observations that the oncology social worker must either qualify for sainthood or find the work inordinately depressing. This is not a description that most social workers find useful, especially those new to the field of oncology. However, these well-intentioned comments do force one to consider both the positive and negative impacts of the work. Identifying sources of stress and developing strategies to manage the physical and emotional aspects of the work are crucial to maintaining professional and personal balance.

Much has been written over the years about the burnout associated with the helping professions. Burnout has been a term frequently used to describe the long-term responses of persons on the front lines in social service agencies and health care settings. A more recent expression to describe this phenomenon is "compassion fatigue," but the syndrome has not changed. It can occur when physical and psychological resources are depleted by the constant demand for a person's energy, expertise, and compassion. People are most vulnerable when they set unrealistically high expectations for themselves and for those with whom they work. Oncology social workers are prime candidates for energy depletion, especially when their empathy is not balanced by a flexible approach to the work and the ability to work toward their own goals, not those set by others.

Perhaps a better nomenclature for this is "professional grief" which more accurately reflects our response to repeated loss, a given in oncology social work. In a manual produced by Novartis (1999), it is suggested that oncology health care providers see more death in a year than most others see in an entire career or even in their life-time. Professional grief implies that those dealing with multiple deaths accumulate grief over time. Recognizing one's own develop-mental issues, especially around loss, can help in managing the inten-sity of the work and the resulting grief. For example, a social worker struggling with an aging parent might have difficulty dealing with the elderly, or a worker new to motherhood might find pediatric can-cer distressing. Once the developmental issues are understood, the social worker is better equipped to take appropriate steps to cope.

The first step in developing a self-support protocol is to identify and validate what an individual finds difficult about the work and rec-ognize that it is not useful to generalize; what is particularly distress-ing for one social worker may not be for another. It is precisely the variations in personality, prior experiences with illness and death, cur-rent life situation, training, supervision, and length of time in the field that determine what will create work-related stress for an individual.

It helps to learn early in clinical practice that there are limita-tions to what an individual social worker can accomplish and that setting both limits and realistic goals helps each member of the team, as well as patients and their families, maintain appropriate bound-aries. One of the pitfalls for social workers new to the field is a sense of urgency about helping patients. When this translates into "doing for" patients rather than helping patients do for themselves, workers run the risk of removing even more control from patients and overex-tending themselves in unhealthy and unprofessional ways.

It is not enough to focus on what is difficult about the work. It is equally important to discover what counterbalances the sadness, frustration, and fatigue that inevitably occur. Social workers need to develop supportive networks inside as well as outside of the workplace and to create strategies that consistently nurture and replenish. It is important to find ways to divert attention from the intensity of ongoing interactions with patients and families. By evaluating their own coping strategies and substituting more adaptive ones for those that are less effective, social workers can substantially reduce their vulnerability.

Much has been written about the parallel process involved in oncology work. When the issues faced by patients and their families and their coping mechanisms are examined, it becomes clear that social workers and other members of the health care team experience the same feelings of uncertainty, denial, and the need to sustain hope that characterize the cancer experience. This parallel process has an effect on relationships. Just as it affects the balance within the family, it affects the balance of the team. Understanding this process can help social workers develop their role on the team.

It is not possible to deliver good cancer care in isolation. Recognition of the value of the other members of the health care team contributes to a sense of shared responsibility and can significantly reduce the unwelcome sense of uniqueness that occurs when a person works in relative isolation. Such recognition is not always easy, especially in settings where competition among staff members produces excessive tension. Social workers often play a significant role in enhancing team cohesiveness. Quite frequently, they are expected to assume the role of team leader and conflict mediator. Although not always explicitly stated, social workers are viewed as having the skills necessary to bring the team together. Such leadership has enormous value in settings where the stress is inordinately high, especially when the social worker facilitates mutual respect among the individual members of the team.

COPING STRATEGIES

This section is not intended to provide a list of every adaptive coping strategy used by social workers in cancer care; however, a few should be highlighted.

In addition to achieving a skill level at which social workers feel competent, understand what is difficult in the work, and learn to set priorities and limits, the worker new to oncology must also learn how to balance the commitment to the job with a satisfying life outside. Just as one cannot look directly at the sun for very long without turning away, oncology social workers must find ways to divert their attention from their work. As well, it helps to discover when to take brief and extended breaks from work. The more indispensable social workers allow themselves to feel on the job, the more difficult it becomes to take care of themselves in a healthy way. Staff members who are unable to let go of the job, even for a well-deserved day off or a vacation of reasonable length, may find themselves so depleted that the only recourse they see is to make a premature permanent job change.

Any discussion of coping would be incomplete without mentioning the effectiveness of humor. For some, this may be the most adaptive way to cope with the demands and stress of the work. In learning to take the work, but not oneself, too seriously there is an opportunity to sit back and put things into perspective. Humor, in its best sense, can be viewed as an expression of caring, for oneself and for others. Like everything else in life, medical settings spawn their own unique brand of humor. Although hospital humor is not meant to be disrespectful, an outsider might consider some of the humor a bit macabre. It is important to remember that there are funny moments even in cancer.

In order for social workers to be effective in this work, they must possess self-awareness. Learning to identify their own patterns of stress and evaluating typical responses for managing the stress helps them seek alternatives to less-adaptive responses. Learning when it is time to make a change is equally important. Many oncology social workers remain in the field for years. Others may find that dealing with the boundary issues and the impact of progressive disease is too taxing. It is far better to consider a job change than run the risk of compromising your job satisfaction. It is perfectly acceptable to want to be happy in one's career.

ADVOCACY

Advocacy has been the hallmark of social work practice since the field's beginning days. Social workers are experts in advocating for patients and families, especially when care is denied or barriers to access exist. However, social workers, in general, traditionally have exhibited less competence in advocating for themselves. When we speak of advocacy a number of arenas come to mind: advocacy on behalf of patients or case advocacy, self-advocacy, institutional advocacy, organizational and public advocacy. Case advocacy is self-explanatory. Self-advocacy has been mentioned above but it bears repeating. Social workers historically have been better advocates for patients and families than for themselves. Contrary to the notion that social workers by definition are not entitled to advocate for themselves emotionally, spiritually, and financially, doing so ultimately benefits both the worker and the client. In fact, one might argue that the self-advocating, assertive social worker is better able to model self-advocating behavior for the patient (Smith, Walsh-Burke, & Crusan, 1998).

The importance of personal and professional self-advocacy cannot be stressed enough. The additional stresses imposed by managed care, especially those created by downsizing and changing social work roles, call for greater understanding of how an individual social worker responds to the challenges and limitations of practice.

Social workers also become involved in institutional advocacy as they fight for resources. It is easier to accomplish this if the social worker is familiar with the unique qualities of the various settings in which oncology social work is practiced. Obviously, it is crucial to understand and feel comfortable with the philosophy of one's workplace whether it be a hospital, oncologist's office, or public or private community agency. Institutional advocacy includes increasing the patient's effective use of the medical system and his or her ability to communicate needs. The social worker in this instance can serve as a catalyst.

Another component of advocacy is public advocacy. Oncology social workers can use their expertise and clinical experience to affect public policy that leads to policy change. Such efforts have a legislative impact. Oncology social workers should be encouraged to publicly articulate what cancer patients need from the health care system and its providers. When these efforts are successful the oncology social worker is left with an immense sense of satisfaction. Organizational advocacy refers to those times when several organizations with similar goals join together to collaborate on a specific problem-solving project. The old adage of strength in numbers is frequently upheld as collaborative efforts produce a stronger voice.

INFLUENCING POLICY DEVELOPMENT ON A LARGER SCALE

As social workers committed to the needs and rights of cancer patients and their families, it is easy to become immersed in direct service without considering that there is a role for individual workers and their professional organizations in the political sphere. A number of organizations are involved in advocacy for cancer patients. The American Cancer Society not only stays abreast of current issues affecting this population, but it also publishes up-to-date information on pending legislation, some of which it has initiated. The National Coalition for Cancer Survivorship also actively works to change the situation regarding issues such as discrimination, employability, and insurability for cancer survivors. The AOSW and the Association of Pediatric Oncology Social Workers (APOSW), with their steadily increasing memberships, have the potential to become powerful political voices for the rights of cancer patients. Through the efforts of these organizations, it is relatively easy for any social worker to learn about current issues and legislation affecting all cancer patients. One can also learn how to become involved as an individual and as a member of a growing constituency with the potential to be a strong lobbying force.

Every social worker, once adequately informed about the issues, can participate in the process. Writing to legislators urging support for specific bills is an effective yet relatively easy way to get involved. This activity can be extremely empowering, as it enhances professional credibility. Just as patients achieve a sense of mastery and control of their situation, professionals who care for them may benefit from becoming advocates. Political activism regarding cancer-related issues might also be considered another coping strategy and it is consistent with the role of the social worker as an agent of change.

CHANGES IN THE HEALTH CARE SYSTEM

Changes in the delivery of health care across the country have significantly affected social work practice, both in hospitals and community agencies. Social workers are required to work more quickly or provide condensed service to patients who are trying to sort through options as well as feelings. Managed care has prompted shorter hospital stays shifting the focus from inpatient to outpatient care. Patients are frequently denied admission or are discharged sicker. At the same time that social workers are expected to maximize continuity of care for patients and coordinate community resources for them, communities continually battle the financial constraints that prevent them from providing optimal services. Even when community resources exist, the large number of people lacking adequate insurance coverage compounds an already difficult situation. This demands enormous creativity and perseverance on the part of social workers and tests their advocacy skills, as well. Social workers often may find themselves promoting or developing new community resources. This can be both exciting and extremely rewarding. Acting as a liaison with community agencies has become an essential component of practice. At times, the social worker's role is to help patients and families access whatever resources are available and to advocate for those that are clearly needed, but do not yet exist. Patients, encouraged to become activists, often gain a sense of mastery in advocating, not only for themselves, but also for others with similar needs.

Since so much care is now being given outside of the hospital, there is a need for community-based professionals to have some education about cancer, its treatment, and its impact on the family. Some community professionals are reluctant to accept cancer patients because they lack basic information, do not know what to expect, and question their ability to manage their own reactions. The social worker who is familiar with cancer is in an excellent position to act as a resource to community agencies and schools.

THE SOCIAL WORK CLINICIAN WHO IS ALSO A CANCER SURVIVOR

When the oncology social worker is also a cancer survivor a number of special professional issues come into play. The feelings of sadness and grief discussed earlier in this chapter now are compounded by the feelings of fear and terror that accompany a diagnosis of cancer. The challenge here is learning to control the terror when working with one's patients. A recurrence in one of those patients exacerbates the fear for one's own future health (Hill, 1989).

Any oncology social worker quickly learns that boundary issues are somewhat less rigid than the way they were presented during graduate school in the context of therapeutic alliance. This does not mean that maintaining appropriate professional distance is not important. The social worker must always consider whether an interaction with or on behalf of the patient is in the best interests of that person. In some ways, interactions with certain patients over the course of lengthy cancer treatment can begin to feel like friendship. This is not necessarily a bad thing, but the social worker must be especially observant and clear as to whose needs are being served. As always, it must be the patient.

When the clinician is also coping with a personal cancer diagnosis, there is the very real threat that boundaries can become blurred. It is crucial to address the question of whether or not to disclose one's own diagnosis to patients. This issue comes up for discussion at every meeting of the AOSW support network for social workers in this situation. Different ways of handling this are suggested and no consensus has been reached apart from a general agreement that one's motives must be clear in choosing to disclose your own diagnosis to patients. While it is true that your credibility might rise with the patient if you are perceived as a "fellow traveler," there is always the risk that the patient will be burdened by the need to take care of you. Before you disclose to a patient, be sure that you have discussed this with the appropriate colleagues, supervisor, and perhaps therapist.

Finally, there is the question of where to receive treatment. For some the convenience of being treated in their place of employment might be desirable. Certainly, there is built in support as well as familiarity with the setting. On the other hand, that same familiarity might interfere with the desire for privacy or at least some anonymity. Some social workers have found it uncomfortable to be confronted by their patients in the clinic or oncologist's office. Others have found this to be less problematic.

SUMMARY

Oncology social work is a vital specialty in the psychosocial care of the cancer patient. In the earlier days of its practice, oncology social workers found themselves caring for patients whose life expectancy was measured, at most, in months. Today, the focus is increasingly on survival and long-term effects of treatment, while still attending to the needs of patients who are in a terminal phase. The systems that care for patients have become intensely complex, placing new demands on everyone involved. Social work has responded by creating a highly respected niche in oncology and by working collaboratively with other disciplines to bring a broad range of practice skills and innovative approaches to the provision of mental health and concrete services for cancer patients and their families. The professional issues are both numerous and complex. At times, it seems that more questions are raised than are answered, especially in the rapidly changing health care climate. Social workers are intrinsically involved, however, and are in a unique position to affect, directly and indirectly, the care of patients and their families.

References

Association of Community Cancer Centers. (2000). *Standards for Cancer Programs*. Rockville, MD: Author.

Association of Oncology Social Work. (1997). *Standards of Practice in Oncology Social Work*. Baltimore, MD: Author.

Association of Oncology Social Work. (1995). *Managed Care: A Survival Kit for the Oncology Social Worker*. Baltimore, MD: Author.

Ferrell, B. R., Rivera, L. M. (1995). Ethical decision making in oncology: A case study approach. *Cancer Practice, 3(2)*, 94-99.

Hermann, J. F., Hilderley, L. J. (1993). Teamwork: A blessing or a burden? *Cancer Practice, 1(4)*, 329-330.

Hill, H. L. (1989). To fill a heart: Oncology social work over the long haul. *Journal of Psychosocial Oncology, 7(3)*, 1145-1152.

Novartis Oncology. (1999). Managing professional grief. *In Words well spoken: Effective communication strategies for oncology healthcare providers* [Workshop Leader's Guide]. East Hanover, NJ: Author.

Smith, E., Walsh-Burke, K., & Crusan, C. (1998). Principles of training social workers in oncology. In J. C. Holland (Ed.), *Psycho-oncology* (pp. 1061-1068). New York: Oxford University Press.

CHAPTER 11

SPECIAL POPULATIONS

PART A: WORKING WITH ADOLESCENTS: PATIENTS, CAREGIVERS, AND SIBLINGS

Amanda L. Sutton, CSW
Jennifer Keller, CSW
Allen Levine, ACSW

ADOLESCENCE: A TIME OF TURMOIL AND DISCOVERY

During adolescence, a young person moves from being a child to developing an identity in the adult world (see Table 1 on page 234). This is a time of discovery, opportunity, and excitement. At the same time, an unconscious process of grief begins. Adolescents must give up their childhood comforts in order to venture into a new and sometimes disappointing world. Coping with the impact of a cancer diagnosis or dealing with the illness of a relative is difficult for any child, but it has particular impact during this crucial developmental stage. This section discusses the common needs and issues that arise when an adolescent confronts a cancer diagnosis, either as patient, caregiver, or sibling. Emphasis will be given on how to approach the young person and the errors adults often make when trying to communicate with this special population. It is important to remember, of course, that generalizations are always dangerous. While some adolescents may reflect the prevalent peer culture, others do not.

TABLE 1

Phases and Tasks of Adolescence

EARLY ADOLESCENCE: 10.5–14 YEARS OLD
- Discover physical and emotional changes
- Conceptualize and explore new identities
- Realize new abilities and opportunities
- Seek increasing freedom from family
- Take on new responsibilities/recognize peer competition

MIDDLE ADOLESCENCE: 14–18 YEARS OLD
- Adjust to changes in mind, body, and spirit
- Search for vocational, sexual, and personal identity
- Experience and acknowledge loss of childhood
- Reexamine values to either ally with parents or revolt
- Withdraw primary focus from family
- Reinvest energy in peer groups

LATE ADOLESCENCE: 18–22 YEARS OLD
- Adjust to adult life and discover personal ideology
- Establish vocational, sexual, and personal identity
- Continue developing independence from family

Adolescents may be mature or immature; serious students or school dropouts; competitive athletes or developing artists or musicians; agnostic, atheistic or deeply spiritual; alienated from parents or closely tied to parents and family. Social workers understand the need for assessing an adolescent's individual personality, relationships, support system, and life circumstances before planning interventions.

WHEN AN ADOLESCENT HAS CANCER

In the Beginning

Before diagnosis, there may be great uncertainty and increased levels of anxiety on the part of the adolescent, parents, and siblings. A major task is to maintain some balance between the serious illness and the possibility of death, and the denial of that reality that allows for the continuation of everyday life (Rolsky, 1992). An adolescent may naturally turn to peers as a main source of support, since peer acceptance is of prime importance for many. If the cancer patient feels or is rejected, feelings of isolation and compromised self-esteem can grow.

The Diagnosis

Once a diagnosis is made, the patient is plunged into the world of hospitals and medical treatment. Information about the particular cancer and its treatment may seem overwhelming. Young people are drawn into the rapid decision making that is necessary, although the legal responsibility may remain with parents. The young person who had been spending time developing a social identity in the world becomes temporarily more dependent on family. Newly achieved freedoms may be modified or lost as patients prepare for treatment and allow others to be involved in their care.

As Treatment Continues

During the diagnostic and early treatment phase, many adolescents feel the loss of control, particularly if medical staff and parents do not involve them in the decisions about the treatment course. Including the adolescent in choices about care and daily activities also is important. Small decisions about food, clothing, room deco-rations, and how to spend free time can have great impact on reclaiming some control and sense of autonomy. It is important to encourage the adolescent to plan fun and pleasurable activities to lighten the difficult days, weeks, and months of treatment.

Hair loss, weight loss or gain, mouth sores, and increased fatigue take on new meaning for the adolescent patient because they frequently compare their physical appearance with that of friends. Peers may become less of a support source when they are uncom-fortable with the changes resulting from the disease or treatment. The idea of cancer may frighten some peers who worry that their friend will die. For others, it is easier to put distance between them-selves and the patient rather than struggle with uncomfortable fears and feelings.

Other Adult Figures

Adolescents strive to be independent, yet the cancer usually forces them to become physically and emotionally dependent on their parents. It is not uncommon for some adolescents to choose not to show emotional upset and not to share many of their fears and uncertainties with parents in order to protect them. It is also common for them to direct the normal anger they feel about their diagnosis and the discomfort and restrictions of treatment at parents and siblings. In these situations, a significant adult, other than parents, can be helpful. Adolescents often form strong attachments to members of the multidisciplinary team. Professional caregivers must be careful to avoid usurping the role of parents, even in those situations where they seem able to relate and communicate better than parents with the adolescent.

Questions About Illness

It is important to recognize that difficult, sometimes unverbalized, questions may be going through an adolescent's mind. Why me? Am I being punished for something that I've done wrong? Is there someone to blame for this? Am I going to die? When young people ask these questions they are looking for answers and hoping to regain control. It is important to encourage them to explore their own thoughts and to put conflicting feelings into words rather than into destructive behavior (Perschy, 1997). Many questions remain unanswerable and parents and professionals are not responsible for finding answers. However, in addition simply to listening and remaining present at times, they also must guide and direct discussion of these questions, helping the adolescent to achieve some resolution or set them aside, and to redirect energy to other important tasks.

Reactions to Illness

Coping with diagnosis and treatment, adolescents can easily lose their fragile sense of self and identity. Adding to this struggle is a loss of opportunity to socialize. In hospitals, daily contact is with adults. Most adolescents receive treatment in pediatric units or outpatient clinics where younger children are the majority of the patients. This can exacerbate the feeling of a backward step to child-hood, especially for the older adolescent. The side effects of treat-ment often leave adolescents unable or reluctant to socialize even if there are other patients their age present. When the adolescent returns home, side effects and fatigue may prevent full participation in school activities, hobbies, and interests. This may fuel resent-ment, shame, or anger. Social workers and other team members intervene in a variety of ways to help adolescents and parents address these and other age-related issues. They work closely with the adolescent, educate siblings and peers, discuss common needs of adolescents with parents, visit schools and talk with teachers and classmates, and provide adolescent groups and activities.

The Dying Process

If the cancer progresses to a point where death is likely, the adoles-cent faces many challenges in considering his or her own death. One is struggling to understand the spiritual and philosophical issues of life and death. Defining a concept of death, exploring beliefs and values of an afterlife, and finding meaning in the present are paramount (Corr & Balk, 1996). Some are enraged that life for them will end before they have even begun to live. Some find com-fort in a strong belief in God and a life after death. Some are dis-traught at the thought of separation from those they love. All are anxious about the unknown. Like all human beings, adolescents are frightened about what they may experience in the final days, weeks, and months of life. Some are worried that they will have unbearable pain. They need reassurance that there are effective ways to manage pain. Patients and parents need information to help them anticipate whatever else may happen. Patients also need some opportunity to exercise control and decision making around how they want to experience the end of life. Helping the patient preserve relationships with loved ones while preparing to say good-bye is also of prime importance. Parents also should be encouraged to help adolescents review the good experiences of their lives, the accomplishments they value most, and the ways in which they want to be remem-bered. Social workers and other team members assist each dying adolescent and family by drawing on the knowledge and skills that comes from professional experience. No matter how experienced, however, it is always anguishing to witness the awareness and sadness of the adolescent for whom life is ending.

WHEN A PARENT IS DIAGNOSED WITH CANCER

Separation/Individuation

One main task of adolescence is to separate from the family of origin in order to create an individual identity in the adult world. When a parent has cancer, the adolescent wrestles between the desire to continue having a life apart from the family and the wish to help and be involved in care of the ill parent (Harpham, 1997). The adolescent can be fearful that daily life will change or, in the case of those with single parents, that there will be no one to care for them if their parent dies. This can be a major concern in cases where the "well" parent is mentally ill, abusive, in jail, or has serious problems in functioning. It is common for adolescents to feel anger and resentment toward the ill parent for getting sick and toward the well parent for imposing new rules and responsibilities. Adolescents also can be jealous of those whose parents are not ill or ashamed of worrying what peers will think of an ill parent. Shame and anger towards the parent with cancer can cause guilt, as can the desire to be away from the family and spend time having fun with friends. Adolescents need the active help of parents, other family members or professionals to help them deal with these concerns.

Depression

Depression in an adolescent can occur because the ill parent is not able to provide positive acknowledgment of accomplishments and the support and reassurance that helps to foster healthy self-esteem. Without this reflection, adolescents are at risk of losing their confidence and sense of self. Depression can result also from the adoles-

TABLE 2

Symptoms of Clinical Depression

Five or more of the following symptoms have been present during the same 2-week period and represent a change from previous functioning: at least one of the symptoms is either (1) depressed mood or (2) loss of interest or pleasure.

- Depressed or irritable mood most of the day, nearly every day
- Markedly diminished interest or pleasure in activities
- Significant weight loss or weight gain
- Changes in sleep (too much, too little)
- Psychomotor agitation or retardation
- Fatigue or loss of energy
- Feeling of worthlessness or excessive guilt
- Diminished ability to think or concentrate, or indecisiveness
- Recurrent thought of deaths or suicidal ideation

Note. Reprinted with permission from the *Diagnostic and Statistical Manual of Mental Disorders* (4th ed.). Copyright 1994 American Psychiatric Association.

cent having inappropriate responsibility for the ill parent or for family tasks. Not all families or adolescents function well before a parent is diagnosed with cancer. It is very important, therefore, for professionals to assess the causes of any perceived depression in an adolescent and not assume that it is a reaction to the parent's cancer (see Table 2).

Changes in Roles and Responsibilities

When a parent is diagnosed with cancer, new time demands arise as parents work treatment routines into their schedules. Side effects can render the ill parent unable to fulfill usual responsibilities that now fall to the adolescent. Young women can be asked to become the surrogate mother and young men the surrogate father, caring for younger children and seeking employment to make up for financial shortages. In families where English is not the primary language of the parents, adolescents can be used to translate, to communicate with the doctor, and to make medical decisions. When these tasks are accomplished successfully, self-worth is enhanced. However, at times young people are given responsibilities they cannot manage. This can damage self-esteem and increase feelings of depression.

It can be confusing to have adult responsibilities and at the same time have to adhere to rules that restrict freedom. If the ill parent breaks promises or is unavailable for important events, or if an activity is eliminated to ease family financial burdens, adolescents can become resentful. Whenever possible, professionals should identify common issues of adolescents and help parents consider the impact of changes in family life on the adolescent. Parents or professionals may need to help the adolescent articulate thoughts and feelings and work on solving problems that arise.

If family responsibilities increase, it can be difficult for the adolescent whose parent has cancer to find time to concentrate on schoolwork, engage in sports and other activities, or be with friends. This can be a distressing and worrisome experience. It is important for parents to encourage young people to attend their usual tasks and activities and to have fun (Harpham, 1997). Being a member of an adolescent support group and listening to others in similar situations can help diminish feelings of loneliness and isolation.

Common Questions Seldom Spoken

There are several questions that adolescents may have but not express when a parent is diagnosed with cancer. Did I cause it? Will it happen to me? Who will take care of me? How will my life change? Will my parent die? These particular questions usually vary with age. For example, younger adolescents are more likely to worry that their past behavior might have contributed to a parent's diagnosis (Simon, Johnson, & Drantell, 1998). Many think back on instances when they were angry and wished for terrible things to happen to their parents. When a parent becomes ill, the adolescent often feels guilty and wonders whether these earlier sentiments caused the cancer. It is not helpful to discount these beliefs. Adolescents need encouragement to voice their questions and receive answers or discuss concerns.

Adolescents often wonder if they will get cancer. This question has special impact when the cancer site is a reproductive or sexual organ. If a young woman's mother has breast cancer, for example, while she herself is developing breasts, her fears may be exacerbated. Parents and professionals should anticipate and address such fears in order to offer realistic reassurance.

Distress Signals

Excessive drug and alcohol use, sexual promiscuity, eating disorders, propensity to use violence with peers and authority figures, a drop in school performance, and self-mutilation are all ways that some adolescents demonstrate their difficulties with life experiences. The adolescent often has little realization of the powerful emotions behind such self-destructive behaviors and actions. Overachievement, withdrawal, and perfectionism are other methods used to manage out-of-control feelings. If a parent or professional suspects an adolescent is at risk for or engaging in these behaviors, it is important to seek the help of a professional who can provide assistance or guidance.

WHEN A SIBLING IS DIAGNOSED WITH CANCER

The Invisible Bystander

When a sibling is diagnosed with cancer, healthy adolescents may be left at home for long periods of time with no adults present to help process emotional and practical changes. Unlike younger children, for whom care is arranged and explanations provided, the healthy adolescent's concerns sometimes are unrecognized or underestimated by parents because they appear to be able to care for themselves. "I'm fine, everything is cool," can be a typical response which keeps inner world experience hidden in order to protect obviously stressed parents from an additional burden. Most social workers in pediatric oncology are alert to sibling needs and offer help to parents in acknowledging and dealing with them.

The Sibling Bond

Siblings serve as a mirror to one's early life experiences and partly define their identities in relation to each other. A diagnosis of cancer can pose a threat to this important bond if the patient's treatment occurs in a distant cancer center and siblings are separated for prolonged periods. Fears that a sibling will die from cancer create a more permanent threat to this important bond. Ambivalence and rivalry often mark sibling relationships (Corr & Balk, 1996). The well adolescents can experience tremendous guilt for not being sick and at the same time feel the relief that they do not have cancer. They also may fear that previous sentiments spoken to the sibling have caused the illness. To diminish self-blame, the healthy sibling needs detailed information on the diagnosis and treatment plan. They should be included in the planning sessions regarding care of the patient and be allowed to decide how to help. The sick child often requires significant parental attention. The well adolescent can feel angry, jealous, and deprived. Often they experience a heightened sense of death anxiety as manifested by somatic health complaints that resemble symptoms of the cancer patient (Corr & Balk, 1996). In some instances, adolescents' siblings can put their death fears to the test by assuming behavior that threatens mortality. It is important for parents and professionals not to diminish or dismiss what usually is an expression of strong feelings. The well adolescent may be calling out for attention. Parents and professionals should express interest in adolescents' experiences and help them feel seen and heard.

"Not Good Enough"

Unknowingly, parents and close adult family members sometimes idealize the sick child (Corr & Balk, 1996). This activates feelings of sibling rivalry in which the well sibling views the sick child as the favorite. When well adolescents are unable to make their parents feel better or fail to get attention, it may result in feelings of being "not good enough." They may begin to believe that adult family members wish them ill instead of the sick child. Again, the role of the parent or professional is not to dismiss feeling, but instead to reassure the patient's siblings that they have a special place in the family that only they can fill. It can make significant difference in self-esteem if parents assign another adult family member or friend to pay special attention to the well sibling. Professionals can also supplement this nurturing role by taking special interest in hobbies, accomplishments, and day-to-day activities of adolescents whose siblings have cancer.

DYING AND BEREAVEMENT

When a parent or sibling's cancer becomes advanced and death is imminent, the adolescent needs information about what is happening. Most witness the physical changes of the patient and report feeling relieved when there is a chance to discuss their concerns and fears. A common complaint of adolescents is that of feeling left out. Openness in communication will decrease isolation. Adolescents should be allowed to decide how they want to handle their good-byes, their participation in family rituals, and their expression of grief. Some will choose to be involved actively, while others will withdraw. It is essential that they make these decisions independently. When a parent is dying, it helps the adolescent to know what plans the parents have made for the family's financial and emotional well-being. When possible, adolescents should be involved in these plans and allowed to articulate their wishes. If a sibling is dying, the well adolescent may need to express guilt for surviving. Whether a parent or sibling dies, the surviving adolescent needs reminding often by parent, adult family members, and professionals that grief is an individual experience in which all feelings are valid and respected (Worden, 1996). Adolescent bereavement groups can be particularly helpful in decreasing isolation and stigma (Perschy, 1997). Traisman (1992) has also developed a useful tool for teenagers who have experienced a loss.

SUMMARY

Adolescence is a time of physical, emotional, cognitive, spiritual, and moral/philosophical development. For the young person dealing with the experience of cancer—either as patient, caregiver, or sibling—this developmental phase affects the ability to cope with the changes brought about by diagnosis and treatment. Giving clear and detailed information about what to expect from cancer and its treatment and validating the complex and often contradictory feelings

TABLE 3

Do's and Don'ts of Communicating with Adolescents

DO	DON'T
• Listen with full attention	• Speak in their language or wear their clothes
• Ask direct questions and be straightforward	• Expect instant responsiveness
• Acknowledge difficulty of cancer experience	• Share your own experience
• Validate all feelings	• Use euphemisms for death
• Communicate that it's OK to be an adolescent	• Give message you can't handle the discussion
• Encourage discussion about their lives	• Look at your watch or fidget
• Diminish self-blame	• Sit in silence
• Involve them in planning	• Take yourself too seriously
• Remind them of their uniqueness	• Forget to have fun

that arise can help the adolescent feel more involved and in control (see Table 3). It is important to include adolescents in any plans that affect them directly. Emerging adolescents have the ability and desire to grapple with existential questions and find meaning and significance in their unique experience. During the cancer experience, they need the adults around them to express interest in their feelings, encourage articulation of unspoken emotions, and remain a patient and consistent presence as they develop identity.

REFERENCES

American Psychiatric Association. (1994). *Diagnostic and statistical manual of mental disorders* (4th ed.). Washington, DC: Author.

Corr, C., & Balk, D. (1996). *Handbook of adolescent death and bereavement.* New York: Springer Publishing Company.

Harpham, W. (1997). *When a parent has cancer: A guide to caring for your children.* New York: Harper Collins.

Perschy, M. K. (1997). *Helping teens work through grief.* Philadelphia: Taylor & Francis.

Rolsky, J. (1992). *Your child has cancer: A guide to coping.* Philadelphia: Committee to Benefit the Children.

Simon, L., Johnson, J., & Drantell, J. J. (1998). *A music I no longer heard: The early death of a parent.* New York: Simon and Schuster.

Traisman, E. (1992). *Fire in my heart, ice in my veins: A journal for teenagers experiencing a loss.* Omaha, NE: Centering Corporation.

Worden, J. W. (1996). *Children and grief: When a parent dies.* New York: Guilford Press.

SPECIAL POPULATIONS

PART B: CULTURALLY SENSITIVE ONCOLOGY SOCIAL WORK: CHINESE CULTURE AS A CASE EXAMPLE

Evaon C. Wong-Kim, PhD, LCSW, MPH

Areport recently released by the Institute of Medicine called "The Unequal Burden of Cancer" substantiated the fact that many ethnic minority and medically underserved populations face cultural, socioeconomic, and institutionalized barriers to cancer prevention and treatment, and experience poorer cancer survival rates than whites. Other identified barriers were stigmatism and fatalism regarding a cancer diagnosis in some ethnic minority communities, isolation, a lack of social support, and mistrust of the medical and scientific establishment (Haynes & Smedley, 1999).

Working with ethnic minority cancer patients and their families is becoming increasingly important for oncology social workers due to the growing diversity of the population living in the United States and the continuing influx of immigrants (Sue & Sue, 1999). Culturally sensitive and competent social work intervention has become an important part of the profession as well as a crucial component of social work education. Leigh (1997) states that a culturally competent social worker "is aware that any helping situation must be consistent and consonant with the historical and contemporary culture of the person, family, and community,

[and] take into account the nature of the exchange relationships which characterize and give objective and subjective meanings to helping encounters" (p. 173). Cultural competence and social diversity are also included in the *Code of Ethics* (Section 1.05) of the National Association of Social Workers (2000, p. 9):

(a) Social workers should understand culture and its function in human behavior and society, recognizing the strengths that exist in all cultures.

(b) Social workers should have a knowledge base of their clients' cultures and be able to demonstrate competence in the provision of services that are sensitive to clients' cultures and to differences among people and cultural groups.

(c) Social workers should obtain education about and seek to understand the nature of social diversity and oppression with respect to race, ethnicity, national origin, color, sex, sexual orientation, age, marital status, political belief, religion, and mental or physical disability.

The challenge of social work practice with ethnic minorities is that there are so many different cultures, and it is difficult to be sensitive to all the beliefs and value systems. However, as suggested by Lieberman (1998), cultural sensitivity can be understood as a form of interpersonal sensitivity, "an attunement to the specific idiosyncrasies of another person" (p. 104) and finding out what we do not know.

It is beyond the scope of this chapter to explain specific social work interventions with each race or ethnic group in the United States, nor is it appropriate to generalize all racial and ethnic minorities into one group. Therefore, the immigrant Chinese population will be used as a case example. This is mainly due to the author's experience in practicing oncology social work with this population during eight years in a metropolitan public hospital. Some of the issues confronting the Chinese population reflect similar issues confronting other recent immigrant populations such as Latin American and Southeast Asian immigrants and refugees (Daniels, 1990).

CHINESE PATIENTS AS CASE EXAMPLE

At the time of the 1990 U.S. Census, Chinese Americans, at more than 1.6 million, were found to be the largest Asian Pacific American group, making up 22.6% of the Asian Pacific American population. Between 1980 and 1990, the Chinese American population doubled, with most of the growth due to immigration. Currently, more than 63% of Chinese Americans are foreign-born (Bureau of the Census, 1993). According to the 1990 census, the Asian American and Pacific Islander population will increase from the present 2.9% to 11% by the year 2050.

ISSUES CONFRONTING CHINESE IMMIGRANT CANCER PATIENTS

Like many other life-threatening illnesses, cancer causes both physical and emotional distress. One of the most difficult and problematic issues for anyone diagnosed with cancer in the United States is the lack of health insurance coverage. According to the 1985 survey conducted by the Boston Redevelopment Authority, Asian and Pacific Islanders (API) and Hispanics were much more likely than whites to be without health insurance. While 12% of the white population and 19% of blacks were uninsured, 27% Hispanic and 27% of API lacked health insurance (Gold & Socolar, 1987). Newly immigrated Chinese patients are uninsured mainly due to problems such as unemployment and underemployment. Patients with no health insurance often learn about their cancer diagnoses in the emergency room when they experience severe symptoms such as bleeding, pain, or extreme weight loss. These symptoms frequently are an indication of either the spread of the disease or a more advanced stage of the disease.

Language Barriers

Besides the lack of health care insurance and, as a result, limited access to preventive care, the language barrier is another reason

Chinese immigrant cancer patients are not receiving the health care services they need. Due to limited resources, many hospitals and health care facilities do not employ full time professional interpreters, and because of the lack of interpreters at health care facilities, Chinese patients who do not speak English either have to delay or reschedule their appointments until an interpreter is available. For cancer patients, the delay of diagnostic work-up and intervention is very likely to affect the prognosis of the patient.

The language barrier can also affect patients' treatment options. Recent immigrants from Mainland China do not understand the reason for medical research. This problem is worsened by research protocols written only in English, and by providers who lack the language and cultural ability to explain the benefits of biomedical research. The lack of Chinese patients enrolled in clinical trials and research studies translates into a lack of data available regarding this population, which is true for other minority groups as well. For example, some cancers, such as nasopharyngeal cancer, although common among Chinese males, is rare in the general population in the United States and few studies have been conducted in finding ways to effectively treat this kind of cancer.

Oncology social workers assisting patients who do not speak English need to take the role of advocate. Besides advocating for quality translation services so that patients can understand their treatment options and rights, oncology social workers also need to explain the Western medical system to the patients so they understand why certain research opportunities are presented. Oncology social workers also need to assess whether patients understand their diagnosis, treatment options, and prognosis. Counseling cancer patients on emotional issues such as loss and grief through an interpreter can be difficult. Besides being patient and encouraging, oncology social workers need to prepare themselves to work with an interpreter. It is not possible to be emotionally detached when translating; therefore interpreters should be informed of the purpose of the counseling session to be aware of the nature of the session before the session begins.

Cultural Barriers

A cultural barrier in this context may be defined as the difference between ethnic minority patients and mainstream health care providers or gaps between patients and the mainstream health care system. Gaps in specific knowledge, attitudes, beliefs, and values may inhibit patients from seeking preventive screening and may result in the delay of detection of cancer. For example, the cultural bias of Chinese females against inserting objects into the vagina has discouraged women from getting annual preventive screening, such as the pap smear to detect cervical cancer. This cultural barrier could prevent women from being diagnosed at an early stage. Because self-touching is considered unacceptable in the Chinese culture, breast self-examination is difficult for Chinese immigrant women to practice. This cultural attitude discourages Chinese women from detecting breast cancer early by doing monthly breast self-examinations. For male Chinese patients, seeing a female physician may prohibit them from expressing any discomfort or pain related to the reproductive organs. Health care providers have to be sensitive to these cultural differences and find creative ways to encourage patients to seek preventive care.

Another cultural barrier experienced by Chinese immigrant cancer patients is the issue of using alternative therapies. Many Chinese cancer patients seek alternative medical consultation from an herbalist when they are receiving chemotherapy. Most of them do not want to disclose that they are seeing an herbalist because of fear of disapproval by their oncologist. In Chinese culture, seeking a second opinion is considered disrespectful. Chinese cancer patients also do not want to disclose this information to their oncologists because they may feel that their oncologists do not understand Chinese herbs. Chinese patients who seek alternative therapies often gather information on their own. This can be dangerous because using herbal therapy along with chemotherapy can have adverse effects. Oncologists, nurses, and social workers can solicit this information within a more accepting conversation where the patient feels more inclined to reveal the use of herbs. For example, they can ask, "What other things are you doing in addition to standard treatment?"

Chinese patients also often expect to be told by their physicians what kind of food they should avoid when they are diagnosed with cancer. Certain foods that are too cold or too hot are considered to upset the balance of the yin and the yang of the body. This knowledge gap between the patient and the provider often creates patients' distrust of the Western medical system. Health care workers may address this by asking, "What questions do you have about your diet?" They can also explain how certain foods can impact treatment tolerance or results.

Issues of Informed Consent

In Chinese culture, according to Hsu (1985), "the meaning of being human is found in interpersonal relationships" (p.27). Chinese culture is characterized by the strong ties that permanently unite closely related human beings in the family and clan. In the Chinese relational system, the most important kind of relationship is the father-son relationship, while the husband-wife relationship is the most crucial in the American system (Ho, 1993). Family is considered to be one of the most important institutions in Chinese culture. Chinese children are taught early to be filial and obey and take care of their parents. Therefore, taking care of their sick parents and making decisions for them are often considered to be a normal part of the culture.

It is not uncommon for Chinese family members to request health care providers to withhold medical information from the patient, especially when the patient is elderly. The reason is that families do not want to "burden" patients with the bad news. Yet in mainstream culture, patients have the right to make their own decisions and to take control of their lives, which are the main tenets of informed consent (Pellegrino, 1992). This kind of cultural emphasis on informed consent is very difficult for Chinese patients and their families to understand when they do not share the same Western cultural values.

In other countries, such as Japan and Italy, it is also common for physicians not to disclose a grim prognosis to their patients (Surbone, 1992). According to a more recent study conducted in

Japan (Elwyn, Fetters, Gorenflo, & Tsuda, 1998), selective disclosure has become more common in Japan than nondisclosure. A patient's age is a statistically significant predictor of nondisclosure. This means that the older the patient, the more likely the physician will not disclose the diagnosis to the patient.

Similarly, according to a study done in a West Coast clinic (Orona, Koenig, and Davis, 1994), both the Chinese and Mexican cultures value the importance of family members taking care of the elderly. Therefore, very often the family felt that they should be informed of the cancer diagnosis and prognosis instead of the patient. The study also found that the issue of informing patients of their terminal illness is controversial. In fact, in Chinese culture, disclosing information such as a poor prognosis is often considered unethical (Orona et al., 1994). This is especially true when treating patients with terminal illness when families believe that the stress and depression caused by knowing this information may be too painful for the patient (Tanida, 1994).

For the Chinese, interdependence is considered more important than autonomy (Koenig & Gates-Williams, 1995). When Chinese patients defer to the family for decision making or when families request that oncologists withhold information from patients, this creates an ethical dilemma for the physician (Muller & Desmond, 1992). It is difficult for the physician to decide what is more important, informed consent by the patient or honoring the patient's wishes of letting the family make important decisions (Abramson & Black, 1985). There is no right or wrong solution when dealing with this ethical dilemma. The oncology social worker's role in this situation is that of a cultural broker. Being a cultural broker means bridging the patient-family-provider gap by providing education and information about cultural differences. This can facilitate open communication and promote a team spirit among all parties in order to achieve the best quality of care for the patient.

When there is such a wide divergence between what a particular culture is used to and how the modern medical system operates, it can be useful for social workers to work toward developing their own philosophy of care. This can help them be more comfortable with the conflict between what physicians feel they need to do and what a particular cultural group would prefer that they do. Social workers can facilitate outreach and collaborative planning by helping the institution develop some sort of policy or procedure in dealing with value conflicts that are this divergent. For example, social workers can suggest that hospitals invite consultation with representatives of particular minority groups so that their expertise can be solicited about some of these issues.

Summary

Social workers have always worked with disadvantaged and underserved clients in oncology, but what may be lacking is an understanding of cultural differences and the impact that these differences can have on the therapeutic exchange (Seeley, 2000). Culturally sensitive social work intervention is not being an expert on each culture, but being open minded about working with clients from other cultures as well as the willingness to learn from our colleagues and our clients.

Armed with advocacy skills and an understanding of cultural diversity and biomedical ethics, social workers can influence health care with ethnically diverse cancer patients in many ways. In addition to providing direct services and consultation to the health care team on issues of importance to ethnic minority cancer patients, oncology social workers can also provide recommendations and intervention strategies for specific populations. Social workers should also be active in conducting research and participating in research activities with diverse populations because this expertise will help other professional disciplines better understand cultural issues that are germane to the research process. With the increasing diversity in our society, social workers need to position the profession to become the leader in providing culturally sensitive services to ethnic minorities and underserved populations.

REFERENCES

Abramson, M., & Black, R. B. (1985). Extending the boundaries of life: Implications for practice. *Health and Social Work, 10*, 165-173.

Bureau of the Census (1993). *We the American Asians.* Washington, DC: U.S. Department of Commerce.

Daniels, R. (1990). *Asian America: Chinese and Japanese in the United States since 1850.* Seattle, WA: University of Washington Press.

Elwyn, T. S., Fetters, M. D., Gorenflo, D. W., & Tsuda, T. (1998). Cancer disclosure in Japan: Historical comparisons, current practices. *Social Science & Medicine, 46*, 1151-1163.

Gold, B., & Socolar, D. (1987). *Report of the Boston Committee on Access to Health Care.* Boston: Boston Committee on Access to Health Care.

Haynes, M. A., & Smedley, B. D. (1999). *The unequal burden of cancer: An assessment of NIH research and programs for ethnic minorities and the medically underserved.* Washington, DC: National Academy Press.

Ho, D. Y. F. (1993). Relational orientation in Asian Social Psychology. In U. Kim & J. W. Berry (Eds.), *Indigenous psychologies* (pp. 240-259). Thousand Oaks, CA: Sage.

Hsu, F. L. K. (1985). The self in cross-cultural perspective. In A. J. Marsella, G. DeVos, & F. L. K. Hsu (Eds.), *Culture and self: Asian and Western perspectives* (pp. 24-55). New York: Tavistock.

Koenig, B. A., & Gates-Williams, J. (1995). Understanding cultural difference in caring for dying patients. *Western Journal of Medicine, 163*, 244-249.

Leigh, J. W. (1997). *Communicating for cultural competence.* Needham Heights, MA: Allyn & Bacon.

Lieberman, A. F. (1998). Culturally sensitive intervention with children and families. *Child and Adolescent Social Work, 7*, 101-120.

Muller, J. H., & Desmond, B. (1992). Ethical dilemmas in a cross-cultural context. A Chinese example. *Western Journal of Medicine, 157*, 323-327.

National Association of Social Workers. (2000). Code of Ethics of the National Association of Social Workers. Washington, DC: NASW.

Orona, C. J., Koenig, B.A., & Davis, A. J. (1994). Cultural aspects of nondisclosure. *Cambridge Quarterly of Healthcare Ethics, 3*, 338-346.

Pellegrino, E. D. (1992). Is truth telling to the patient a cultural artifact? *Journal of the American Medical Association, 268*, 1734-1735.

Seeley, K. M. (2000). *Cultural psychotherapy: Working with culture in the clinical encounter.* Northvale, NJ: Jason Aronson.

Sue, D. W., & Sue, D. (1999). *Counseling the culturally different* (3rd ed.). New York: Wiley.

Surbone, A. (1992). Truth telling to the patient. *Journal of the American Medical Association, 268,*1661-1662.

Tanida, N. (1994). Japanese attitudes towards truth disclosure in cancer. *Scandinavian Journal of Social Medicine, 22,* 50-57.

SPECIAL POPULATIONS

PART C: SPECIAL ISSUES FOR GAYS AND LESBIANS WITH CANCER

Ellen Levine, LCSW

It is important that skilled oncology social work clinicians examine their own values and attitudes when working with lesbians, gays, bisexuals, or transgendered patients[1] as they would with any patient whose personal situation does not necessarily mirror their own. They should be acutely aware of the impact of transference and countertransference in their clinical work with gay men and lesbians. Clinicians should also be aware of the larger societal context within which gay men and lesbians live where homophobic attitudes are still common. Homophobia is the fear or hatred of anyone or anything connected with homosexuality. Such attitudes may be present in institutions and among caregivers in overt or covert ways. Fundamentally, gay men and lesbians who are diagnosed with cancer go through similar physical and emotional reactions and should be offered the same psychosocial support services as heterosexual men and women diagnosed with cancer.

---

[1] For simplicity, the terms "gay men" and "lesbians" are used throughout this section.

INCIDENCE, BEHAVIORS, AND RISK BEHAVIORS

It is estimated that gay men and lesbians may constitute as many as 10% of the United States' population. Despite this fact, until the AIDS epidemic in the mid-1980s, there was little research data available on gay men's health. Unfortunately, there is still very little research data available on lesbian's health issues. Among the limited studies which have been carried out in the lesbian population, only a narrow segment has been surveyed, reflecting primarily a homogeneous subpopulation of lesbians who are white, young, middle class, well educated, and open about their sexual orientation. Even less is known about the health issues of older lesbians who are an "invisible" group and who are considered to be a triple minority because of their age, gender, and sexual orientation (Denenberg, 1992; Deevey, 1990).

While there are no data to suggest that gay men and lesbians are inherently at greater risk for cancer, there is a subgroup of the gay community whose sexual behavior choices may put them at a higher risk for certain types of cancers due to specific behaviors, often referred to as "risk factors." For example, there are two sexually transmitted viruses that have been linked to cancer: the human immunodeficiency virus (HIV), which causes AIDS, and the human papilloma virus (HPV), which causes genital warts. An individual who contracts HIV or HPV during sexual activity may increase his or her risk of developing certain types of cancer. For people with HIV, there has been an increased risk of Kaposi's sarcoma, non-Hodgkin's lymphoma, testicular cancer, and squamous cell cancers of the anus or cervix. The HPV virus has been shown to cause cancers of the cervix and vulva in women and possibly to contribute to the cause of cancer of the penis (Schover, 1997). Again, these data reflect studies done among a very narrow segment of the gay and lesbian communities and are not indicative of the many men and women in stable, long-term relationships.

Lesbians may be at a higher risk for breast or ovarian cancer because research indicates that many of them have either never completed a full-term pregnancy or have their first child after the age of 30. Lesbians may also be at a higher risk for endometrial cancer if they have never used birth control or have had no full-term pregnancies. In addition, lesbians in general appear to have a higher incidence of tobacco and alcohol consumption than heterosexual women and some data suggest that they, on average, may have a higher body mass than heterosexual women. All of these characteristics and behaviors are considered to be added risk factors for the diagnoses of breast, ovarian, and colon cancer (Howe, 1994; Longnecker, 1994).

BARRIERS TO HEALTH CARE

Lesbians experience all of the same barriers to health care common to women in general. These include lack of financial resources (including transportation and childcare), racism, sexism, ageism, and socialization that teaches them to place the needs of others before their own. Some lesbians may also neglect having annual cancer screenings, including mammograms and pap smears, because of the misconception that their sexual practices do not put them at risk for gynecologic or breast cancers (Bradford, Ryan, & Rothblum, 1994; Stevens & Hall, 1988). Research also suggests that lesbians do not seek routine health care services because of a fear of homophobia (Roberts & Sorenson, 1999). The burden of AIDS in our society can make coping with a cancer diagnosis even more problematic for a gay man. If he is HIV positive, his immune system may be compromised, making it more difficult for him to fight the cancer effectively which adds to his burden of perceived responsibility for his situation. Thus, a gay man with HIV potentially faces the dual social stigma of both HIV and cancer, with all the associated myths, fears, and stereotypes. Even when a man is HIV negative, others may still imply blame for his cancer due to his lifestyle choice (Schover, 1997).

While women as a whole are underinsured, both gay men and lesbians have the added barrier of not being able to be placed on a partner's health insurance policy. Other barriers for both groups include invisibility, marginalization, and fear of discrimination. Past negative experiences in health care settings which might affect gay men and lesbians' choices of health care include intimidation, hostility shown toward the patient or partner, breach of confidentiality, neglect, denial of care, undue roughness in the physical examination, or even sexual assault by a staff member (Bradford, et al., 1994; Stevens & Hall, 1988). These factors may, in turn, lead to a gay man or lesbian seeking fewer screening exams, thus resulting in later diagnosis, should a cancer occur.

These perceived barriers by gay men and lesbians are supported by surveys done in the medical community. In one survey of lesbian physicians, 52% had observed denial of care or provision of reduced care to gay or lesbian patients and 88% had heard physician colleagues disparage gay or lesbian patients because of their sexual orientation (Schatz & O'Hanlan, 1994). Although 98% of these same physicians felt it was critical that patients inform their doctors about their sexual orientation, 68% believed that patients who did so risked receiving substandard care. Some recent studies, however, have shown that gay men and lesbians who were "out" to their health care practitioners felt more satisfied with their care, were more receptive to psychosocial interventions, and went more regularly for screening exams (Gruskin, 1999).

INTERVENTION TECHNIQUES

Social workers are well trained in working with a wide range of clients. Nonetheless, clinicians who have experience working with gay patients offer guidelines to refine good basic oncology social work practice (Abrams, 1993; Mautner Project, 1997).

History Taking
- Ask open-ended, gender neutral questions which do not assume heterosexuality.
    Examples include:
    With whom do you live? What is their relationship to you?

Is there someone you would like to include in the discussions about your treatment?

Gender neutral language allows patients to disclose the gender of their partners and to give information on their own terms, without having to fight, resist, or deny the health care provider's assumptions. Use the language that patients use to describe their relationships.

- Ask patients to define their family unit to allow them to describe their partner, children, family of origin, and members of their family of choice if they so desire.

- Provide opportunities for patients to disclose sexual orientation but be aware that they may choose not to do so. The office environment can promote an open atmosphere. For example, having some books on shelves that deal with sexual orientation issues can communicate that it is an acceptable topic to discuss (Bruss, Brack, Brack, Glickauf-Hughes, & O'Leary, 1997).

- If patients do disclose that they are gay, ask if they want this information put in the medical chart. Tell them about the institution's confidentiality procedures.

- Involve patients' partners in discussions of patients' experiences and institutions' procedures. For example, ask patients if they prefer their partner or another family member be the primary recipient of information.

Sexuality-Related Questions

- Gather basic information about sexuality. Discussing sexuality during a first interview serves two purposes. It tells patients that the social worker considers sexuality an important and valued aspect of their life and it clearly conveys the message that it is acceptable to discuss sexuality. Include open ended questions like:

    Are you sexually active? Do you have intimate relations with men, women, or both?

    Has your cancer diagnosis affected these intimate relations? Would you like to discuss this?

- Address issues of infertility and parenting. Many gay men and lesbians either already are or hope to become parents in their future. Some have children from previous heterosexual relationships while others may continue to be bisexual. Gay men may adopt a child or have a child with a surrogate mother. Lesbians may adopt or choose to have a child by artificial insemination. A gay parent who has been diagnosed with cancer should be advised to seek legal counsel to address issues of guardianship or custody of children (Schover, 1997).

- Evaluate the impact of the cancer diagnosis on the patient's body image and sexuality and provide sensitive interventions. The physical disfigurement caused by some cancer treatments may be more difficult for gay men for whom physical appearance may be a higher priority. While our society now gives women more support if they lose a breast or become bald from treatment, men are expected to be stoical and not show any sign of difficulty with their corresponding physical changes. The focus on sexuality as the defining characteristic of homosexuality by some strata of gay male society, and by most of the larger society, may also increase the impact of losing sexual function.

Assessment and Counseling

- Provide interventions which respect the lifestyle choices of patients and their need to maintain privacy.
- Demonstrate some knowledge of gay cultural issues and norms as well as the ability to ask when in doubt.
- Become familiar with the stages of sexual identity formation, the meaning of related terms, and the process of "coming out." There are many models which attempt to describe the processes by which gay men and lesbians understand their sexuality, come to identify as gay or bisexual, and disclose this information to others (Carrion & Lock, 1997; Wilson, 1999). All of these must be viewed within the larger context of societal stigma that potentially affects every aspect of the developmental process.

Sexual identity refers to the label one gives oneself. Men or women who choose same sex partners may choose to call themselves "gay" or "lesbian" or "homosexual." Men or women who sometimes have sex with the opposite sex may call themselves "gay" or "bisexual." Sexual identity is not the same as sexual behavior or sexual orientation. Sexual behavior does not always follow from sexual orientation. For health care providers, it is more important to know about sexual behavior than only knowing someone's sexual identity or orientation.

In addition, as with any premorbid personality traits, a person's stage of sexual identity will have an impact on his or her emotional response to cancer. The health professional should consider the psychosocial issues faced by cancer patients at the different stages of the cancer experience and develop ways to help gay men or lesbians cope with the cancer, considering where they are in the development of their gay identity. For example, if a patient is going through an earlier stage of their gay identity development, he or she may be very isolated and have a limited support system. If the patient has not "come out" publicly, a cancer diagnosis may serve as a catalyst to do so as a way to gain greater social support. Such a patient might need additional psychosocial support and could potentially be under increased financial pressure due to negative reactions of the family of origin or employer. If a patient is more "out" about being gay, he or she may be at a greater risk for discrimination and hate violence (Gruskin, 1999).

• Consider where the patient is in his or her life cycle and be especially aware of issues affecting gay adolescents and older gay men and lesbians.

For adolescents who may be struggling with their sexual identity, there has traditionally been little awareness by health care personnel of the issues, which they are confronting. Research suggests that gay, lesbian, and bisexual youth (i.e., ages 14–21) are at increased risk for mental health problems, such as major depression, generalized anxiety disorder, and suicide (Fergusson, Horwood, & Beautrais, 1999). In fact, they are two to three times more likely to attempt suicide than other adolescents and may comprise up to 30% of completed youth suicides (Garofalo, Wolf, Wissow, Woods, & Goodman, 1999; Remafedi, 1999). Clinicians should watch for behaviors which include depression, poor school performance, alcohol and substance abuse, acting out or suicidal thoughts. Issues of sexuality are best addressed in the context of ongoing care and a good relationship with a health care provider. When an adolescent is diagnosed with cancer, he or she may be able to use the opportunity of regular treatment visits as a time to address sexual identity concerns. It is also important to help gay youth to connect with others like them and identify appropriate community resources (Harrison, 1996).

Many of the problems facing older gay men and lesbians are similar to those faced by older heterosexual patients. These include declining health, fixed incomes, death of significant others, and the effects of ageism in our society. Issues of particular concern for older gay men and lesbians might include fears about discrimination in the health care system, employment, housing, and long-term care. These concerns may compound their anticipated losses associated with the normal aging process (Quam & Whitford, 1992).

- Assist in mobilizing the patient's support system and make referrals to both gay and non-gay community resources. These might include gay-friendly medical settings, clergy, or civil rights organizations. Help patients and their partners to fully participate in medical decisions as a family unit. Discuss power of attorney and health care proxy with gay patients. Because gay relationships do not have the same legal status as marriage, a gay patient's partner may not be given the same rights as a spouse to visit, participate in discussions with health care professionals, have access to a patient's medical records, or make decisions about a partner's health care if a patient is very ill. It is therefore essential that legal documents be signed and entered in a gay patient's medical records and that the partner maintains copies of these documents. Legal counseling is frequently available through gay community organizations.

Institution-Wide Interventions

While the issues of homosexual patients are more openly discussed today, it is important to remember that it was only in 1973 that the

American Psychiatric Association (APA) voted to change the listing of "Homosexuality" in the *Diagnostic and Statistical Manual of Mental Disorders*, Second Edition (DSM-II) as a sexual deviation for everyone who was homosexual. They replaced it with a new term called "Sexual Orientation Disturbance" which applied only to those who were "disturbed by, in conflict with, or who wished to change their sexual orientation" (APA, 1980). In 1980, the DSM-III was published, and the term was changed to "Ego-Dystonic Homosexuality." Finally, in the DSM-III-R which was published in 1987, the category was eliminated altogether because it was not considered a mental disorder. However, many medical professionals who are currently practicing were trained at a time when homosexuality was considered to be a mental illness and was illegal (Gruskin, 1999).

The skilled oncology social worker needs to serve as a role model of acceptance for the health care team in responding to the needs of gay men and lesbians coping with a cancer diagnosis. Interventions in support of such a role include:

- Responding to homophobic reactions on the part of staff or colleagues with advocacy and information to help dispel negative myths about homosexuality. This also includes educating them about heterosexism, which is the belief that heterosexuality is better than or more natural than homosexuality.
- Advocating to all medical caregivers the rights of patients and partners to fully participate in medical decisions as a family unit.
- Serving on institution-wide committees on outreach, patient diversity, patient education, and medical ethics to address such issues as the development of gender neutral patient registration forms and visible non-discrimination policies which include sexual orientation.

Unless an institution has had a particular reason to become sensitized to the needs of gay and lesbian patients, these issues are rarely in the minds of clinical staff and probably less so in those of administrative staff responsible for policy development. Oncology social workers may be able to advocate more effectively for this population due to their understanding of human behavior and attention to collaborative relationships among team members and policymaking staff. Certainly oncology social workers struggle with the same negative effects of homophobia as other team members, but it may be one of a few disciplines that is still educated about the impact of personal self awareness on professional competence and behavior. This is not to say that social workers function as the conscience of the institution. Social work has a long tradition of advocacy for those out of the "mainstream" and it is that expertise that needs to be utilized in the interests of gay and lesbian patients.

REFERENCES

Abrams, S. (1993). *Coming out with cancer: Issues for lesbians and gay men with cancer.* Paper presented at the annual conference of the Association of Oncology Social Work, New York.

American Psychiatric Association. (1980). *Diagnostic and statistical manual of mental disorders* (3rd ed.). Washington, DC: Author.

Bradford, J., Ryan, C., & Rothblum, E. D. (1994). National Lesbian Health Care Survey: Implications for mental health care. *Journal of Consulting and Clinical Psychology, 62(2),* 228-242.

Bruss, K. V., Brack, C. J., Brack, G., Glickauf-Hughes, C., & O'Leary, M. (1997). A developmental model for supervising therapists treating gay, lesbian, and bisexual clients. *Clinical Supervisor, 15(1),* 61-73.

Carrion, V. G., & Lock, J. (1997). The coming out process: Developmental stages for sexual minority youth. *Clinical Child Psychology & Psychiatry, 2(3),* 369-377.

Deevey, S. (1990). Older lesbian women: An invisible minority. *Journal of Gerontological Nursing, 16(5),* 35-39.

Denenberg, R. (1992). Invisible women. Lesbians and health care. *Health PAC Bulletin, 22(1),* 14-21.

Fergusson, D. M., Horwood, L. J., & Beautrais, A. L. (1999). Is sexual orientation related to mental health problems and suicidality in young people? *Archives of General Psychiatry, 56(10),* 876-880.

Garofalo, R., Wolf, R. C., Wissow, L. S., Woods, E. R., & Goodman, E. (1999). Sexual orientation and risk of suicide attempts among a representative sample of youth. *Archives of Pediatric Adolescent Medicine, 153(5),* 487-493.

Gruskin, E. P. (1999). *Treating lesbians and bisexual women: Challenges and strategies for health professionals.* Thousand Oaks, CA: Sage.

Harrison, A. (1996). Primary care of lesbian and gay patients: Educating ourselves and our students. *Family Medicine, 28(1),* 10-23.

Howe, G. R. (1994). Dietary fat and breast cancer risks: An epidemiologic perspective. *Cancer, 74,* 1078-1084.

Longnecker, M. P. (1994). Alcoholic beverage consumption in relation to risk of breast cancer: Meta-analysis and review. *Cancer Causes Control, 5,* 73-82.

Quam, J. K., & Whitford, G. S. (1992). Adaptation and age-related expectations of older gay and lesbian adults. *Gerontologist, 32 (3),* 367-374.

Remafedi, G. (1999). Sexual orientation and youth suicide. *Journal of the American Medical Association, 282(13),* 1291-1292.

Roberts, S. J., & Sorensen, L. (1999). Health related behaviors and cancer screening of lesbians: Results from the Boston Lesbian Health Project. *Women and Health, 28(4),*1-12.

Schatz B., & O'Hanlan, K. (1994). *Anti-gay discrimination in medicine: Results of a national survey of lesbian, gay, and bisexual physicians.* Report from the Gay and Lesbian Medical Association, San Francisco, CA.

Schover, L. R. (1997). *Sexuality and fertility after cancer.* New York: Wiley.

Stevens, P. E., & Hall, J. M. (1988). Stigma, health beliefs and experiences with health care in lesbian women. *Image–The Journal of Nursing Scholarship, 20(2),* 69-73.

The Mautner Project for Lesbians with Cancer. (1997). *Tools About Caring for Lesbian Health.* Available at: http://www.mautnerproject.org. Accessed June 27, 2000.

Wilson, I. (1999). The emerging gay adolescent. *Clinical Child Psychology & Psychiatry, 4(4),* 551-565.

SPECIAL POPULATIONS

PART D: CANCER AND THE ELDERLY POPULATION

Carol P. Marcusen, LCSW, BCD
Elizabeth J. Clark, PhD, ACSW

Age is the single greatest risk factor for cancer with 60% of all cancers and 69% of all cancer deaths occurring among persons over the age of 65. This means that 2 out of every 100 Americans 65 years of age or older are diagnosed with cancer each year. Yet, there are few cancer screening and staging guidelines for the older patient, little relevant toxicity research, few appropriate clinical trials, and much erroneous treatment bias based on ageism (Calabresi & Freeman, 1997).

Ageism is when someone discriminates against another person solely on the basis of age. Like racism or sexism, ageism is a negative view that desires, fears, or concerns of older people are somehow different from, and not as important as, those of other people. This can mean that the needs of older patients do not get the same attention as the needs of younger patients (Alliance for Aging Research, 1995; Bernabei et al., 1998). For example, among clinicians there seems to be an underlying assumption that older persons cannot tolerate aggressive treatments. Similarly, many older cancer patients are automatically excluded from eligibility in clinical trials because of chronological age, when physiologically they might meet the requirements (Castellucci, 1999).

UNDERTREATMENT OF PAIN

The treatment of pain presents another example of ageism in medicine. Chronic pain is common in older persons, and it often goes
undetected. This particularly has been found to be true in nursing
home populations. It is estimated that 45%–80% of nursing home
residents have substantial pain that is untreated (American
Geriatrics Society, 1998).

One reason for the lack of adequate pain treatment is that the
majority of elderly persons have co-morbidities (multiple medical
problems) that make assessment and management difficult. Another
reason is that the elderly themselves often fear taking too much
medication out of concern that they will become addicted to the
drugs. Many older persons have not received adequate education
about the use of their medications and they take them improperly,
or "stretch" their pills by taking fewer than prescribed or by skipping
doses or days. Others use pain medication only when the pain
becomes acute.

LACK OF HEALTH LITERACY SKILLS

An added concern in pain and disease management is the low level
of health literacy skills among the older population (Gazmararian et
al., 1999). When you adjust for education and cognitive functioning, it is not surprising that many older patients do not understand
the directions for taking their medications or managing their care
regimens. Many elderly never learned to read, or they speak English
as a second language. They are embarrassed by this fact and try to
keep it hidden. As a result, the health care team may be unaware of
their inability to understand informed consent forms, follow instructions, read informational brochures, read the instructions for pre-
operative procedures or tests, or even understand the written flyers
that pharmacists include with their prescriptions.

To address these issues, the health care team, in addition to
doing a thorough assessment of health status, must also assess

chronic pain, medication usage (how and when used), the use of over-the counter remedies or complementary therapies, and the health literacy level of their older patients. It is also important to ask what is happening in the individual's social life.

SEXUALITY IN THE ELDERLY

Sexuality and self-image issues are common examples of ageism in medicine. A common assumption among many clinicians is that the older person may not want or need breast reconstructive surgery, treatment for impotence, or other procedures that may restore sexual functioning or pleasure. The message translates that the elderly are asexual. A person reaches a certain age and therefore, sexual behavior is no longer important or practiced. Although sexual behavior and ability may decrease during the aging process for some, this does not mean that self-image and sexuality are any less important for others. The loss of a breast, the loss of one's hair, or the loss of an erection can be devastating to the older person who has already experienced losses in self image such as receding hairline, sagging skin, multiple wrinkles, and aging spots. American culture does not recognize beauty in the manifestations of age. How devastating it must be to be dealt additional blows to one's self-image by the treatment for cancer. The importance of an erection that can penetrate or the ability to counteract a dry vagina may be very important to the elderly person. These issues should be consistently explored and options given to the older person so that they may continue living their lives as fully as possible.

GENERATIONAL DIFFERENCES

Generational differences for the older person being treated for cancer are also often ignored by the health care team due to lack of awareness of these issues. With the move in health care to involve patients more in their own management, older persons who have been accustomed to leaving all of the decision making in the hands of their physicians are disadvantaged. The older person may rely totally upon a family physician for all information related to disease detection and management. The family physician may not have all the information needed. Their disease, then, may not be managed optimally. Education and information are important in dealing with the differences in the provision of health care by different generations. The older person may not be comfortable with the many specialists needed in their care. They may see the physician as an authority figure who is not to be questioned. Consumerism in health care is new to the current older generation. How to be a good consumer must be learned and the older person with cancer will need to learn the skills necessary to navigate the health care system of today. Social work intervention can, and should, include education and skill training.

There are also generational differences in caregiving. Who in the family is supposed to give care or coordinate the care given? Is the elderly grandparent comfortable with a granddaughter giving him his bath? If the "older son" lives at a distance, can other children assist in making important decisions and providing hands on care? Is the older person accepting of alternative long-term care options such as convalescent care when the children are all working and cannot physically be available to provide the care needed? Is the elderly parent willing to have a stranger provide care in their home? These are just a few of the many questions needed to be addressed in providing the care to an older person. Clinicians who are aware of these questions will be able to provide their senior patients with optimal care giving options.

LOSS AND THE ELDERLY

Loss is a constant theme in the lives of older persons. The longer one lives, the more losses one is likely to experience. For the elderly, losses may accumulate suddenly, be sequential, or occur with repetition. Some losses, such as the loss of employment due to retirement, may result from choice. Other losses, such as loss of hearing, diminished eyesight, or loss of some aspect of bodily functioning may occur due to the aging process. Still other losses result from the death of spouses, family members, and friends.

These losses can have a snowball effect for the individual. The loss of income when a person retires may decrease income to the point that it is necessary to change living arrangements. Maybe an older couple is forced to move from the family home to an apartment. Diminished health may lead to a loss of independence. Reduced eyesight may require older persons to give up their driver's license. This, in turn, may mean that they cannot attend their usual social functions. An elderly woman who becomes widowed (loss of a loved one) loses her social role as wife (loss of some aspect of self), and may no longer be able to maintain her home (loss of external object).

Cancer and Loss

When cancer is added to the loss equation, the results can be devastating. The elderly spouse may be physically unable to care for the loved one with cancer. Watching an adult child or a grandchild struggle with cancer is overwhelming for many older persons, and when the older person also is the cancer patient, the losses may be great. In addition to physical losses such as loss of a breast or other body part, loss of hair, or loss of stamina, there may be financial losses as the individual struggles to pay for outpatient medications. If they do not feel well enough to get out, they may begin to feel isolated and lonely, and social loss, the loss of interacting with their friends, occurs. Others may begin relating to them differently, assuming that they are terminally ill and that recovery is not possible. This has serious emotional consequences for the person with cancer.

DEPRESSION AND THE ELDERLY

When you consider the frequency of loss, increasing isolation, and chronic pain or fatigue, it is not surprising that many older persons experience depression. The symptoms may be apparent or hidden. It is estimated that 5%–10% of the elderly who visit primary care physicians have major depression, but only one in six of these persons gets adequate attention (Rimer, 1999).

There are many barriers to treatment of elderly depression. One is the myth that depression (like loss) is natural in old age. Other barriers are high cost of psychotherapy, lack of trained geriatric psychiatrists, psychologists, and social workers, and the lack of coverage for outpatient anti-depressant drugs, which can cost between $60 and $100 per month. Additionally, some persons with depression are misdiagnosed with dementia. Finally, there is the elderly generational resistance to the idea of emotional illness and seeking help.

Loss, chronic pain, and depression contribute to a diminished quality of life for older persons with cancer. Social work intervention at a variety of levels is indicated.

FINANCIAL CONCERNS AND THE ELDERLY

The financial impact of cancer is great and may be devastating to anyone facing cancer. The elderly tend to be at significant risk due to such factors as fixed incomes, possible loss of some income with death of spouse, and lack of available adequate resources. Financial concerns can be looked at as those related to direct medical costs and non-medical expenses, such as transportation, home care products, home maintenance, and custodial care (Hoffman, 1998). Many in our society feel that Medicare provides a comprehensive health care program for seniors. Medicare does not do this. Among benefits Medicare does not cover are routine physical examination, prescription drugs, hearing aids, or custodial care in nursing or board and care homes. Beneficiaries are required to pay various deductibles and co-payments.

Some options being used by the senior population in taking

care of direct medical costs include a Medicare HMO or a Medicare supplemental health insurance policy. An HMO provides a specific set of health care services to its enrolled members. Members are required to use the facilities and medical personnel of the HMO. Medicare supplemental policies are designed to go along with Medicare. There are numerous designated plans in compliance with federal law. All plans must include some basic benefits and then may offer one or several additional benefits. The plans range in price based upon benefits provided and geographical area of the country where the beneficiary resides.

In order for the senior to make appropriate decisions with regard to insurance coverage, much information is required. Those clinicians working with this population can be most effective if they are informed of the benefits, regulations, eligibility, costs, and protections available to the elderly.

Non-medical costs tend to be very high for seniors who because of co-morbidities (multiple medical problems) also tend to have multiple needs in this area. Transportation for treatment, housekeeping assistance, nurse's aides, wigs or prostheses, and nutritional products are not covered by any general insurance policy (and not by Medicare.) Again, knowledge of resources is crucial in assisting the senior population in this area.

Medicare Hospice Benefits

A Medicare beneficiary who chooses hospice care receives non-curative medical and support services for his or her terminal illness. Hospice uses a team of people to deliver care. The team usually consists of family, a nurse, physician, social worker, dietitian, and clergy, all working together to plan and coordinate care. Other trained caregivers are available as needed. The family member is very important to the team because they provide care for the patient on a daily basis, 24 hours a day, every day. The other team members make regular home visits to support the person in the home. A nurse and physician are on-call 24 hours a day, seven days a week to provide advice over the telephone and to make visits whenever necessary. The elderly person with cancer may have an elderly spouse in the home who is not able to provide the care necessary for hospice to be an option for this person. Other adult children and family members may not be available due to their own family and work responsibilities. In choosing hospice, the Medicare beneficiary gives up the right to standard Medicare benefits only for treatment of the terminal illness. Again, the elderly person needs to be educated to this hospice benefit and options for other possible choices.

LEGAL AND ADVOCACY ISSUES FOR THE ELDERLY

Autonomy is an important concept in western culture, and we have learned to value this principle. The older person seems to be faced daily with threats to personal autonomy. Their ability to maintain independence with increasing age and the effects of illness and aging need exploration. Again, the clinician who is sensitive to these issues and is aware of the information and resources available to the elderly can be instrumental in providing the quality of life care that is needed at this time. Two areas of planning can be helpful in maintaining autonomy for the older person with cancer. They are personal planning and financial planning.

Personal Planning–Advance Directives

In order to maintain independence and personal autonomy, a person might explore advance directives. Advance directives are signed legal documents that inform family and physicians of personal choices for future medical care, including whether life supporting measures are wanted. There are multiple forms of advance directives such as the durable power of attorney for health care, a living will, and a physician directive. Each state has laws recognizing advance directives. Multiple resources and information crucial for the older person in making these decisions are readily available.

Financial Planning–Property Assets

Important to the elderly and anyone facing a life-threatening disease is the issue of preparing one's estate and "putting one's house in order." The older person needs and will appreciate receiving information on estate planning, wills, trusts, and powers of attorney. The older person also needs information on planning for burial and funeral arrangements. This type of planning can provide older persons with a sense of control, completeness, and security. All of these are important components of the autonomy concept.

SUMMARY

Cancer is a common problem for many elderly people. Being older should not add to the burden of the disease. Social work intervention can be instrumental in overcoming many of the burdens placed on older persons by the disease and their age. The social worker can educate and model for the rest of the health care team attitudes and approaches that will lessen the impact of age on the overall management of a person's disease.

REFERENCES

Alliance for Aging Research. (1995). Attitudes and preferences of American women concerning treatments for early stage breast cancer. Washington, DC: Author.

American Geriatrics Society. (1998). The management of chronic pain in older persons. AGS Panel on Chronic Pain in Older Persons. *Geriatrics, 53* (*Suppl*), S8-S24.

Bernabei, R., Gambassi, G., Lapane, K., Landi, F., Gatsonis, C., Dunlop, R., Lipsitz, L., Steel, K., & Mor, V. (1998). Management of pain in elderly patients with cancer. SAGE Study Group. Systematic Assessment of Geriatric Drug Use via Epidemiology. *Journal of the American Medical Association, 279* (23), 1877-1882.

Calabresi, P., & Freeman, H. (1997). Concerns of special populations: Cancer and the aging population—A meeting of the President's Cancer Panel, July 31, 1997. *Cancer, 80* (7), 1258-1260.

Castellucci, L. (1999). Better fundamentals—not "Razzle Dazzle"—needed in cancer research on the elderly. *Journal of the National Cancer Institute, 91,* 14-16.

Gazmararian, J., Baker, D., Williams, M., Parker, R., Scott, T., Green, D., Fehrenbach, S., Ren, J., Koplan, J. (1999). Health literacy among Medicare enrollees in a managed care organization. *Journal of the American Medical Association, 281* (6), 545-551.

Hoffman, B. (1998). *A cancer survivor's almanac: Charting your journey.* Minneapolis, MN: Chronimed Publishing.

Rimer, S. (1999). Gaps seen in the treatment of depression in the elderly. *The New York Times,* September 5,1,18.

CHAPTER 12

SEXUALITY AND FERTILITY

Les Gallo-Silver, CSW, ACSW
Lissa Parsonnet, PhD, ACSW

Kinsey (1953) and his team of researchers provided startling information about sexual practices, concerns, and behaviors in the United States in the late 1940s and early 1950s. Forty years later, Laumann, Michael, Gagnon, and Michaels (1994) revisited many of the same sexual issues reported in Kinsey's original studies, finding that while some practices have changed, much has remained the same. The age of first sexual experience appears to be younger, oral intercourse for heterosexuals seems to have become more prevalent, more woman report that they masturbate, and adolescent pregnancy rates are higher. Though disappointing, it is not surprising that neither of these early investigations included the medically ill population in their research.

In the early part of the century, few survived a cancer diagnosis; today it is expected that over 50% of those diagnosed with cancer will be long-term survivors. With the heightened possibility of survivorship come questions related to the *quality* of survivorship. Quality of life issues include an array of psychosocial components ranging from emotional adjustment, to workplace concerns, and include interpersonal relationships, changes in body image and function, and the ability to establish a sense of identity, which incorporates, but is not solely determined by, the cancer diagnosis. Unfortunately despite increased focus on quality of life among cancer survivors, in much of the country, it is still not commonplace for the medical community to address issues of sexual adjustment and fertility with patients before, during, or after cancer treatment.

Ganz, Rowland, Desmond, Meyerowitz, and Wyatt (1998), Yarbo and Ferrans (1998), Monga, Tan, Ostermann, and Monga (1997), and Foley (1995) are a few of the authors who have contributed to the body of knowledge which indicates that sexual functioning and the maintenance of intimate relationships are important aspects of quality of life for people treated for cancer. While one might expect that a culture that accepts television commercials about erectile dysfunction and vaginal lubricants would also frankly address the sexual issues of special populations, neither our experience nor the literature supports this assumption. Discomfort with sexual issues continues to be a major barrier preventing oncology social workers and other health professionals from addressing the issue of sexual functioning and the changes caused by cancer and cancer treatment as an integrated part of practice.

ISSUES OF INFORMED CONSENT

Issues of fertility are sometimes raised because oncology professionals are legally and ethically bound to address issues of fertility prior to initiating treatment for cancer. In addition, the potential dangers posed by chemotherapy agents to an unborn fetus are frequently part of the written consent forms for patients being enrolled in clinical trials. Patients may be cautioned to refrain from sexual activity due to concerns about their platelet count or suppressed immune system and to use condoms as a protection against pregnancy. At times, the effects of treatment on fertility are addressed as if conception did not require or relate to a sexual act. This situation can cause misunderstandings of a highly problematic nature. This is demonstrated by Bobby, a 19-year-old man undergoing treatment for lymphoma. He happily announced to his oncology social worker and nurse that they were wrong about his potential ability to have children. He recently experienced an erection and had intercourse with his girlfriend without using a condom. He believed that discussions about his diminished fertility were related to an inability to achieve an erection. When he discovered that in between chemotherapy cycles he was able to be sexually aroused, he believed his health care team's concerns and warnings were unwarranted. Similarly, Delia, an 18-year-old woman undergoing treatment for Hodgkin's disease, admitted to having unprotected sex in order to become pregnant before she "lost" all her "eggs." She felt that since she became aroused by her boyfriend during petting and became lubricated, that she was still potentially fertile. Both of these examples demonstrate how the reluctance to address sexual functioning and sexual activity directly, in language that patients can understand and relate to, could cause just the types of situations that consent forms attempt to advise patients against.

When not explicitly mandated by protocol or consent form, mention of threat to fertility is often neglected in patient–physician communication. Schover's pilot study of survivors' attitudes toward having children after cancer treatment found that only 65% of those surveyed could remember discussing the topic of fertility with health care providers (Schover, Rybicki, Maritin, & Bringelsen, 1999). When discussion does occur, it is often clinical and impersonal in nature, discouraging patients from asking questions. Patients may feel that they are not justified in asserting concerns about fertility when their health care team is focussed on saving their lives.

Information about the impact of cancer treatments on sexual functioning and fertility is crucial for patients, and needs to be addressed in a timely and sensitive manner. Sadly, people with cancer who are perceived as "beyond" their childbearing years may be provided with even less information than "younger" patients. This was the case for Emily, a 75-year-old woman diagnosed with ovarian cancer. She struggled with intense feelings of loss and defeminization following her hysterectomy. She reported feeling uncomfortable sharing her feelings with her health care team who indicat-

ed that since she could no longer have children "anyway," the surgeon removed "useless" organs. Given this communication, it is not
surprising that Emily believed she could not share the fact that she
was a sexually active lesbian. She felt no one could help her and her
partner of 30 years with this important part of their lives. Similar difficulties occur for patients who are considered "too young" to be
given information about changes in sexual functioning or fertility.

The Role of Oncology Social Workers

Oncology social workers are challenged to assist people with cancer
and their partners with the issues of sexual functioning and fertility.
The types of communication problems described above occur when
oncology professionals find it difficult to manage issues of sexuality
and sexual functioning due to their anxiety and discomfort with the
subject, lack of training, and limited instruction on how to use educational materials.

Nishimoto (1995) reports that people with cancer and their
partners, faced with the emotional and physical issues related to
their changed bodies and concerns about their ability to function
sexually, may be fearful about resuming or attempting to have intimate relationships. Schover (1997) reports that issues concerning
treatment-related sexual difficulties, infertility, or an unknown
potential fertility issue can complicate the journey of healing following the end of treatment and diminish a person's overall psychological adjustment. Oncology social workers can have enormous
impact in this area of practice by becoming sensitized and giving
voice to these often unspoken issues, and by learning how to use
educational materials, psychoeducational interventions, and cognitive behavioral techniques to assist patients and their partners with
their concerns about sexual functioning and fertility.

THE PHASES OF SEXUAL FUNCTIONING

Oncology social workers need to integrate a basic knowledge about
sexual functioning in order to feel confident in exploring the issue

and offering assistance through education and intervention with people with cancer. Understanding the phases of sexual functioning, as developed by Masters and Johnson (1970) and Kaplan (1983), readily enables oncology social workers to use the basic social work technique of partialization to help patients address issues. Once difficulties are partialized, they can appear more accessible to problem solving interventions and resolution. Problems in sexual functioning can then be isolated while areas of healthy functioning can be identified. The phases identify four elements of the human sexual response.

Desire, or *libido*, is defined as interest in sex as well as an emotional and physical accessibility to sexual thoughts and feelings. *Excitement*, or *arousal*, is defined in part by changes in the sexual organs caused by stimulation. *Orgasm* is defined as the culmination and release of the body's responses to increasing stimulation. *Resolution*, or the *refractory phase*, is defined by the physical changes and emotional reactions that occur following orgasm.

Using the Phases of Sexual Functioning When Working With Patients

Using the phases of sexual functioning in oncology social work practice can only be accomplished by addressing sexual issues within the psychosocial assessment process. Including questions about sexual activity, past and present, is comfortably done by including the questions as part of the assessment of a patient's social supports. Oncology social workers may overlook the fact that, for many people, the relationships which share physical intimacy are often the most emotionally intimate as well. Placing the issue of sexuality into the context of interpersonal relationships may not capture every patient's history or life situation but it can be a comfortable way to begin to integrate the issue into a standard psychosocial assessment. Studies by Young-McCaughan (1996), Burke (1996), Flay and Matthews (1995), and others of cancer survivors have documented the impact of cancer-related surgery, chemotherapy, hormone therapy, and immunotherapy on the specific phases of sexual functioning. The phasic approach to evaluating sexual functioning has helped researchers identify many areas of impaired functioning for cancer patients which vary depending upon the specific treatment. This information is presented in an accessible and readable format in the American Cancer Society's (ACS's) pamphlets, "Sexuality and Cancer: For the Woman Who Has Cancer and Her Partner," and "Sexuality and Cancer: For the Man Who Has Cancer and His Partner." These pamphlets, originally prepared for the ACS by Leslie Schover, can be readily used as an active teaching tool. Oncology social workers can address issues with patients and their partners by reviewing the material together and highlighting sections that pertain to the patients' situation.

Using educational materials in an active manner is demonstrated by the approach taken with Gerald, a 58-year-old man recovering from prostate cancer surgery. The ACS pamphlet was used to help Gerald understand that he could experience desire and orgasm even though he would likely have difficulty in the excitement or arousal phase as his surgery may have created an inability to have an erection. This information liberated Gerald from the overwhelming label of being "impotent." Gerald was then more open to a referral to a sex therapist who encouraged him to explore his ability to respond to sexual stimulation by giving him "homework" which was essentially permission to masturbate. While Gerald could not achieve an erection, his physical enjoyment of his "homework" gave him confidence to pursue more physical contact with his wife, Jane. Gerald remembered that as a young man he had experienced orgasm without a full erection. As he and Jane became physically comfortable with each other again, he did experience orgasmic feelings without becoming erect. The oncology social worker's intervention was crucial in empowering Gerald to seek further help in a confident and proactive manner.

A similar approach was used with Marie, a 59-year-old woman who underwent a colostomy as a treatment for her colon cancer. She was anxious and frightened about the impact of her surgery on her boyfriend, Peter. Marie and Peter were both divorced and without partners for many years. They were introduced by mutual friends and fell in love. Marie was overwhelmed as she struggled to adjust to her new ostomy. She felt unattractive and indicated that her days of being sexually active were "at an end" even though Peter was reassuring and supportive. Her oncology social worker used this statement as an opportunity to use the ACS's pamphlet as a working "lesson plan" in their individual supportive counseling sessions. Marie was pleasantly surprised by the information that women having her type of surgery could still feel desire and experience orgasm. Marie was encouraged to experiment with a vaginal lubricant as vaginal dryness was a problem for her. On her own initiative, she began using it to assist in massaging and stimulating her breasts and inner thighs. Marie viewed discussions about sexual issues as an appropriate topic to share with her oncology social worker because reviewing the ACS pamphlet together proved to be such an effective intervention. These exercises with the vaginal lubricant later became the focus of joint counseling with a sex therapist who helped Marie and Peter return to their intimate relationship in a mutually satisfying manner. In the case of both Gerard and Marie, significant relationships included sexual relations as important part of remaining emotionally intimate. Educational materials were used in an active and collaborative manner to help these patients willingly explore their altered bodies.

HELPING PATIENTS ACCOMMODATE CHANGES IN BODY IMAGE

Dramatic changes in weight and muscle mass, hair loss, and for some patients, loss of an apparent body part, surgical scars, and ostomies have an intense impact on the individual's body image. Feeling attractive and desirable is a part of a person's self-perception as much as it is a result of how others interact with them. For people with cancer who do not have sexual partners as well as people who do have partners, their personal impressions of how they "look" or appear to others is a crucial element to sexual experimentation and ultimate functioning during and after treatment. Referrals to programs which focus on make-up and hair styling, such as the "Look

Good Feel Better®" program (sponsored by the ACS and the National Cosmetics, Toiletries, and Fragrancy Association), creating opportunities for people with cancer to obtain low cost assistance in this area, and encouraging patients to purchase clothes that fit them regardless of size, are concrete ways to help patients gain confidence in their appearance. This type of intervention helped William, a 27-year-old gay man who was being treated for head and neck cancer, which affected his jaw and cheek bone. This left his face looking obviously asymmetrical. Counseling with his oncology social worker focused on his feelings of self-loathing when he looked in the mirror, and his anger and sadness when he perceived that people were staring at him. The oncology social worker located a men's hairstyling business, which was willing to help William at a cost he could afford. William wore his hair long, pulled back into a ponytail. He hid his face by looking down and avoiding eye contact. The hairstylist suggested giving William a body wave as well as highlighting his hair in a subtle manner. The increased body of his long hair created the illusion of symmetry and the highlights attracted the attention of the eye away from his face. His new "theatrical look" gave him new confidence. His posture and the manner in which he approached people changed in a positive and engaging way. William then met a partner and had his first long-term relationship since his illness.

A different type of intervention is demonstrated in the case of Angela, who at forty-six was struggling to cope with breast cancer, breast reconstruction, infections, and swelling in her arm. She shuddered whenever her husband Jim came near her; fearful he would touch her in a way that would increase her discomfort. Angela felt mutilated and out of control, so she asked Jim to sleep in another room. Angela was frightened that she was damaging a strong and loving marriage in which physical closeness had been mutually enjoyed. Joint supportive counseling enabled Angela to offer Jim "rules for touching," which helped her feel more in control but also less lonely and ugly. Her oncology social worker suggested she and Jim go to a lingerie specialty store and buy several different matching silk bedclothes. This seemingly superficial and concrete suggestion along with the "rules for touching" resulted in Jim being invited back into their shared bedroom and prepared them for a referral for sex therapy.

UNDERSTANDING SEXUAL REHABILITATION INTERVENTIONS

As described by Gallo-Silver (2000), sexual rehabilitation counseling is an aspect of sex therapy which is focused on helping a person to return to base line sexual function or to accommodate a new base line functioning in keeping with the physical limitations posed by illness or injury. Sex therapists help patients by identifying which phase of sexual functioning is problematic and then create "homework" exercises that might enhance or improve functioning for the patient. This approach to sex therapy is based on the work of Masters and Johnson (1970), and Helen Singer Kaplan (1988). Essentially the "homework" interventions are based on three activities, which can be adapted to a patients' and partners' specific situation and problem. These three activities are self-stimulation/masturbation (self-pleasuring), sensual massage (sensate focus), and changes in coital (sexual intercourse) positions. Understanding how these interventions can help people with cancer and their partners can perhaps enable and empower oncology social workers to make appropriate referrals with confidence and increased comfort.

Laumann et al. (1994) reported that although large numbers of men and women have masturbated at some point in their lives, masturbation remains a taboo sexual activity. Sex therapists use masturbatory "home work" assignments as a way of encouraging patients to explore the changes in their bodies and become more aware of how their bodies react to sexual stimulation. "Self-pleasuring" is a cognitive reframing of masturbation in order to make the activity more accessible, for the purpose of sexual rehabilitation. Self-pleasuring enables an individual to explore the body's response to sexual stimulation without the added pressures of performance anxiety and concerns about their partner's reactions, concerns, and fears. Exercises are often centered around bathing, an activity in which people are more comfortable touching their own bodies. Once people become more aware of their body's pleasurable response, they can become more willing to explore further and experiment. The use of fantasy and erotic materials helps to nurture and increase feelings of desire and ultimately heightens the physical experience.

For people whose bodies have been altered by surgery and chemotherapy, self-pleasuring provides an opportunity to gain more knowledge about the areas of functioning that remain intact. This was the case for Tariq, a 29-year-old man treated for testes cancer, and recovering from a bone marrow transplant. He complained of always feeling tired and weak. He worried about his loss of stamina and was self conscious of his body, which he saw as emaciated and scarred. Tariq married an 18-year-old woman selected by his family when he was 26 years old. His wife was sexually naive and did not communicate comfortably in English. Tariq and his wife were devout Moslems. Sex therapy could not begin until the therapist consulted with the family's Iman (Islamic clergy). Some of the techniques used in sex therapy are based on sexual practices that are often unacceptable or taboo for devout Moslems, Jews, and Christians. The Iman agreed to permit the use of these sexual practices as a way of preserving and supporting this young couple's marriage. Tariq's self-pleasuring homework exercises instructed him to massage the area between his scrotum and his rectum (the perineal region) with the tips of his fingers while lying in a warm bath. As he became better acquainted with how his body responded to this stimulus, he was willing to do the exercises on his bed using a lotion for lubrication. He was then given permission to continue these exercises while viewing erotic videos. Although he was instructed not to touch his penis, he noticed that the skin became pinker and his penis lengthened and thickened. Feeling more hopeful about his erectile potential, he felt more confident about having physical contact with his wife. Tariq's wife was frightened and overwhelmed by the prospect of resuming their sexual relationship. Appropriate self-pleasuring homework exercises were written down in English and given to her bilingual aunt. Her aunt then translated the exercises to her. Although the therapist never had a formal counseling session with Tariq's wife, through the use of her aunt as an intermediary, her own insecurities and misgivings were addressed. Tariq and his wife were then ready for the next series of homework exercises which are based on sensual massage techniques, developed by Masters and Johnson (1970) called "sensate focus."

Sensate Focus

Sensate focus is an organized series of exercises based on the principles of sensuous massage techniques, which structure non-coital foreplay. The goal of these exercises is to provide couples with a way of being physically close and intimate without the pressure and anxiety that can be evoked by attempting sexual intercourse. Kaplan (1988) provides a step-by-step guide on how to teach and use these exercises. The structure and ground rules of sensate focus help to diminish the worries, self doubts, and concerns which can be an obstacle to sexual relations. Even though sensate focus was originally designed to assist couples whose sexual difficulties were more psychogenic in nature, they have been easily adapted to assist people with cancer and other medical problems. The exercises can eliminate or decrease the acute self-consciousness and self-evaluation that some people experience during sexual intercourse. These feelings of acute awareness, which can diminish the body's responsiveness, is referred to in the literature as "spectatoring." The person experiences a sensation of viewing rather than participating in love making which tends to result in a loss of contact with one's body, pleasurable physical sensations, and with one's partner. People with cancer, anxious about their sexual performance, abilities, and attractiveness often struggle with "spectatoring" even after completing the self-pleasuring exercises. Sensate focus exercises provide concrete and practical behaviors that can diminish "spectatoring" by acting as a distractive technique.

Spectatoring was an issue for Karen, a 53-year-old woman, who was surgically treated for an early stage lung cancer. She was struggling with post-operative discomfort and frightened by her shortness of breath. Karen had been married to her husband David for 10 years. They were both recovering from difficult divorces when they met and married. Their sexual relationship was an important aspect of their close and mutually devoted marital life. Their first attempt at sexual intercourse following her surgery was unsuccessful and upsetting for her and David. Karen was taught how to better modulate her breathing by practicing more effective exhale breaths during self-pleasuring exercises. When she felt more confident, they began sensate focus exercises tailored for their needs. Three times a week, on Monday, Wednesday, and Friday during the late morning hours, Karen was instructed to slowly and gently massage her husband's body (front only) avoiding his genitals and breasts. She was told to do this for fifteen minutes. David was instructed to do the same to Karen, but avoiding her rib cage area as well as her genitals and breasts. They became playful with each other and both grew less conscious of Karen's breathing. The slow pace of the exercises helped Karen gradually increase her stamina for physical intimacy.

Sensate focus seems to be more effective when following an organized schedule. Becoming aroused or experiencing orgasm are not the stated goals of the initial phases of these exercises, and are expressly discouraged. This technique can diminish anxieties about performance and worries about one's partner's expectations. It is best to recommend scheduling sensate focus sessions when the person affected by cancer may be at a higher energy point. The late morning is often an effective time for sexual activities because people with medical problems usually have more energy earlier in the day. Couples need to be instructed to avoid the genitals and breasts so that the degree of excitement/arousal is controlled. In addition, couples are instructed to avoid the most problematic and emotionally sensitive areas of the body. For Karen this was her rib cage area. After several weeks of "training," Karen and David were able to return to sexual intercourse.

Position Changes

Sex therapists often suggest that couples change the typical position they once used during sexual intercourse to minimize physical and emotional discomfort, while enhancing closeness and enjoyment. For women with an ostomy or who have been treated for breast cancer, a side-by-side position in which the man is behind the woman can avoid rubbing or leaning against sensitive areas of the body. The side-by-side position and the female superior position, gives the woman partner more control over the extent of vaginal penetration and facilitates replacing vaginal penetration with rubbing against the thighs, buttock (side-by-side) or abdomen (side-by-side while facing each other and female superior). For men with an ostomy, the female superior position can be adapted so the woman does not lean against his upper torso. For men who experience a partial erection, the female superior position can help enhance their erectile abilities. When the woman straddles her male partner's lower torso, he can "stuff" his partially erect penis into her vagina. This creates a partial vacuum effect, which can increase blood flow to the penis. Couples feel empowered to experiment with position changes following the completion of self-pleasuring and sensate focus exercises. They can feel more comfortable with each other and are then able to enjoy experimenting with different positions.

FERTILITY ISSUES AFTER A CANCER DIAGNOSIS

The drive to procreate is central to the human core, evoking instincts to nurture and cherish, and promoting in some sense the quest for immortality. Seen as a pivotal milestone in coming of age, childbearing is viewed by some as a developmental accomplishment representing maturity and normalcy. Recent trends toward delayed childbearing create an older population of childless couples, whose dreams may still include children. Though cancer is to a very great degree a disease of aging, it has been estimated that at least 54,500 Americans treated for cancer each year risk future difficulties in childbearing (Meistrich, Vassilopoulou-Sellin, & Lipshultz, 1997). This striking figure, paired with postponed childbearing, suggests that a number of those being treated for cancer in their reproductive years will have difficulty beginning their family.

The issues in considering childbearing after a cancer diagnosis are many, ranging from treatment induced infertility, to the medical safety of pregnancy, and including the psychological issues of loss, recovery, sexual functioning, healing, self and body image, and choice. As a childless, 33-year-old woman who was advised to undergo surgery to remove her ovaries following treatment for breast cancer poignantly remarked, "First I had to fight for my life, and now to protect it I have to sacrifice another life."

Lost Dreams

Gabrielle was 42 years old and single at the time her breast cancer was diagnosed. She underwent a lumpectomy and lymph node dissection, and was scheduled to receive adjuvant chemotherapy and radiation. A successful professional, Gabrielle enjoyed sports, music, and art, as well as the company of a large circle of friends. Because she was self-employed, she was able to arrange her schedule to accommodate both her vigorous exercise routine and one of her favorite activities: weekly "play dates" with her young godsons. All that was missing was a significant relationship and a child of her own. At forty-two, Gabrielle was beginning to hear the ticking of her biological clock, yet she remained optimistic that the right man would come into her life, and together they would raise children of their own. Anything Gabrielle had wanted in life had required hard work and patience, but with both of these she had attained most of her life goals. Gabrielle had confidence in her physician's assurance that her prognosis was good; however, her concern was preserving her fertility throughout chemotherapy. Physicians estimated that Gabrielle had a 50% likelihood of maintaining or regaining menstruation at the end of treatment. To increase the odds, Gabrielle explored the world of complementary medicine; she took herbs and supplements, as well as regular acupuncture and massage sessions, all aimed at preserving fertility. In the months before her final chemotherapy treatment she stopped menstruating, but two months following the cessation of chemotherapy, her cycle began again.

Gabrielle credited the complementary therapies she had used, as well as God, for her good fortune. Before treatment was completed she met a wonderful man, fell in love, and the following year married. Gabriella thought that all her dreams had come true until at age forty-five, she learned that despite her continued menstruation, she was unable to conceive a child of her own. Gabrielle was devastated. The many blessings in her life, she felt did not compensate for the loss of this special dream. She became angry with her husband for having a daughter by an earlier marriage. She became angry at her 11-year-old stepdaughter, and at any pregnant woman she encountered. Most of all, she became angry at cancer, at the disease that robbed her of her most cherished wish. The losses associated with cancer can be many, but to some the inability to bear children, especially to those who have not yet had children, can be the most devastating loss of all.

Particularly unhelpful to Gabrielle and others facing infertility after cancer, are the well-intended reminders that "at least you're still alive to face this problem," "you should be glad to be alive," or "at least you found a man who was willing to marry you without knowing for sure that you could have children." These and other platitudes, which minimize their experience, can make survivors feel more isolated and misunderstood. The loss of a dream, as any other significant loss, must be mourned before one can move on.

Self-Image

Cancer can be a powerful assault on one's sense of self, changing how one looks and feels physically, and altering one's perspective on life. To some, the loss of fertility confirms what the cancer diagnosis suggests, that they are not "normal," "healthy," or "as good as" their peers. For others, there is a sense of being unlucky, or a feeling of being punished. For those who are single, infertility can convey a sense of being "damaged goods," perhaps making one seem less marriageable. Even those who are partnered may worry that their partners may leave them if children had been part of their plans for the future. Specialized support programs, such as Resolve, can help individuals and couples to cope with both the practical and emotional issues connected with infertility.

The Meaning of Having Children After Cancer

Facing a life-threatening illness may stimulate thoughts about the meaning of life. For some, children, or the hope to have children, provide that meaning, offering a reason to endure the rigors of treatment. Dow (1994) found that having children after cancer had four key meanings. Children can serve an *anchoring* function, giving one a reason to get up in the morning, and drawing one's attention away from illness. Some survivors credit their children with *helping them to get well*. Others felt that having children enabled them to *look forward to the future*. After a cancer diagnosis, this future orientation is very difficult for many survivors to achieve. Finally, Dow's study found that having children enabled survivors to *feel complete*. In the face of losses, both physical and emotional, this feeling of being complete can be elusive. For many, having children is an opportunity to feel normal again, and to reconnect with their peers.

For those working with cancer survivors, it is important to be sensitive to the many meanings childbearing can have. Survivors can be helped to understand the nature and meaning that infertility or possible infertility has to them. This understanding can be helpful in making decisions about options in reproductive assistance.

Uncertainty Regarding Fertility

In addition to the many areas of uncertainty related to treatment side-effects and outcomes, the maintenance of fertility is an aspect that may not be fully known until one attempts to bear children. Schover et al. (1999) found that about one-quarter of those surveyed reported strong anxiety about potential infertility. Many survivors reported being quite concerned about unknown risks to future offspring, including both an inherited predisposition to developing cancer, and possible birth defects resulting from the survivor's cancer treatments.

OPTIONS IN ASSISTED REPRODUCTION

When a treatment has the known potential to damage sperm production, a man should be informed of sperm-banking as an option for maintaining the ability to genetically father children. This term refers to the collection of sperm through masturbation. Collection takes place at a sperm bank, so that sperm cells can immediately be flash-frozen. Once frozen, sperm can be stored for up to 50 years. Generally there is an annual storage fee (Schover, 1997). Sperm can be inserted directly into a woman's uterus through a process known as intrauterine insemination.

For married women, embryo banking may be a possibility. Unfortunately this technique is not only expensive, but has yielded disappointing results (Schover, 1997). In many cases this technique requires a delay in the initiation of treatment, which may be problematic from a cancer-treatment perspective.

Options for parenthood when a patient has been rendered infertile by cancer or its treatment can include sperm or egg donation, surrogate parenting, and adoption. Organizations such as the American Society for Reproductive Medicine, the Organization of Parents through Surrogacy, Resolve, and Adoptive Families of America can help inform patients of their options, and direct patients to local resources.

SUMMARY

As cancer has increasingly become a curable or chronic disease, it becomes incumbent upon oncology professionals to understand the effects that both the disease and its treatment can have on those affected. Though at times difficult to discuss, sexuality and fertility issues are as vital a part of life to cancer survivors, as they are to those who have never experienced illness. By remaining silent about these life-enhancing topics, oncology social workers risk conveying the message that survival should be enough, and that cancer survivors should not strive to maintain the priorities that may have sustained them prior to their illness. For most adults, sexuality is an important part of close and loving relationships. Following cancer treatment, this expression of intimacy may be important to emotional healing as well as to ongoing quality of life. Similarly maintaining the dream of bearing children may seem more urgent to those who have faced a life-threatening illness. Because sex still seems to be a taboo subject among the medically ill, it is often difficult for cancer survivors to discuss their sexual functioning or ability to bear children. Oncology social workers need to be sensitive to the importance of sexuality and fertility among cancer survivors. Questions and dialogue about these components of life should be integrated into our psychosocial assessment, thus opening an important door to communication, and conveying an understanding and willingness to discuss this intimate part of life, and the hopes, dreams, and realities attached to it.

REFERENCES

Burke, L. M. (1996). Clinical sexual dysfunction following radiotherapy for cervical cancer. *British Journal of Nursing, 5(4)*, 239-244.

Dow, K. H. (1994). Having children after breast cancer. *Cancer Practice, 2(6)*, 407-413.

Flay, L. D, Matthews, J. H. (1995). The effects of radiotherapy and surgery on the sexual function of women treated for cervical cancer. *International Journal of Radiation Oncology, Biology and Physics. 31(2)*, 399-404.

Foley, G. V. (1995). Sexuality—a forgotten issue. *Cancer Practice, 3(5)*, 273.

Gallo-Silver, L. (2000). Sexual rehabilitation of persons with cancer. *Cancer Practice, 8(1)*, 10-16.

Ganz, P. A., Rowland, J. H., Desmond, K., Meyerowitz, B. E., & Wyatt, G. E. (1998). Life after breast cancer: Understanding women's health related quality of life and sexual functioning. *Journal of Clinical Oncology. February: 16(2)*, 501-514.

Kaplan, H. S. (1983). *The evaluation of sexual disorders: Psychological and medical aspects.* New York: Brunner/Mazel.

Kaplan, H. S. (1988). *The illustrated manual of sex therapy.* New York: Brunner/Mazel.

Kinsey, A. C., Pomeroy, W. B., Martin, C. E., & Gebhard, P. H. (1953). *Sexual behavior in the human female.* Philadelphia: Saunders Publishing.

Laumann, E. O., Michael, R. T., Gagnon, J. H., & Michaels, S. (1994). *The social organization of sexuality: Sexual practices in the United States.* Chicago: The University of Chicago Press.

Masters, W. H., & Johnson, V. E. (1970). *Human sexual inadequacy.* Boston: Little, Brown, & Company.

Meistrich, M. L., Vassilopoulou-Sellin, R., & Lipshultz, L. I. (1997). Gonadal dysfunction. In V. T. DeVita, S. Hellman, & S. A. Rosenberg (Eds.), *Cancer: Principles and practice of oncology* (5th ed., pp. 2758-2773). Philadelphia: Lippincott, Williams, & Wilkins.

Monga, U., Tan, G., Ostermann, H. J., & Monga, T. N. (1997). Sexuality in head and neck cancer patients. *Archives of Physical Medicine and Rehabilitation, 78(3),* 298-304.

Nishimoto, P. W. (1995). Sex and sexuality in the cancer patient. *Nurse Practitioner Forum, 6(4),* 221-227.

Schover, L. R. (1997). *Sexuality and fertility after cancer.* New York: Wiley.

Schover, L. R., Rybicki, L. A., Maritin, B. A., & Bringelsen, K.A. (1999). Having children after cancer. A pilot survey of survivors' attitudes and experiences. *Cancer, 86(4),* 697-709.

Yarbo, C. H., & Ferrans, C. E. (1998). Quality of life of patients with prostate cancer treated with surgery or radiation therapy. *Oncology Nursing Forum, 25(4),* 685-693.

Young-McCaughan, S. (1996). Sexual functioning in women with breast cancer after treatment with adjuvant therapy. *Cancer Nursing, 19(4),* 308-319.

CHAPTER 13

END OF LIFE ISSUES

Susan C. Hedlund, MSW, LCSW
Elizabeth J. Clark, PhD, ACSW

A century ago, most adults died fairly quickly from infections or accidents. Death was a relatively normal part of life. Now, dying has become a complex phenomenon. Death may come more slowly, either because medical advances slow the progression of disease, or the moment of death is postponed as a result of medical technology that allows the body to stay alive in situations that in the past would have resulted in certain demise. Dying is now influenced by medical technology, social science, and economics. In fact, there is no universally accepted medical definition of what "dying" or "terminal" is, or how soon before death one should be considered dying.

The dying process has been elongated as a result of medicine's growing effectiveness. For those whose quality of life remains high, or at least satisfactory, this can be a good outcome. For those whose quality of life is poor, or who are suffering greatly, it has become harder and harder to die. Through antibiotics, transfusions, artificial feedings, and other interventions, dying can be extended well beyond the point where living has much meaning, either for the individual or the family.

Alternatively, for those who are dying "well," those whose

symptoms are well-managed, and for whom the dying process can offer a time of introspection, resolution, and meaning, dying may be a time of wonder and exploration, for saying goodbye to family and friends, and for achieving the completion of life's tasks (Byock, 1998). Because of changes in medicine and its technology, determining when the dying process actually begins is increasingly difficult. Many physicians, therefore, are reluctant to actually confirm that a patient is dying, or is in the last stages of life. The oncology social worker can act as both advocate for the patient and liaison to the health care team. This involves clarifying the needs of the patient and family and facilitating communication with the physician.

Still, death will be a personal reality for all of us. The first wave of the Baby Boom Generation is now reaching fifty. Many in this "sandwich" generation are faced with raising their own children while also caring for aging parents. They are confronted with difficult decisions about illness, death, and caregiving. By the year 2011, the oldest Baby Boomers will reach 65, and the elderly will make up a large proportion of the population. Each year, more people will die than the year before. Society is being pushed to deal with the medical, economic, and social aspects of an aging population.

ADVANCE DIRECTIVES/HEALTH CARE SURROGATES

Some authors suggest that a "good death" has largely to do with the decisions we make about our medical treatment and terminal care, and with our psychological preparation, than it does with good or bad fortune (Webb, 1999). Making decisions about terminal illness in advance is important. There are several ways to do this.

An advance directive is a legal document through which patients provide instructions for the kind of care that they do or do not want to receive, or else name another person to make such decisions for them. The patient's preferences include decisions about life-sustaining treatments including artificial fluids and nutrition.

Advance directives generally take effect when the patient becomes incompetent to make health care decisions during the course of a terminal illness, or else becomes permanently comatose. These preferences are elicited in the event of specific clinical conditions common at the end of life, including close to death, permanently unconscious, advanced progressive illness, and extraordinary suffering. Decisions are based on the values of the individual patients as expressed in advance directives or through the appointment of a health care surrogate or representative to act on their behalf. An alternative representative can be appointed in the event that the health care representative is unable to participate in the decision making process. The use of an advance directive is regulated differently in each state. There are three types of advance directives: a living will, a durable medical power of attorney or health care proxy, or the family consent (or surrogacy/succession) law (Cassel & Field, 1997).

A living will is a type of advance directive that puts a person's wishes about medical treatment in writing so that if that person cannot communicate, his or her desires are clearly stated and recorded. State laws may define when a living will goes into effect, and may limit the treatments to which the living will applies. A person's right to accept or refuse treatment is protected by constitutional and common law. Living wills can be specific, addressing the patient's wishes regarding procedures such as cardiopulmonary resuscitation, mechanical ventilation, surgery, the use of artificial hydration or nutrition, blood transfusions, or antibiotics. The more specific the living will, the less chance there will be for family conflict or confusion among members of the health care team.

A durable medical power of attorney is a legal document that allows patients to appoint someone they trust to make decisions about their medical care when they cannot. This type of advance directive may also be called a health care proxy or appointment of a health care agent. The person appointed by such a document may be called a health care agent, surrogate, attorney-in-fact, or proxy. In many states, the person appointed through a medical power of attorney is authorized to speak for the patient any time that patient

is unable to make a medical decision, not only for end-of-life decisions. The third kind of law—the family consent (or surrogacy/suc-
cession) law—requires no document to be signed prior to the loss of
competence. As of 1996, between 24 and 36 states (depending on
how various state statutes are interpreted) have passed family succession laws; these states have simply set up a system whereby particular family members, in a designated order of succession, are to be the
ones to make treatment decisions for an incompetent patient. Such
laws do not preclude living wills or health care proxies, but if such
documents have not been signed, the patient is still protected.

Advance directives work in tandem with conversations held
with health care providers, patients, and their families about what the
future might hold. Advance care planning also may include a "values"
questionnaire to assist the patient in clarifying values, attitudes about
death, and spiritual perspectives. Discussions between the health
care team and patient and family members can be of great benefit
when considerations about the wise use of life-sustaining treatment
occur in the future. It is now a mandate of the federal government
that hospitals must ask inpatients if they have an advance directive,
and, if not, offer information about preparing one if desired.

ISSUES WITH STOPPING TREATMENT

The legal debate over right-to-die issues began over 20 years ago and
dealt with the withdrawal of medical treatment. Decisions by state
and federal judges over the years led to changes in national and state
legislation. Historically, the patients' rights movement has focused
on the right of an individual to refuse unwanted medical treatment.
Recently, debates about medical futility, treatment rationing, and
managed care have caused patients' rights advocates to examine the
flip side of patient autonomy—the right to request treatment.

There are some ethicists and health care professionals who
believe that patient autonomy has gone too far and should be limited. According to these professionals, people should not have the
right to request treatment that is inappropriate or futile. Some argue

that difficult decisions should be left in the hands of the patient or those closest to the patient. Others argue that it makes no sense to aggressively treat patients when the outcome will be medically futile. In the future, society will be faced with difficult decisions regarding patient autonomy versus medical futility (Cassel & Field, 1997). In the meantime there will be many patients who struggle with decisions about the appropriate point to limit or stop treatment, and the way to consider such decisions.

As with all medical treatments, the benefits and burdens should be weighed against one another when deciding about stopping treatment (Quill, 1996). Treatments may be started because there is still hope that the patient will improve. Even in the last stages of life, some treatments are started in the hope that the patient's comfort will be enhanced, or that a patient will recover from a temporary setback. Deciding to use these treatments in the course of a serious illness requires careful consideration because once these treatments have begun, it can be hard to decide to stop. Examples of such treatments include artificial nutrition (tube feeding), intravenous (IV) hydration, chemotherapy, antibiotics, and ventilators.

Artificial treatments can be very effective, and some authors encourage a time-limited trial if treatment could improve comfort or quality of life (Lynn & Harrold, 1999). Some worry that once a treatment is started, they will not be able to discontinue it. Both legally and ethically, not starting and stopping are seen as equal actions. Thus, if treatment is not improving comfort or quality of life, then it can be discontinued.

Other issues that arise as patients or families are making decisions about discontinuing treatment are issues regarding the perception of "giving up." Patients may struggle with concerns about disappointing loved ones, or giving up too soon. Families may fear that by stopping treatment for a loved one, they somehow will be responsible for killing them. The law, however, does not see stopping these treatments as raising questions of homicide or suicide. An adult patient is under no obligation to take any medical care.

Discontinuing treatment may simply allow the natural progression of the disease to take its course. The important principles to consider when deciding about stopping treatment involve knowing what stopping treatment will accomplish, and what, if any, burden it will cause. It is a highly individualized and personal decision for both patients and their loved ones. Similarly, social workers new to oncology also may struggle with the discontinuation of treatment. This struggle usually resolves as more clinical experience is gained and the social worker clarifies personal and professional values in relation to oncology.

Patients in their final months of life have a variety of needs including family support, comfort, and spiritual counseling. Most benefit from care or consultation with an interdisciplinary team such as that offered by comfort care, palliative care, or hospice. While these terms are often used interchangeably, comfort care, palliative care, and hospice are defined separately in state and federal laws governing health care benefits and reimbursement.

COMFORT CARE AND PALLIATIVE CARE

Comfort care and palliative care, as opposed to care oriented toward cure or remission of the disease, are medical and related services designed to help alleviate pain and other symptoms of an illness. The major difference is that while palliative care has the goal of providing comfort and maintaining a high quality of life, the patient's prognosis, while grave, may not be terminal. Therefore, therapy aimed at remission or cure may still be desired. Comfort care does not include diagnostic or cure-oriented therapy or active treatment that is intended to prolong life.

Comfort care (but not hospice) may be provided by home health agencies and physicians or physician groups. Comfort care, palliative support, or pre-hospice teams who consult to reduce the pain and suffering of patients with serious or life-threatening illnesses are available through some hospitals and most hospices.

Comprehensive palliative care programs provide for mental health and spiritual needs in addition to physical comfort. The Health Care Financing Administration (HCFA) has recently created a diagnosis related group (DRG) that will allow payment for end of life care for people who die in hospitals or require hospitalization for palliation of symptoms (Cassel, 1996).

Comfort Care

Comfort care, as defined by many state programs, includes the combination of medical and related services that will make it possible for a terminally ill individual to die with as much comfort as possible given the nature of the illness. Comfort care includes hospice and palliative care, but is not limited to care provided through a hospice program.

Palliative Care

Palliative care focuses on reducing or abating physical and other symptoms of a terminal illness. For purposes of reimbursement, a distinction is often made between active and symptomatic palliative therapy. The goals of active palliative therapy are to prolong survival and arrest the progression of the disease. Active palliative therapy is not usually covered under a hospice or comfort care benefit. The goals of symptomatic palliative therapy are to achieve comfort, to manage symptoms, and to improve the quality of life. A short course of radiation therapy to achieve comfort by reducing the size of a tumor is an example of symptomatic palliative therapy. Side effects that compromise comfort may rule out therapies such as full-dose radiation or chemotherapy as symptomatic palliative therapy.

Hospice

The word "hospice" comes from the same root as hospitality. In early Western civilization, it was used to describe a place of shelter and rest for weary or sick travelers on long journeys. Earlier this century, hospices evolved into religiously inspired centers dedicated to caring for seriously ill or dying patients. The early notion of service for the dying evolved and was joined with the modern science of pain management, symptom control, and grief counseling by Dame Cicely Saunders, founder of the first modern hospice, St. Christopher's, which opened in a London suburb in 1967.

Hospice today refers to a concept of comprehensive palliative care for terminally ill patients, not necessarily a place (Buckingham, 1996). Using a combination of skilled symptom management, aggressive treatment of pain, psychosocial support, and attention to spiritual and emotional concerns, hospice teams and physicians work to offer patients the possibility of a comfortable, peaceful, and dignified death. Dying at home is what many people say they would want to do, and hospice offers that possibility. Hospice is distinguished from home care, which is a more generic term for the wide variety of health care services that can be provided in the home setting to people who are sick but likely to recover from their illness. Hospice care focuses on the comprehensive care of dying patients. Hospice establishes pain and symptom control as the principle clinical goals. When patients can no longer benefit from curative treatment, they may be offered hospice care if their physicians believe they have less than six months to live (although usually when a patient is referred to hospice they have far less than six months to live). Late referrals to hospice are problematic because patients and their families may not have sufficient time to prepare for death. It is also difficult for the hospice team to develop meaningful relationships in a short time. Oncology social workers often act as patient advocates in helping the health care team make the transition from a curative to a palliative approach.

Over 90% of hospice care is provided in the patient's home. However, some dying patients cannot use this option because they live alone or with someone who is unable to care for them, or because their care needs are too great to manage at home. In such cases, inpatient hospice care may be offered through a contracting hospital, a skilled nursing facility, or the hospice's own inpatient facility.

There are some patients and families whose desperation about continuing to live makes the hospice option impossible. In these situations, oncology social workers often find themselves offering support to the health care team as well as providing supportive care and assistance to the patient. Psychosocial support, resources, and symptom management can be provided without the election of hospice.

SPIRITUALITY AT THE END OF LIFE

A common theme for people at the end of life is the attempt to find meaning in how they have lived their lives, and meaning in what is happening to them in the process of dying (Cassel & Field, 1997). The connection between spirituality and end of life may seem obvious to people who have strong roots in organized religion. Religion gives believers a pathway with clear road signs and expected activities. For those whose faith is an active part of life, there may be comfort in achieving religious milestones in the process of coping with illness and facing death. For those who have been actively addressing spiritual issues throughout life, with or without formal religion, the end of life may feel like the natural conclusion of life. However, for many, the end of life forces people to face many issues, including unanswered spiritual questions, and the search for meaning.

Life-threatening illness often requires a redefinition of "self," and forces us to think about what really matters. Often, people discover that what really matters are relationships with others, with the world around them, and with making peace within a spiritual perspective. For some people with life-threatening illness, as well as for those who love them, the illness may magnify questions of faith previously unresolved and may require a revisiting of conflicts with religion or faith. Life-threatening illness may also raise questions for those whose faith is strong, yet who find themselves challenged by the realities of serious illness and the suffering that may exist in its context.

Spirituality goes beyond readily defined social roles and relationships (Sharp, 1997) and focuses on one's relationship with the interior "self" or the "soul" as well as with the possibility of a life or existence beyond the finite world. Relationships with others, God, and the universe may be of concern as death approaches and the question of meaning becomes paramount. Some authors suggest that the search for meaning becomes an important "task" at the end of life. For many, it is the most important, and potentially rewarding, aspect of the dying process, and overshadows the importance of spending all of one's energy on medical treatment or on relatively unimportant tasks.

ANTICIPATORY GRIEF

Anticipatory grief is the term used to describe the process of "grief rehearsal," or the experience of grief prior to the occurrence of death itself. Many people with life-threatening illnesses and their loved ones begin the process of grieving as the illness changes life, and many losses are experienced. The person who is sick must contend with the reality that life is ending, face saying goodbye to those they love, and contend with finding meaning in life and in dying.

Families and friends of the dying person may begin the process of anticipating life without their loved one, both physically and emotionally. At times this can be a difficult and confusing process. They may experience guilt in anticipating their loved one's death, or, at times, wishing for death to come so the suffering can end. For others it can be a time of preparing for life beyond the loved one's illness and death. It should be understood that anticipatory grief does not replace the normal grieving process that takes place after death occurs. Many believe, however, that it serves to cushion the impact of acute grief and therefore may be less painful than the grief experienced by a sudden death.

Anticipatory grief allows loved ones to say goodbye, to rehearse for the future, and to anticipate leave-taking. It also provides the opportunity for the reconciliation of previous conflicts, and for involving the dying person in making some decisions about the future.

Anticipatory grief can have some negative consequences, however. It might lead to increased isolation of the patient as family members begin to withdraw and plan for life without their loved one. Also, on occasion, it may force patients to confront the reality of death before they are ready or rob them of the hope they so badly need to sustain them through the final days of life.

MAINTAINING HOPE AT THE END OF LIFE

Despite stage of illness, hopefulness and a positive future outlook are important components for quality of life. Many wonder how it is possible for someone to remain hopeful when their prognosis is terminal. Yet, we realize that persons who are dying are also still living, and they may need emotional assistance to live as fully as possible until they die.

Hope is a complex concept, and defining it is not easy. Part of the difficulty is that there are numerous types of hope, and people define hope differently. In general, we can say that hope is a way of thinking, feeling, and acting. It is a cognitive-affective resource that is a psychological asset. Hope enhances quality of life, and it is a prerequisite for taking action.

Hope can be generalized and based on something conceptual and broad. An example might be a patient hoping to live fully in whatever time is remaining. There also is particularized hope. This type of hope is more specific and defined such as hoping to live long enough to see a new grandchild born.

In oncology, health care professionals are most familiar with therapeutic hope, hope that is based on therapy and related to the cure or remission of disease (Nuland, 1995). What they often fail to realize is that patients use various types of hope and often use them interchangeably. The other important point is that hope changes as situations and circumstances change. Hope is not a static concept, and it always involves a consideration of the future.

Many hopes are not realized. For example, when first diagnosed, an individual may hope for a cure. If a cure is not possible, a hope for a long period of remission might become the dominant hope. If this new hope cannot be maintained, hope will once again need to be refocused.

Hope can transcend reality, but hope does not equate with denial. Cancer patients need and desire accurate information about their disease, their treatment options, and their prognosis. If this information is presented with compassion and with assurance of continuing support, even approaching terminal illness can be accepted, and new hopes can be established for the time remaining.

Perhaps the most important things we can do for our patients is to maintain a community of hope in our treatment settings. We need to allow for individual differences in how, and for what, our patients and their loved ones hope. No matter what the disease stage, every person has the right to be hopeful (Clark, 1997a).

LOSS AND GRIEF

The United States has been described as a death denying or death avoiding society. We use death to sell books, newspapers, and magazines, and we use death to advertise movies and television shows, yet, we are very uncomfortable dealing with personal loss.

Part of our discomfort comes from the fact that we are unfamiliar with death. Many Americans now reach adulthood without losing a loved one to death. Also, despite the hospice movement, most people still die in institutions–hospitals or nursing homes. Technology has extended both living and dying.

Societal norms about dying also have changed. At the turn of the century, there were proscribed norms for grieving. When a loved one died, relatives wore mourning clothes and curtailed social activities for one year. There were rituals for managing death and bereavement.

The temporal norms for mourning also have changed. Today we are given 3–5 days leave from work to bury our loved ones and do our griefwork. There is a trend toward cremation and memorial services. We feel awkward and ill-at-ease if we need to attend a viewing or funeral, more so if the body is present. We send purchased sympathy cards instead of writing personal notes to the family. In short, we do not know how to mourn. Grief has become deritualized, and we no longer know what to do or how to act when a loved one dies. Even patients sometimes state that there are no guidelines for dying well. They do not know what to do or what is expected of them by family, friends, or health care professionals. Despite this lack of practical guidelines there is a uniform and recognizable syndrome of acute grief that individuals experience when faced with the death of a loved one. Most people are unfamiliar with this syndrome and unprepared for it (Rando, 1993).

Symptomatology of Acute Grief

The symptomatology of acute grief was identified in 1944 by a psychiatrist who studied survivors of the tragic Coconut Grove fire in Boston (Lindemann, 1944). Depending on a variety of factors such as whether the death was sudden or expected, acute grief may induce an initial feeling of numbness, an inability to grasp fully what has happened, for the first two or three weeks after the death. This appears to be a protective psychological mechanism; the psyche cannot absorb the enormity of the event and the subsequent emotional pain.

The acute phase of grief includes episodes of bodily distress and intense emotion that seem to occur in time waves lasting from 20 to 60 minutes. There is a feeling of tightness in the throat, a choking sensation with shortness of breath, an empty feeling in the abdomen, a lack of muscular strength, intense mental pain, and a need for sighing. Other symptoms of acute grief include crying and sobbing, restlessness, loss of appetite and sexual drive, and sleep disturbances.

These physical symptoms are combined with sadness, depression, and an inability to concentrate. There also may be what is known as searching behavior—where the bereaved searches for the dead loved one's presence and is preoccupied with thoughts of the deceased. Additionally, responses similar to auditory or visual hallucinations, where the bereaved is certain they hear their loved one's voice or see their face in a crowd, may occur.

One of the most important things a social worker can do for a bereaved client is to normalize the acute bereavement response (Clark, 1997b). This means describing what is currently happening and what they may experience in the future, and offering reassurance that they are not having an emotional breakdown, but that this is the acute grief syndrome.

Despite the intensity of acute grief, our society demands that we put our grief aside quickly, that we hide it and "get back to normal" in as short a period as possible. Hiding grief means that, in public at least, the bereaved attempts to carry on, to keep busy, to act as if nothing has happened. Denial of the significance of the loss and the inability to openly express one's grief may extend the grief process.

When does grief end? How long does it last? The answers to these questions are unclear. We know that grief cannot be resolved in the week that one is excused from work for the death and the funeral. We also know that for the first year, there will be anniversary reactions that seem to magnify the grief response on certain significant dates such as the birthday of the deceased, wedding anniversaries, and even the anniversary of the death itself. Experts now believe that 2–3 years may be a more realistic time frame for completing the four tasks of mourning: accepting the reality of the loss; experiencing the pain of grief; adjusting to a changed environment; and relocating the loss emotionally and moving on (Worden, 1991).

Professional Loss and Grief

Most oncology social workers have received basic training in grief counseling and are able to assist both patients and families with end of life issues. What so often is lacking is training for dealing with their own professional loss and grief. Many oncology social workers are employed in what can be described as high loss settings, and they may see more death in a year than others see in a lifetime. Witnessing suffering is very difficult.

While professionals are trained to put aside their own emotions in times of crises and emergencies, they do have personal and profound feelings about the deaths of their patients and about the hurt that their families experience. One tenet in grief theory is that for every loss, there is an accompanying grief. Additionally, we know that loss, like stress, can accumulate.

Cumulative grief, sometimes called bereavement overload, is precipitated by multiple losses with little time allowed for grieving, or even acknowledging, the loss. In high-loss, high-stress environments, social workers and other helping professionals can find themselves feeling vulnerable and irritated. They may find it harder to maintain hope for themselves and for their patients, and they may exhibit signs and symptoms of burnout.

Burnout is a syndrome of emotional exhaustion that occurs among individuals who work closely with others under conditions of chronic tension and stress (Schaufeli, Maslach, & Marek, 1993). Numerous books and articles have been written on the subject, and few health care professionals complete their training without some exposure to boundary setting, transference issues, and the need to maintain balance between one's personal and professional lives. Too often, though, professionals do not recognize the signs and symptoms that signal stress overload and potential burnout.

The physical symptoms of burnout are fairly easy to identify. These include symptoms such as fatigue, feeling run down, headaches, sleeplessness, and gastrointestinal disturbances. The behavioral and psychological symptoms may be harder to identify because they are intermingled with work demands such as working harder and accomplishing less; coming to work earlier and staying later; feeling unappreciated and resentful; avoiding patient contact; and being unable to make decisions. New oncology social workers can experience these same symptoms in the beginning of their work with patients. They usually pass with more clinical experience and attention to boundary issues that can complicate the adjustment process to work in oncology.

One additional sign of burnout should be highlighted—feeling indispensable. Too often, as professional caregivers become more and more overloaded, they tend to think they cannot take breaks or days off or vacations because they are "too needed" at their place of employment. Eventually, the balance between personal and professional life becomes unequal, and family concerns and complaints add to the stress overload. While exhibiting some of the signs or symptoms above does not indicate that an individual has "burned" out, but it should be a signal that a personal (and professional) assessment is warranted.

ADDITIONAL END OF LIFE ISSUES

Organ Donation

For some people, the prospect of organ donation after death occurs may add to a sense of perceived meaning at the end of life. This is particularly true in the case of sudden, unexpected death. The idea of donating organs of the deceased can be perceived by loved ones as the opportunity to make something "good" come from a tragic event: the possibility that the end of one life may offer continued life for someone else. Many states have laws that enable adults of sound mind to make their wishes for becoming an organ donor known by carrying a "Uniform Donor Card" or asking to have their driver's license encoded with a "D" to identify them as prospective donors.

For certain illnesses, a transplant offers the best chance of survival or an improved quality of life. Anatomical donations are not bought or sold, nor will they result in further expense beyond normal hospital or funeral expense. Removal of donated organs does not produce disfigurement or interfere with customary funeral services. Certain diseases, such as malignancies or communicable diseases, may preclude the possibility of organ donation (in some states, corneal donation is a possibility). It is wise to consult one's physician, or others familiar with the medical and legal aspects of organ donation in one's state.

Viatical Settlements

Social workers need to be aware of a fairly new financial resource for their patients who are nearing the end of life. Called viatical settlements, this option can be an important part of estate planning (Calder & Card, 1996).

In a viatical settlement, the patient sells a life insurance policy to a viatical company and receives a percentage of the face value of the policy. The company pays all future premiums and then collects the policy's benefit when the patient dies. The patient and family are free to use the money received for medical expenses or in any way they deem necessary or desirable. There are some companies that offer what is called a secured no-payment loan against the policy. This is like a line of credit; you borrow only what you need.

There are some restrictions. Not all insurance policies may be sold. The patient also has to have a life expectancy of 5 years or less. If less than 2 years, the patient will not have to pay taxes on the settlement. There are no age requirements, and patients do not need to be disabled.

The social worker can help patients explore whether or not a viatical settlement is a possibility, and they can help locate a reliable viatical company. Before proceeding, however, the patient should have an attorney review the viatical contract. Each state's insurance commission can provide information about viatical companies in that state.

SUMMARY

The role of oncology social workers in end of life care is multifaceted. The knowledge and expertise that social workers bring to the oncology setting have a positive and important impact on the care of persons with cancer from the time of initial diagnosis to end of life care and bereavement follow-up. Oncology social workers can assist with both practical and existential concerns. This can be a tremendous reassurance to patients and families facing loss and experiencing grief. The ability to offer a calm and reassuring presence and to normalize the grief process at end of life can significantly influence healthy recovery from grief.

To be able to work effectively in this field, social workers must also understand the impact that social work has in their personal lives, and they must engage in regular self-assessments and healthy self-care. Witnessing suffering is very hard, but the sharing of such significant events enriches rather than diminishes the caregiver. As C. Murray Parkes (1986), one of the foremost experts on loss and grief so eloquently noted, "With proper training and support, we shall find that repeated grief, far from undermining our humanity and our care, enables us to cope more confidently and more sensitively with each succeeding loss" (p. 7).

REFERENCES

Buckingham, R. W. (1996). *The handbook of hospice care.* Amherst, NY: Prometheus Books.

Byock, I. (1998). *Dying well: Peace and possibilities at the end of life.* New York: Riverhead Books.

Calder, K., & Card, I. (1996). Straight talk about insurance and health plans. In B. Hoffman (Ed.) *Cancer survivor's almanac* (pp. 167-201). Minneapolis, MN: Chronimed Publishing.

Cassel, C. K. (1996). Letter to colleagues about Medicare palliative care. *Millbank Memorial Fund.* July 20, 1996.

Cassel, C. K., & Field, M. J. (Eds). (1997). *Approaching death: Improving care at the end of life.* Washington, DC: National Academy Press.

Clark, E. J. (1997a). *You have the right to be hopeful* (2nd ed.). Silver Spring, MD: National Coalition for Cancer Survivorship.

Clark, E. J. (1997b). The end of the continuum: Bereavement care for the adult. *Cancer Practice, 5(4),* 252-254.

Lindemann, E. (1944). Symptomatology and management of acute grief. *American Journal of Psychiatry, 101,* 141-148.

Lynn, J., & Harrold, J. (1999). *Handbook for mortals: Guidance for people facing serious illness.* New York: Oxford University Press.

Nuland, S. W. (1995). *How we die: Reflections on life's final chapter.* New York: Vintage.

Parkes, C. M. (1986). The caregiver's griefs. *Journal of Palliative Care, 1,* 5-7.

Quill, T. E. (1996). *A midwife through the dying process: Stories of healing and hard choices at the end of life.* Baltimore: The Johns Hopkins University Press.

Rando, T. A. (1993). *Treatment of complicated mourning.* Champaign, IL: Research Press.

Schaufeli, W. B., Maslach, C., & Marek, T. (1993). *Professional burnout: Recent developments in theory and research.* Washington, DC: Taylor & Francis.

Sharp, J. (1997). *Living our dying: A way to the sacred in everyday life.* New York: Hyperion.

Webb, M. (1999). *The good death: The new American search to reshape the end of life.* New York: Bantam Books.

Worden, J. W. (1991). *Grief counseling and grief therapy: A handbook for the mental health practitioner.* New York: Springer Publishing Company, Inc.

CHAPTER 14

HOW TO ACCESS ONCOLOGY RESOURCES

John W. Sharp, MSSA

Much of what oncology social workers do can be described as empowerment. We empower cancer survivors to gain control over what seems to be uncontrolled so they can regain a sense of order and coping in their lives. Much of what creates a sense of shock and aloneness in the experience of cancer is the strange terminology, making life and death choices about treatment and knowing how to cope emotionally with an unfamiliar and frightening life challenge. Access to the proper resources is key to creating this sense of empowerment.

Fortunately, the quantity of resources available to cancer survivors has expanded in the past decade. Both in print and electronic media, information about treatment and support continues to grow. For instance, several autobiographical books by cancer survivors are published each month. Online cancer information has experienced exponential growth from cancer organizations and cancer centers. Parallel with the growth in the quantity of resources is the speed at which new resources appear. This is most evident in the area of electronic information, as cancer information has been part of the explosive growth of the Internet.

This chapter will address how oncology resources can be accessed by social workers utilizing current communication tools:

- print materials including books, newsletters, and journals
- audio and video materials
- telephone access through toll-free numbers and teleconferencing
- radio and television including talk shows and news
- the Internet including the World Wide Web, email, chat rooms, and other tools.

The chapter will conclude with future communication mechanisms, which have the potential to enhance access to resources.

PRINT MEDIA

The printed page has been the traditional means of gaining access to information and support for cancer survivors. Books on diagnosis and treatment of various cancers from the American Cancer Society (ACS) and the Leukemia and Lymphoma Society to mention only two, have been important to cancer survivors to read and reread as a means of gaining an understanding of their disease and treatment options. Comprehensive cancer reference books like *Informed Decisions*, provide an overview of cancer biology, the four major treatment modalities (surgery, chemotherapy, radiation, and biologicals) and side effects to answer almost any question about cancer (see Table 1). Other reference books, such as, the book *Childhood Leukemia*, provide guides to specific kinds of cancer. Books on personal experiences of cancer abound. Some books of this genre are most helpful for those with the same type of cancer. Other books, such as, Scott Hamilton's biography, provide a more general sense of coping with the cancer in the context of one's life. Advice books are available and provide another medium for cancer survivors to enhance their knowledge and coping. *A Cancer Survivor's Almanac* is a good example of a handbook on coping.

Newsletters from cancer organizations and cancer centers provide updates on new cancer treatments, treatments for side effects, and personal experiences of others. Cancer-related magazines are a unique type of resource. Since the magazine *Coping* was introduced in the 1980s, it has been the model for other cancer periodicals. *Coping* provides a balanced combination of timely news and person-

TABLE 1

Print Materials

RECENT BOOKS ABOUT CANCER

- *A breast cancer journey: Your personal guidebook.* (2000). Atlanta, GA: American Cancer Society.
- *American Cancer Society's guide to complementary and alternative cancer methods.* (2000) Atlanta, GA: American Cancer Society.
- Bast, R. C., Kufe, D. W., Pollock, R., Weichselbaum, R. R., Holland, J. F., and Frei, E. (2000). *Cancer medicine (5th Ed.).* Atlanta, GA: American Cancer Society and Toronto: B. C. Decker.
- Bostwick, D. G., MacLennan, G. T., & Larson, T. R. (1999). *Prostate cancer: What every man— and his family—needs to know (Rev. Ed.).* New York: Villard.
- Hamilton, S., & Benet, L. (1999). *Landing it : My life on and off the ice.* New York: Kensington.
- Hoffman, B. (1998). *A cancer survivor's almanac.* Minneapolis, MN: Chronimed Publishing.
- Houts, P., and Bucher, J. (2000). Caregiving: A step-by-step guide for caring for the person with cancer at home. Atlanta, GA: American Cancer Society.
- Keene, N., & Lamb, L. (1999). *Childhood leukemia : A guide for families, friends & caregivers* (patient-centered guides). Sebastopol, CA: O'Reilly & Associates.
- Lenhard, R. E., Osteen, R. T., & Gansler, T. S. (2001). *Clinical oncology.* Atlanta, GA: American Cancer Society.
- Levin, B. (1999). *Colorectal cancer: A thorough and compassionate resource for patients and their families.* New York: Villard.
- Murphy, G. P., Morris, L. B., & Lange, D. (1997). *Informed decisions: The complete book of cancer diagnosis, treatment, and recovery.* New York: Viking Press.
- Runowicz, C. D., Petrek, J. A., & Gansler, T. S. (1999). *Women and cancer: A thorough and compassionate resource for patients and their families.* New York: Villard.
- Schimmel, S. (1999).*Cancer talk: Voices of hope and endurance from 'the Group Room,' the world's largest cancer support group.* New York: Broadway Books.
- Spingarn, N. D. (1999). *The new cancer survivors: Living with grace, fighting with spirit.* Baltimore: Johns Hopkins University Press.
- Wilkes, G. M., Ades, T. B., & Krakoff, I. (2000). *Patient education guide to oncology drugs.* Toronto: Jones & Bartlett.

MAGAZINES

- *Cancer & You,* P.O. Box 1605, Royal Oak, MI 48068; Phone: 800-746-0355; www.cancerandyou.com.
- *Coping,* P.O. Box 682268, 377 Riverside Dr., Suite 111B, Franklin, TN 37068-2268; Phone: 615-790-2400; Fax: 615-794-0179; e-mail: copingmag@aol.com.
- *InTouch,* 48 South Service Road, Suite 310, Melville, NY 11747; Phone: 631-777-3800; e-mail: intouch@cancernetwork.com.
- MAMM Magazine, 349 West 12th Street, New York, NY 10014; Phone: 888-901-MAMM; www.mamm.com.

NEWSLETTERS

- *Blood & Marrow Transplant Newsletter* (formerly BMT Newsletter), 2900 Skokie Valley Road, Suite B, Highland Park, IL 60035; Phone: 847-433-3313, toll-free: 888-597-7674; Fax: 847-433-4599; www.bmtnews.org.
- *NABCO News,* National Alliance of Breast Cancer Organizations, New York, NY. 9 East 37th Street, 10th Floor, New York, NY, 10016; Phone: 212-889-0606, toll-free: 888-80-NABCO; Fax: 212-689-1213; www.nabco.org.

al interest stories which are helpful to cancer survivors. There is information about new treatments, about coping with specific struggles in cancer from sexuality to talking to children. There are celebrity stories, which are told in a non-exploitive manner. There are resource listings of specific cancer organizations and resources, which are constantly updated. Other magazines have a different focus. The magazine *MAMM* focuses on breast cancer with a sophisticated approach, which is directed at women. The newsletters of the National Alliance of Breast Cancer Organizations (NABCO) and the *Blood & Marrow Transplant Newsletter* are excellent examples of the written communication tool. Medical journals provide a source of the latest treatment information, but the technical language makes these a less preferred resource for cancer survivors. Medical journals are usually only available in medical libraries connected with medical schools or teaching hospitals and may limit access to health care professionals. Many medical journals are now making at least their abstracts available online. Searchable databases, such as Medline and Cancerlit, also provide online access to journal article titles and abstracts.

Other print resources are readily available. Booklets on specific cancers and their treatments are available from the ACS and other cancer organizations, usually free of charge. Many cancer centers order stocks of these helpful booklets (such as "Nutrition for the Person with Cancer" and "Understanding Chemotherapy") and make them available in treatment areas or in packets of information given at the initiation of treatment. Public libraries and cancer center resource centers or wellness communities (community-based cancer support programs) have many of the cancer resource books and personal experience books available. The cancer-specific libraries in cancer centers and wellness communities may be staffed by volunteers with library experience or resource professionals while public libraries have professional librarians willing to find appropriate materials in their holdings. The key issue in print material on cancer is currency since treatment advances change the treatment options and psychosocial resources. For the cancer survivor, convenience of these resources is essential. Having books, booklets, and newsletters specific to their experience available where they receive treatment and support and with the assistance of knowledgeable resource professionals conserves their energy for other needs, especially during the crisis at the beginning of cancer treatment.

VIDEO AND AUDIO MATERIALS

Audiotapes have become an important resource for cancer survivors. These provide an adjunct to print material in the form of personal stories, training in relaxation and imagery, and patient education material. The most significant audiotapes recently developed are the "Cancer Survival Toolbox®" created by the National Coalition for Cancer Survivorship, the Association of Oncology Social Work (AOSW), and the Oncology Nursing Society. This tool provides a set of audiotapes, which are low key discussions about the skills needed to cope with cancer. This comprehensive program has a leader's manual to use with the tapes in the context of a support or education group. Relaxation tapes are another significant audio resource. These are designed to be used in teaching the survivor guided imagery, progressive relaxation, or affirmations to enhance coping with cancer. A popular set of tapes are by Belleruth Naperstak who has developed a series called "Health Journeys" including a general tape on cancer and one specific to chemotherapy. Audiotapes of patient stories can be actual books-on-tape or briefer examples of coping with cancer.

Videotapes have become popular tools to enhance coping as most homes now have VCRs and cancer centers have VCRs available in group rooms and waiting rooms. Videotapes follow a similar pattern to print and audio medium; however, some unique resources are available. For instance, two resources to help parents help their children deal with their cancer are available (see Table 2). Videos on relaxation have the additional advantage of presenting calming scenes of nature. Videos have been underutilized as a resource because of their production costs and limited distribution. Most successful videos are produced and distributed in partnership with industry, particularly the pharmaceutical companies.

It should be noted that audio and video are increasingly becoming available over the Internet. This, combined with the availability of digital cameras, will reduce production costs and enhance distribution. To date, there are only a few examples of information for people with cancer on CD-ROM, such as the *Breast Cancer Lighthouse* (Gold Standard Multimedia Inc. and Michigan State University, 1999) and *Easing Cancer Pain* (Karen Ogle, Michigan State University,

TABLE 2

Audiotapes and Videotapes

TITLE	SUMMARY	SOURCE/LENGTH
Cancer Survival Toolbox®	Audio: A series of nine programs For learning self-advocacy skills	National Coalition for Cancer Survivorship, 1998, 30 minutes per program
Getting Well Again with Carl Simonton	Video: Chemotherapy guided imagery. Nature scenes and affirmations	SmithKline Beecham Oncology 35 minutes, 1996
Kids Tell Kids What It Is Like When a Family Member has Cancer	Video in two parts: 1) Teen sibling whose brother has a brain tumor. Goes to camp. 2) Interviews with 6 children whose parents have cancer	Pharmacia & Upjohn and Cancervive, 1998 30 minutes
Coping with Workplace Issues: A Guide for Cancer Patients and Their Families	Video: Social worker, physician, nurse, and attorney talk about return to work	Cerenex Pharmaceuticals (Glaxo), 1993, 20 minutes
Helping to Control Cancer Pain	Video: Encourages patients to report pain and addresses fears and questions from caregivers	Purdue Frederick 1994, 20 minutes
Claiming Our Lives, Telling Our Stories	Video: Lesbians with cancer tell about their own experiences	ACS, Minnesota Division, 1998 22 minutes
Patient to Patient: Cancer Clinical Trials and You	Video: Discussion of clinical trials in lay language by patients	National Cancer Institute 1998, 14 minutes
On with Life: Practical Information on Living with Metastatic Breast Cancer	Video: Includes treatment options and stories of cancer survivors	National Alliance of Breast Cancer Organizations and Chiron Therapeutics, 1996, 30 minutes
Talking About Your Cancer: A Parent's Guide to Helping Children Cope	Video for parents on talking to their children about their cancer	Fox Chase Cancer Center, 1996, 18 Minutes
My Mom Has Breast Cancer: A Guide for Families	Video: Psychologist presents information and interviews with children	KidsCope 1996, 33 minutes
Hear How I Feel	Video: Young adults talk about their parents' cancer	Northeastern Ontario Regional Cancer Center, 1996, 30 minutes
Recognizing the Impact of Anemia-Related Fatigue in Oncology Patients	Video: A self-learning program for case managers	Oncology Nursing Society. Parsippany, NJ: Ortho Biotech, Inc., 1998
Health Journeys for People Undergoing Chemotherapy	Audio: one of a series of tapes on using guided imagery and affirmations	Belleruth Naparstek, Health Journeys, 1994

2000, http://commtechlab.msu.edu/products/index.html). It could be that reference material or interactive games or tools are not suited to the cancer survivor who often prefers the immediacy and currency of the Internet.

TELEPHONE RESOURCES AND TELECONFERENCING

There are several types of telephone resources available, such as one-to-one telephone sessions for the provision of information and referral along with counseling, telephone support groups, telephone education programs, and teleconferencing. In all these methods, the telephone offers a combination of intimacy and safety, and mutual support systems for people isolated by illness or circumstances. It is also attractive to those who may not be comfortable with a more traditional group format, while at the same time, relieving distress as face-to-face groups do. Additionally, the telephone creates an informal atmosphere with participants reporting that they enjoy the anonymity and the relief of not worrying about their appearance. These groups provide continuity in the face of hospitalization, while offering socialization and networking between meetings that provides relief to caregivers.

Disadvantages of telephone groups are the difficulties for the social work leader who cannot take cues from face-to-face contact, and can also overestimate the physical abilities of the participants. Social work leaders report that their level of attention must be very high at all times when leading a telephone support group, and that their traditional methods of involving group members must be adjusted to the telephone format. However, they report high levels of satisfaction with the format, based on their ability to reach people who would have been unable or reluctant to participate in a group. Patient members in telephone groups offered by Cancer Care, Inc., a national non-profit social service organization, report satisfaction in evaluations, saying "We're not inhibited by sitting in a room looking at one another," and reporting that "we like the openness" (Colon, 1996).

Telephones are also a valuable way to provide education to a patient population that is offered choices and expected to manage complicated treatments on their own. With access available to anyone with a phone, telephone education programs can reach large numbers of people in geographically diverse areas. Many of the participants would not have the opportunity to hear organized presentations with up-to-date information on a variety of subjects, including disease overviews, symptom management, and coping skills. Participants in these programs cite the sense of community that comes from listening with hundreds of others, and the chance to learn in the comfortable environment of home without distraction (Glajchen & Moul, 1996).

There are three main resources available by toll-free numbers for cancer survivors: the National Cancer Institute's (NCI) Cancer Information Service, the ACS's toll-free number, and Cancer Care's telephone counseling line. The first two provide information on cancer and its treatment and offer free booklets on various types of cancer. The NCI Cancer Information Service also provides information on cancer clinical trials through its PDQ database. The ACS also provides information regarding programs, services, and local resources. Cancer Care provides the offer of free information on cancer and coping with cancer but also, as the name implies, counseling for the emotional aspects of cancer. In addition, Cancer Care provides referrals to local resources to meet a variety of medical, financial, and emotional needs including referrals to local support groups (see Table 3).

Cancer Care, Inc. of New York City has developed this resource most extensively. Now national teleconferences occur on a weekly basis on a variety of topics, from medical updates on specific types of cancer to coping with different aspects of the cancer experience. Their standard format is to have one or two speakers present on a topic for the first half-hour and then open the phone lines for a question and answer period. The success of this program is evident: 200–600 persons attend these teleconferences, and some-

---

TABLE 3

Telephone Resources

American Cancer Society: 1-800-ACS-2345

Brain Tumor Information Line: 1-800-934-CURE

Cancer Care, Inc.'s Cancer Counseling Line: 1-800-813-HOPE (4673)

(includes information about teleconferences)

National Cancer Institute's Cancer Information Service: 1-800-4-CANCER

Y-ME National Breast Cancer Organization: 1-800-221-4141

---

times, even support groups at cancer centers attend via speaker-phones. One reason for the success is active partnerships with cancer-specific organizations, pharmaceutical sponsors, and cancer centers. Chai Lifeline (www.chailifeline.org), an organization supporting parents of children with cancer, has begun a similar program.

Teleconferencing can be utilized in other formats as well. For instance, virtual support groups can utilize teleconferencing to connect patients with similar diagnoses or situations.

The technology for videoteleconferencing is available at low cost for use over regular phone lines. In the future, more virtual meetings of cancer survivors can occur this way. Videoteleconferencing is also available through the Internet, which has yet to be capitalized on by the cancer community.

RADIO AND TELEVISION

Mass media is the least frequent mode of access to cancer information and support. Occasionally the major networks will present the story of a cancer survivor. News stories of new cancer treatments afford some information about treatment. This includes some important evening news programs, which can examine cancer in more depth. It should be noted from a historical perspective that the concept of The March: Coming Together to Conquer Cancer™ in 1998 was initiated as a result of celebrity cancer survivors appearing on *Larry King Live*, the CNN interview program. And the Relay for Life, National Cancer Survivor's Day®, and Race for the Cure® events provide some coverage to destigmatize the cancer experience and promote a sense of solidarity for viewers. Rarely, a cancer center might air a show on cancer to a local market. One of the only shows in either media that has weekly national exposure is The Group Room®, a radio call-in show from Los Angeles (www.premrad.com/talk/group.html). This show takes calls from cancer survivors and their families, which are screened by social workers and responded to by psychologists and physicians. In this way, the quality and integrity of the show is preserved while providing a unique service. Overall, radio and television are underutilized as a communication tool for cancer. Perhaps as the expense of producing such programs decreases and cable access programming becomes more prevalent, cancer centers and wellness communities can provide more programming. Internet radio may provide more opportunities for these specialized programs in the future. Coalitions of national cancer organizations could provide national programming which would focus on detection, treatment, and survivorship. Radio talk shows, a popular medium for many today, could be exploited to better serve the cancer community.

THE INTERNET

The fastest growing source of information and support for cancer patients is the Internet, which is being used more and more to provide psychosocial services (Pergament, Pergament, Wonderlick, & Fiddler, 1999). As the cancer survivors' movement expanded and the Internet became available and popular for public use and computers became faster, cancer organizations exploited this new tool. On the World Wide Web, Oncolink of the University of Pennsylvania Cancer Center became one of the first comprehensive cancer sites on the Internet and became the prototype for others. From the beginning it included basic cancer information, stories of survivors, news about new treatments, information about alternative treatments, and links to other cancer-related Web sites. Since its inception in 1994, many other Web sites have followed this model and provided a similarly broad range of information and support on specific cancers or to specific segments of the cancer community.

At the same time, the growth of the Internet created problems for the cancer community. Timeliness of information is key to finding appropriate treatment information. Some cancer sites and even cancer centers failed to update their cancer information on a regular basis (Biermann, Golladay, Greenfield, & Baker, 1999). As a result, accuracy of survival statistics and current treatment protocols was compromised. In addition, information about alternative and complementary treatments including the ability to order vitamins and other substances over the Internet exploded. Unsubstantiated health claims could be distributed to a large audience quickly resulting in a boost to these treatments and, in some cases, undermining or questioning traditional medical care. Some cancer survivors, so desperate for a cure, spend hours and days on the Internet searching for some glimmer of hope, doing so without a critical eye. Newer users of the Internet may be deceived or confused by the fact that Web site looks professional and appears to represent a valid medical viewpoint simply because it is on the Internet (Markman, 1998).

Oncology social workers can help their patients navigate the Internet, and seek credible sources of information and support (Sikorski & Peter, 1997). Reputable indexes of complementary and alternative medical sites on the Internet are more recently available along with documents which caution the user and help the layperson to evaluate these treatments (see Table 4). Oncology social workers need to know at least the basics of the Internet and reliable sources of information in order to guide cancer survivors to helpful information and teach their patients healthy skepticism of what they read. Urgency for cancer information should be redirected to trust in their medical team, a healthy lifestyle, and finding supportive environments during and after treatment which can enhance a sense of hope (Sharp, 1999).

TABLE 4

Internet Resources

EXAMPLES OF HIGHLY RELIABLE CANCER WEB SITES

GENERAL CANCER INFORMATION
National Cancer Institute - CancerNet	www.cancer.gov
American Cancer Society	www.cancer.org
Oncolink - University of Pennsylvania Cancer Center	www.oncolink.com
Cancer Care, Inc.	www.cancercare.org
National Coalition for Cancer Survivorship	www.cansearch.org

SAMPLING OF SITES BY CANCER TYPE
National Alliance of Breast Cancer Organizations	www.nabco.org
Prostate Cancer Infolink	www.comed.com/prostate
Leukemia & Lymphoma Society	www.leukemia.org
National Brain Tumor Foundation	www.braintumor.org
Support for People with Head and Neck Cancer, Inc.	www.spohnc.org

SOURCES OF INFORMATION ON NEW TREATMENTS
NCI Clinical Trials	www.cancertrials.nci.nih.gov
American Society of Clinical Oncology	www.asco.org
Cancer Care: Teleconference audio files	www.cancercare.org/audio/teleconferences.htm
Cancer News	www.cancernews.com

COMPLEMENTARY AND ALTERNATIVE MEDICINE (CAM) WEB SITES
National Center for Complementary and Alternative Medicine at the National Institutes of Health	nccam.nih.gov
Oncolink: Complementary Treatments	www.oncolink.com/specialty/complementary
Health Journeys	www.healthjourneys.com
American Cancer Society	www.cancer.org/ and search on alternative
Quackwatch	www.quackwatch.com

SEARCH ENGINES FOR CANCER INFORMATION
Yahoo	www.yahoo.com/health/diseases_and_conditions/cancers
Infoseek Cancer News	infoseek.go.com/webdir/health/diseases_and_ ailments/A_D/cancer
Web MD	www.webmd.com
The Mining Company: Cancer Index	cancer.miningco.com

STATEMENTS ON RELIABILITY OF HEALTH INFORMATION ON THE INTERNET
Oncolink: Source Reliability Issues	www.oncolink.com/resources/reliability
Health on the Net Foundation	www.hon.ch/HONcode/
Internet Health Care Coalition	www.ihc.net/about/mission.html
Association of Cancer Online Resources	www.acor.org/about/mission.html

TABLE 4 (continued)

EXAMPLES OF CANCER LISTSERVS
ALL-L Acute Lymphocytic Leukemia General List
BC-SUPPORTERS: Support List for Husbands of Breast Cancer Patients
CANCER-PAIN: PAIN Associated with Cancer and Cancer Treatments
KIDNEY-ONC The Kidney Cancer Online Support Group
LYMPHEDEMA: The LYMPHEDEMA Online Support Group
PED-ONC: The Pediatric Cancers Online Support Group
SARCOMA: The Sarcoma (Cancer) Online Support Group
TC-NET: The Testicular Cancer Online Support Group

EXAMPLES OF INTERNET COMMUNICATION TOOLS FOR CANCER SUPPORT

Listserv	Association of Cancer Online Resources www.acor.org
Web Forum	Cancer Survivors' Network www.acscsn.org
Private Online Support Groups	Cancer Care, Inc. www.cancercare.org
Ask the Expert or Doctor	BMT Information www.bmtinfo.org/bmt/common/htm/home.htm Americas Doctor www.americasdoctor.com
Personal Stories	Cancer Survivor's Network www.acscsn.org Oncolink www.oncolink.com International Myeloma Foundation www.myeloma.org
Chat Rooms	OncoChat (IRC) www.oncochat.org

Each Internet tool provides a different avenue for cancer resources. The Web sites have traditionally provided information previously available in paper documents. Everything from what to expect from chemotherapy to how to talk to one's children about cancer are at hand. The advantage here is that the need for keeping a library or brochure rack in the cancer center has diminished. The social worker can now point the cancer patient to a Web site address that may specifically address their needs. For instance, a breast center could provide a large package of materials to a newly diagnosed patient including treatment options, reconstruction alternatives, surviving side effects like lymphedema, coping with breast cancer and a listing of local support groups. The exact same information could be available on the breast center's Web site with links to information from the ACS, NCI, and NABCO. The social worker could guide the patient and family through the main features of the Web site while in the clinic area. Once at home, they could select documents to read or print out, follow hyperlinks if they want more information and return to the information several times by bookmarking it in their browser.

Web sites can offer more dynamic features that enhance access to information and support (Sharp, 2000). They also offer search features to help the user find more specific information. For example, if the cancer survivor has been offered interferon as a treatment, she or he may want to search within a **reputable** Web site to gain more information on the effectiveness and side effects of interferon. Or one might search for how others have used their spirituality to cope with cancer. Another dynamic feature is interactivity. This can take several forms including:

- web forums,
- registering for updates or additional information,
- completing surveys or health screening forms,
- requesting more information about a specific topic,
- requesting a match with another survivor for peer support,
- registering to be contacted about clinical trials, and
- audio and video programs.

Web forums are pages where users of the Web site can post a message, often a question, to which other users can add their comments, such as the Cancer Survivor's Network (www.acscsn.org). Many sites offer the opportunity to register for access to special areas and/or to receive regular updates when new information is posted to the Web site (e.g., www.healthjourneys.com). Surveys provide feedback to the web master in enhancing the Web site and health screenings offer a quick way to evaluate health risks, such as risks for hereditary cancers.

Many Web sites now have a "Contact Us" button, a form in which cancer patients can ask questions from cancer experts or cancer centers when the user cannot find the information they need on the Web site. A few Web sites, such as the Support for People with Head and Neck Cancer (www.spohnc.org), offer survivor-to-survivor matching to enhance support. A few places on the Internet give users not only the opportunity to search for clinical trials by disease, treatment, and location, but also allow patients to register and give some information about their disease and health status in order to be contacted by centers doing clinical trials (www.centerwatch.com). Finally, audio and video clips including lectures on cancer treatments (www.asco.org), presentations at survivor conferences (www.oncolink.com) and individual patient stories (www.acscsn.org) all enhance the sense of personal interaction on a Web site.

E-mail will continue to be the most common interactional tool on the Internet. Anyone with e-mail can join Internet discussion groups for cancer through a tool called a listserv. These allow subscribers to interact by sending e-mail questions and comments to a common email address, which then distributes it to all the subscribers. There are more than 70 such cancer groups currently, and these will continue to grow as communities of cancer survivors find the need and desire to utilize this resource. For rare or uncommon cancers, such as sarcoma or kidney cancer, these listservs provide the connection for patients internationally who may not have met another person with their type of cancer at their own treatment center. Two Web sites provide the opportunity to subscribe to a number of these lists: Oncolink (www.oncolink.com/forms/listserv.html) and ACOR, the Association of Cancer Online Resources (http://listserv.acor.org/archives/index.html). In some cases you can subscribe from the specific organization sponsoring the listserv, for instance, www.comed.com/prostate for a prostate cancer listserv. These listservs are usually moderated by an oncology professional or survivor in order to screen subscribers and monitor what is being said.

Unsubstantiated claims may be distributed or the moderator can screen these; many of the groups have sophisticated, long-term survivors who will challenge treatment claims and thereby keep the information on the listserv more reliable. These discussion groups tend to take on unique characteristics, for instance, some breast cancer groups may talk more about their daughters, others may be more focused on new experimental treatments or, in the case of bone marrow transplants, compare notes on the phases of treatment. Usually, there are long-term members of the group who are more active in the discussions and provide a welcoming atmosphere and assist new members in getting their questions answered. Overall, listservs allow the user to read and respond to messages at their convenience with a level of anonymity unless the subscriber reveals more about himself or herself. One caution: the more active cancer listservs with hundreds of members can generate dozens of messages a day, which can become a burden rather than a help to the patient. Oncology social workers should caution cancer survivors about the possible information overload from the Internet and the need to pace oneself.

Other Internet tools include chat rooms and private support groups. Chat rooms are now likely to be Web sites, which allow real time interaction, much like a live support group. More popular among teens and young adults, the chat may be scheduled so that an adequate number of users can be online simultaneously to discuss cancer and coping, usually in short sentences. Some chat rooms require the downloading of additional software such as www.oncochat.org.

Chat rooms tend to be more spontaneous since these are live interactions. Chats can also be scheduled with cancer experts who either have a transcriber responding to questions during the chats or who type the responses themselves. Health Care portal sites like www.americansdoctor.com sponsor these types of chats on a variety of medical topics on a daily basis but only occasionally sponsor a cancer-related chat. Private email support groups are more like closed-membership support groups. These are sponsored by organizations, which have staff who can interview participants prior to beginning the group. The group can be run by chat or e-mail and is usually time-limited. Only the other members of the group have access to the chat or email forum. This kind of group can bring together people from wide geographic areas and provide an additional sense of privacy for the members (see www.cancercare.org/services/online3.htm).

One of the main limitations of the Internet as a resource is that it is not accessible to all. While a growing number of households have computers and access to the Internet, African Americans and other people of color are underrepresented as Internet users. Also, those with lower incomes are less likely to own a computer or have access to the Internet. There are three alternatives for Internet access: public libraries, wellness communities, and cancer centers. Most public libraries now have computers with Internet access. There are often time restrictions and possibly printing restrictions that can create barriers to use; however, librarians are increasingly savvy about web resources and can be helpful to cancer survivors and their families in searching the web. Wellness communities are now available in most large cities and most have resource centers, which include Internet-connected computers. Volunteer and paid staff can be helpful with Internet resources. Many wellness communities have their own Web sites, which assist in finding appropriate cancer resources (www.wellness-community.org).

In conclusion, the Internet is a vast network of tools and resources for cancer survivors. The main drawbacks of using the Internet are information overload, reliability problems, and the lack of universal access. Oncology social workers should have as part of their skill set the ability to guide cancer survivors to appropriate starting points on the Internet and help survivors avoid these pitfalls.

ONCOLOGY SOCIAL WORK RESOURCES

Social workers need access to specific training resources, which are increasingly available. These resources follow those mentioned above for cancer survivors. There is a growing library of books on counseling appropriate for oncology social workers, such as *Helping Cancer Patients*

Cope and *Group Therapy for Cancer Patients*. There is also an array of journals available including the *Journal of Psychosocial Oncology, Cancer Practice*, and *Psychooncology*. Audio and videotapes are becoming available in conjunction with specific programs, such as the caregiver program hosted by Oncolink, "Strength for Caring: An Educational Program for Family Cancer Caregivers" (http://cancer.med.upenn. edu/psychosocial/caregivers/sfc/home.html), and the NCI's "Cancer Clinical Trials Education Program." Web sites for professional organizations provide some important resources (www.aosw.org), as do listservs. The AOSW and the Association for Pediatric Oncology Social Workers (www.aposw.org) both provide listservs for their members. In the future there will be more resources available to support the work of oncology social workers. This will come from a mixture of government support primarily through the NCI, professional organizations, like AOSW, cancer organizations like the ACS and the Leukemia and Lymphoma Society, and from oncology related businesses, such as Orthobiotech's fatigue and family caregiver initiative.

SUMMARY

The sheer quantity of resources for cancer survivors will only continue to grow. The key role for oncology social workers is to guide cancer survivors in finding their way through the maze of information available. More research is needed to evaluate the most effective combination of resource tools for cancer survivors. Each approach needs to be individualized. Some cancer survivors may have a higher threshold for information glut. Getting the right resources at the right time is the most helpful approach. This means getting treatment decision resources early in the cancer experience and coping with long-term side effect resources later in the cancer journey. In the future, technology may help to customize resources for each cancer survivor based on literacy level, language, need for coping, or informational resources and what resources are most useful for their personality and comfort level. Customized web pages and Internet push technology are two possibilities for the future.

Customized Web pages, available through Web portals, allow the user to customize the appearance of the page that first comes up when they connect to the Internet. Some organizations are doing this for other diseases already. This would include an area for cancer news, coping resources, a search for their specific type of cancer from medical abstracts, a calendar of cancer events (local and national), information on clinical trials, and a link to their email messages from a listserv. Push technology is simply pushing information down to users through the Internet. This could be through a customized Web page, through a scrolling marquee or email updates that could be about new treatments or other cancer-related news. More universal access to the Internet, telephone, and other resources in the future must reach underserved populations. With computers or phones in community cancer centers, those receiving treatment would be more likely to gain this access. Others who can be left out of this information boom are those with hearing or sight impairments. Social workers should advocate for resources being accessible to these groups through books on tape, Web pages that can use screen-to-voice technology, and other creative approaches. Finally, in order for social workers to assist their patients in accessing these technology-based resources, they must have access and training themselves. Training in the use of technology needs to begin in college and graduate programs and continue through educational programs at regional and national conferences, such as the AOSW. Only then will oncology social workers meet this challenge and provide maximum benefit to their patients.

REFERENCES

Biermann, J. S., Golladay, G. J., Greenfield, M. L., & Baker, L. H. (1999). Evaluation of cancer information on the Internet. *Cancer, 86,* 381-390.

Colon, Y. (1996). Telephone support groups: A non-traditional approach to reaching underserved cancer patients. *Cancer Practice, 4(3),* 156-159.

Glajchen, M., & Moul, J. (1996). Teleconferencing as a method of educating men about managing advanced prostate cancer and pain. *Journal of*

Psychosocial Oncology, 14(2), 73-87.

Markman, M. (1998). Cancer information and the Internet: Benefits and risks. *Cleveland Clinic Journal of Medicine, 65*, 274-276.

Pergament, J. D., Pergament, E., Wonderlick, A., & Fiddler, M. (1999). At the crossroads: The intersection of the Internet and clinical oncology. *Oncology, 13(4)*, 577-583.

Sharp, J. (1999). The Internet: Changing the way cancer survivors obtain information. *Cancer Practice, 7*, 266-269.

Sharp, J. (2000). The Internet: Changing the way cancer survivors receive support. *Cancer Practice, 8*, 145-147.

Sikorski, R., & Peter, R. (1997). Oncology asap: Where to find reliable cancer information on the Internet. *Journal of the American Medical Association, 277(18)*, 1431-1432.

CANCER IN THE FAMILY: UNDERSTANDING AND USING SUPPORT SERVICES

Joan F. Hermann, MSW, LSW

Director, Social Work Services
Fox Chase Cancer Center
Philadelphia, Pennsylvania

The American Cancer Society is committed to a comprehensive approach to the management of cancer. This appendix is included in *Social Work in Oncology: Supporting Survivors, Families, and Caregivers*, and it is written specifically for patients, their families, and friends. Its purpose is to help you to understand psychosocial support services and how they may be useful to you or to members of your family.

Cancer is a very complicated disease and requires the help of a variety of specialists in managing it. Just as you or other family members have probably needed the services of a surgeon, medical oncologist, or radiation oncologist, there may be times during your experience with cancer that psychosocial support services may be helpful. By psychosocial support services, we mean those services that will help you to cope with the emotional and practical problems that can occur in dealing with a chronic illness. Cancer is often called a "family disease" because it affects more than the person who is diagnosed. Patients and their families have a powerful influence on how each deals with cancer diagnosis and treatment. It is not possible for patients and those important to them to act in isolation from each other and in fact, to try to usually makes the situation even more complicated. Cancer is no longer an inevitably fatal disease; many types are curable and most are treatable, enabling patients to live many long and fulfilling years after their diagnosis. Psychosocial support services may enhance the quality of your life and help you with whatever difficulties and special challenges you may be encountering in dealing with cancer.

WHY WOULD PEOPLE NEED PSYCHOLOGICAL HELP IN DEALING WITH CANCER?

Most people struggling with a new diagnosis feel as if this is the most serious situation they could possibly face. The word "cancer" still evokes images of death and suffering even though heart disease actually is responsible for more deaths than cancer. This rather primitive fear and anxiety that patients describe makes the emotional burden of cancer greater than for many other diseases.

A person's reaction to cancer is influenced by a number of factors. Some of these are age, culture, family beliefs about illness, finances, philosophy of life, and the nature of the cancer itself. Younger people have different struggles than older people; optimistic people may find stress easier to cope with than pessimistic people; people with financial problems may have fewer choices than those with higher incomes. So there may be factors over which you have no control that may make a cancer experience especially difficult.

A cancer diagnosis means learning a whole new body of information to understand what is happening physically and emotionally. Sometimes people forget that they already have skills that have helped them cope with other problems. The skills that have worked for you in the past can be combined with new ones that you will acquire in dealing with cancer.

Many decisions will be made in the first few weeks and months of a cancer diagnosis. In addition to learning and understanding the language of cancer, decisions will be made about where to be treated, choosing a physician, treatment options, and managing treatment side effects. In addition to the medical issues confronting you, it will be useful to learn what you can about emotional responses to cancer so you are in the best position to help you and your family. While many people cope with the cancer experience without formal counseling, most people will benefit by learning about the emotional and psychological stresses associated with having cancer and identifying strategies for themselves in how to reduce their stress. (There is no evidence that stress has anything to do with getting cancer. It also will not make cancer cells travel to other parts of the body.) Support from family, friends, and the health care team will also be important.

WHAT CAN I EXPECT FROM THE HOSPITAL WHERE I AM BEING TREATED?

The availability of support services will depend on where you are receiving your treatment. In cancer centers, university or community hospitals in urban areas, these services are likely to be available. Smaller community hospitals or those in more rural areas may not offer all types of services. In this situation, you may find the services you need from agencies in the community, private counselors, peer support programs, Internet resources, "chat rooms," or telephone support groups.

"Crisis intervention" is the term that describes most of the support services that occur in hospitals. An example is what happens when someone is first diagnosed with cancer. Patients facing a new diagnosis describe feelings of being numb or "in shock." They have trouble concentrating and absorbing medical information so that decisions can be made about treatment. Feelings of anxiety, sadness, and even panic are common. Sometimes patients are so overwhelmed by fears about the future that they have trouble focusing on the "here and now." A cancer counselor will help people absorb accurate medical information so that wise decisions about treatment can be made. They will help patients prioritize their concerns, prepare themselves for treatment, and develop a kind of roadmap to help the patient and family manage the first weeks or months of treatment.

In a large institution or cancer center which treats adults, oncology social workers are usually part of a larger team of people including doctors, nurses, rehabilitation specialists, radiation technologists, nutritionists, etc. Sometimes oncology social workers meet every patient particularly if the patient is being evaluated for a complex treatment, such as a bone marrow transplant. More typically, other members of the treatment team refer patients to oncology social workers. A referral may be made for help with the emotional impact of cancer or for more concrete or practical problems like how to get transportation services or where to buy a wig. Patients and family members may also refer themselves if they need help with family or practical problems.

The oncology social worker can also help you identify community services to which you are entitled. An example might be the Office of Vocational Rehabilitation (OVR). (The name of the agency may vary from state to state.) This office is concerned with helping people whose ability to work has been affected by illness. If cancer treatment has altered your ability to do your job, they might pay for re-training in another field. Young people who have been treated for cancer may be eligible for help with college tuition. The OVR also can help pay for medical equipment. There are a variety of community agencies from which you can receive services if your life circumstances are changed as a result of cancer.

Usually an oncology social worker will start with a "psychosocial assessment" to identify your needs and those of your family. They will want to know how you and those close to you are reacting to the illness and what difficulties you may be encountering in dealing with the situation. This does not mean they think you won't be able to cope with cancer—it is a way for you to be understood in the most comprehensive way. Health care professionals understand that cancer is a complex disease with the potential to cause significant family stress. For this reason you may want to learn what services may be useful to you. Just learning about some of the issues from people who have worked with other families dealing with cancer may be helpful. An example might be how to explain a cancer diagnosis to young children in such a way that fosters confidence and hope.

The treatment approach described above is unfortunately not the norm in all treatment centers across the country. There are many reasons for this, some having to do with the cost of such services and other having to do with attitudes about what people need to cope with illness. Experienced oncology professionals know that cancer can cause unusual stress and the more that people are prepared for the challenges that may occur, the easier it will be to avoid getting into trouble emotionally.

WHAT KIND OF SUPPORT SERVICES SHOULD I CONSIDER?

Support services for people with cancer are usually available as individual counseling, family counseling, support groups, complementary/alternative treatments, and even on the Internet, if you have access to a personal computer. Making a decision about what is best for you depends on a number of factors, such as what services are available from your hospital or community, the cost or location of these services, and what kind of insurance coverage you have. Support services in the hospital where you are being treated are usually free while community agencies or practitioners typically charge a fee. Agencies sometimes have a sliding scale meaning the charge is based on your income. In some communities, there are organizations like the "Wellness Community" or "Gilda's Club" that offer free support services to cancer patients and their families. The hospital where you are being treated should be able to direct you to these services.

Deciding what kind of help to get depends on your understanding of how your reaction to the cancer is effecting you and your family. For example, if you are a young parent and are feeling sad or depressed, it may be hard to find the energy to respond to young children. You may be feeling too preoccupied and worried to deal with all that is going on. Or you may be an older person who is finding it difficult to accept the help of your adult children in managing your illness. Talking with a counselor may help you put a new perspective on the situation and find ways to solve problems that you may not have thought of. Often, feeling more in control of your own feelings and reactions may be all it takes to help your family to get back on track. Sometimes people need to do more than one thing to begin to feel better. For example, counseling combined with an antidepressant medication may be worth a try. The point is that there are many kinds of help available—if what you are doing doesn't seem to be helping, you may need to experiment with other strategies in order to feel better. The vast majority of people are able to learn to cope with cancer.

WHAT CAN I EXPECT WITH INDIVIDUAL COUNSELING?

Individual counseling offers an opportunity for you to talk with a counselor about what is worrying you and to figure out how to tackle those worries. The counselor will first ask questions about you and your family and what, in particular, you are concerned about. You might find that talking about the situation puts a different perspective on things. Finding out how you have dealt with problems in the past may help you to figure out what to do next. The counselor will help you prioritize your needs so greatest needs can be addressed first. You may talk about different ways to approach the situation before deciding what to try first. It is important not to get impatient or frustrated if your first approach does not seem to be working. Problem solving is often a stop and go process—you may try out a variety of possibilities before arriving at an approach which is right for your family.

You may feel much better after one or two sessions with a counselor. While that is a good thing and probably means you have found the right person for you, it does not usually mean that your problems are all solved. It may be that what you are feeling is the relief that comes from sharing your troubles with another person. Human behavior is very complex and not easy to change. Insight into why we do the things we do is sometimes quite elusive. In addition, understanding why we may behave in a certain way does not necessarily mean we will be able to quickly change the behavior pattern. So give the counseling process adequate time in evaluating how useful it is for you.

Problem solving is a complex process and is influenced by a variety of factors. These include your feelings about the situation, personality characteristics and relationships among family members, your ability to be flexible and to try new things, and the effects of other life events. For example, if you are having problems at work, this may interfere with your ability to cope with what is going on at home. If you are experiencing difficult treatment side effects, you may have less energy to cope with a spouse's expectations.

It is easy to be critical of yourself, but when dealing with a diagnosis of cancer it may not be possible to control every thing going on in your life. Understand that you are probably doing the best you can and that it will take time to feel like yourself again. Cancer is both physically and emotionally taxing and people often underestimate the toll it can take on you and the people you care about. Do not be hesitant or afraid to seek the support you need in order for you and your family to begin to feel better.

If you decide that you would like to try counseling, you will probably find yourself talking this over with the important people in your life. Hopefully, those people will be supportive of the idea but sometimes patients are surprised to discover that this may not be so. If you are married or in a long-term relationship, your partner may be resentful and feel that your desire to get help means there is something missing in your relationship together. If you are a young adult still living at home, your parents may feel they have failed in some way. Or it may be that your family wants to be included and you would prefer to sort things out for yourself. These situations can be very stressful, as the decision to try counseling is not an easy one. People have a hard time with the notion that they cannot easily solve any problem that comes along. While this reaction is understandable, it is not necessarily logical or helpful. No one questions the fact that we are not all auto mechanics and cannot take a motor apart to see what is wrong with the car.

If you see a counselor, give it two or three sessions to decide if it is helpful. Also, you should know that services are always confidential. (The exception to this is when someone is suicidal and the counselor has an obligation to try and protect that person.) If you are seeing a counselor who is part of the medical team caring for you, talk to the counselor about what will be documented in your medical record. Usually what is documented concerns how you are dealing with the cancer and whatever else is going on which will help you cope or might make it more difficult. If you have particular worries that you do not want shared, tell your counselor.

The point is that there are many different support services available. If one is not right for you chances are something else will be. The next sections discuss other kinds of counseling that may be helpful to you and to the people you care about.

WHEN MIGHT FAMILY COUNSELING BE A BETTER OPTION?

Some professionals think that family counseling is the best way to cope with cancer because a diagnosis of cancer always affects other family members. Behaviors among family members are influenced by many things—life experiences, personality, feelings, the quality of relationships, family belief systems, the family's stage of development (composed of young, middle aged, or elderly people), cultural and racial characteristics, and finances to name a few. For instance, if a family believes that problems should not be shared with outsiders, that family would have difficulty accepting the need for counseling. If a family believes that children should be spared any exposure to the painful realities of life, that family will probably not be comfortable telling a child about a parent's diagnosis. These two belief systems can make a cancer diagnosis more difficult than it needs to be and counseling may be helpful in trying to think about a problem in a new way.

One of the ways to decide about family counseling is to look at what is going on among the people you care about. Ask yourself the following questions:

- *Can I talk to my spouse about how I feel?*
- *Is my spouse or partner able to listen to what I am saying or does it seem to be too painful for them?*
- *Does it help to talk to the important people in my life when things are going badly?*
- *Do my partner and I always end up in a fight about how we expect each other to be reacting?*
- *Do my children seem more worried, sad, or lonely than before the cancer?*
- *Do they tell me how they feel?*
- *Are my children misbehaving more than usual?*
- *Do we seem unable to enjoy being together as a family?*
- *Are we fighting among ourselves more often?*
- *Are my children backsliding in their development? (For example, having more difficulty separating from you, maintaining toilet training, being unable to play by themselves, or being unusually dependent on you.)*
- *Is my family able to accept help from others?*
- *Do I resent it that people outside of the immediate family seem happy?*
- *Do I feel angry a lot of the time that others do not have this burden to deal with?*
- *Are my constant feelings of sadness or anxiety effecting those people I care about?*
- *Are financial or insurance problems interfering with my ability to deal with the situation?*

- *Am I or my partner less interested in sexual intimacy?*

The issues described above happen in all families, to some degree at different times in our lives. They may be more troublesome now or your attempts to change things or to feel better are not working. In the typical family with its mixture of different personalities and ways of behaving, change is often difficult. Recognizing a problem and understanding why you or family members behave in a particular way are important steps in figuring out how to get along better.

A family counselor will understand how the behavior of individuals affects the family as a whole. The problem may be the way family members communicate with one another. Or it may be a lack of understanding among family members about behaviors that are hurtful or get in the way of people receiving support from each other. Sometimes tension in a family will prevent people from understanding each other so the same hurtful behaviors continue. It is often easier for someone outside the family to help family members look at a situation differently and try new ways of behaving that may make it easier to give and to receive support.

Family counselors work in a variety of ways in how they approach helping people. Some always see whole families together; others may mix up the sessions with some devoted to the whole family and others with an individual. The nature of your problems will influence the approach used. There may be times when your worries are directly related to the experience of having cancer. There may be other times when family relationships are effected by the cancer in ways that make you unhappy. The family counselor will try to help you and your family understand what is going on and what family members need to feel better. As in any kind of counseling, the important thing is to find a counselor that you and your family trust. If that cannot be established within a reasonable time frame (a matter of 1–3 months), it may be that you need to find someone else that you feel more comfortable with.

WHEN SHOULD I CONSIDER A SUPPORT GROUP?

The purpose of a support group is to help people share their concerns with others and to learn new ways of tackling difficulties. Participants can expect to learn more about the disease itself in addition to getting new ideas from others like themselves. For instance, a newly diagnosed person who has never had to share a diagnosis with children can hear from others how children might react. A woman with breast cancer can learn from other women about breast reconstruction. Young adults can hear how others have approached problems with dating from those who have "been there."

Support groups for people with cancer can be organized in several different ways. Some meet in hospital settings, within a community agency like the American Cancer Society, a family service agency, or even in a patient's home.

Open-ended groups are set up to allow anyone with cancer or their family members to attend as many sessions as they find helpful. Or people might attend during periods when the course of the illness is changing, decisions need to be made about new treatment options, or new family concerns come up.

Closed groups are those in which the same group of people meet for a prescribed period of time, like for six or eight sessions. They can be organized for people with the same diagnosis, the same sex or age range, the same stage of disease, or by the kind of treatment people are receiving.

Groups can be organized by topic, meaning different issues will be discussed each week or they can have a free-flowing agenda where participants can discuss whatever topic they choose. Regardless of the kind of group you attend, confidentiality should be discussed by the group facilitator at your first meeting. You should feel free to discuss your concerns with others and know that what is discussed will remain confidential among group participants.

Groups can be organized by professionals or by cancer survivors. Professionals include oncology social workers or nurses, psychologists, psychiatrists, or clergy. Professionals should be licensed in their respective fields and have skills in group "facilitation." This means they will have had training in how to go about setting up a group and how to help members get their needs met. They also know how to deal with group members who tend to monopolize the conversation or with people who are so upset or angry that a group is not working. If a cancer survivor is facilitating a group, that person may or may not be able to accomplish these tasks. Some cancer survivors are very comfortable dealing with difficult behaviors and have had enough life experience to be very effective in a group setting. Others may not or may find themselves getting uncomfortable or overwhelmed by what is being discussed in the group.

People often have strong feelings about the kind of group that they want. Some will feel that only someone who has "been there" will make a good group leader. Others want a professional who might be able to offer more education about cancer or emotional issues. You might consider trying both types of groups to identify what type is right for you. Your "comfort level" is usually a good indication that you have found the right group for you. If you feel comfortable sharing your experiences and are better able to address your problems, the group will probably be helpful. If not, consider another group or another kind of counseling until you figure out what is best for you or your family.

Some people are more comfortable in groups than others. It may be easy to imagine sharing your feelings with others or it could seem like a real invasion of your privacy. There are few "rights or wrongs" about how people feel about participating in a group. Some people find them very useful at the point of diagnosis or changes in treatment because there is so much information to sort through in order to make decisions. Patients with more experience with cancer can help new patients know what to expect and how to avoid troublesome situations.

Sometimes people reject going to a support group because they think that it will be "too depressing" listening to other peoples' problems. This does happen occasionally but for the most part, patients are very good at helping a discouraged group member feel better. Everyone has down times—the trick is to figure out how to stop the negative thinking from taking over. It's all too easy to imagine the worst. Other patients have "been there" and can often offer the kind of encouragement and even 'inspiration' to keep fighting when times are tough. Sometimes new group members are surprised at how much humor is expressed in a support group. Finding something funny in a situation is a very good way of moving past a difficult time.

It may take time to determine how much of yourself to share with others. Some group members will be very talkative while others learn better just by listening. Usually, group members will gradually feel more comfortable in discussing their concerns and will get satisfaction from helping others in the group.

DOES EVERYONE BENEFIT FROM ATTENDING A SUPPORT GROUP?

Sometimes patients will experience pressure from family or friends about attending a support group. This happens because people often don't feel comfortable talking about cancer; they think that they have to say something to "fix" the problem or to help you to feel better, when really they just need to listen. The nature and seriousness of your needs will help you decide whether to try a support group. Some needs lend themselves to being addressed in a support group. Examples are the need for information, such as how children typically react to a parent's diagnosis, how to explain your diagnosis at work, or how to communicate better with your doctor. Other problems, such as severe marital or psychological problems, may seem too "private" to share with others.

The intensity of your feelings about a situation will also help you to decide about attending a group. You may feel so upset about your situation that the idea of discussing it with others makes it worse. Your own distress may make it impossible to listen to the problems of others. In fact, there may be times when the danger of feeling more overwhelmed is too great to consider joining a group.

In this kind of situation, an individual counselor can concentrate on you and help you to feel better more quickly. Once you feel less anxious or overwhelmed, you will be in a better position to benefit from a support group.

Occasionally, people dealing with serious medical problems get so desperate that they think about suicide. This is not a usual response to having cancer but can happen to people who may have other stresses in their lives in addition to the cancer. Sometimes people can feel so depressed and hopeless that they can not imagine how the situation will ever get better. If this is how you or a family member is feeling, you need immediate help. This is not the kind of situation that joining a support group will help. A psychiatrist should be consulted who can evaluate the severity of the situation and recommend medications or perhaps a short hospitalization to help the person feel more in control.

ARE THERE SUPPORT GROUPS FOR CHILDREN?

There are two groups of children who can benefit from a support group. These are children who have cancer themselves or those who have a parent or grandparent with cancer. Many pediatric cancer centers offer groups for children with cancer and their siblings. You can also call the American Cancer Society at 1-800-ACS-2345 to get information on Children with Cancer in the Family: Dealing with Diagnosis, Dealing with Treatment, and Dealing with Progressive Illness. Groups for children with a sick parent are becoming more and more common. The need for children to meet others who are in the same situation as themselves is a very real one. Cancer is different from other problems that children experience. Children who have a parent with cancer are not likely to know others with a sick parent. Divorce is very common in the world of children so they are more likely to know other children whose parents are divorced than those who have cancer. For this reason, children with a sick parent often feel very isolated and different from their peers. When they meet other children who are dealing with cancer in the family, it is very comforting to realize that others have the same worries. Some of these worries include the following:

- *Why has cancer happened to my parent?*
- *Is it something I did that made it happen?*
- *Did my parent "catch" cancer from someone else?*
- *Will my other parent get sick?*
- *Can I get cancer?*
- *How will my life change?*
- *Will my parent still be able to take care of me?*
- *Will my friends at school know about my parent's cancer?*
- *Should I talk to my friends about it?*
- *Will people treat me differently?*
- *Will my parent die?*
- *Who would take care of me if mom or dad dies?*
- *Will I still be able to do things I enjoy?*
- *Will mom or dad still do "fun things" with me?*
- *Will I have to take care of mom or dad?*

While these questions may not be asked directly, we know from experience with other families that these are questions children think about when a family is struggling with cancer. While you will not know the answers to all of these questions, especially when you or your child is first diagnosed, these are issues that need to be addressed at some point in your experience.

Support groups for children should be facilitated by professionals. People like schoolteachers or guidance counselors, art therapists, music therapists, and oncology social workers or nurses with experience with children are examples of possible group leaders. The professional should be knowledgeable about cancer and the issues it raises for families.

The success of a group for children will depend on the professional's use of play therapy or activities to involve children to address tough issues. Adults receive help by talking about a problem whereas children are less able to verbalize their feelings and worries. A professional should be experienced in getting children to open up through play, drawing, and games. A cancer survivor sometimes is able to do this if they have had experience or training in working with children in groups and know how to help children safely talk about scary feelings.

The best kind of support program for children is one that offers a corresponding group for parents. Parents are a child's best teachers and you will learn from other parents about ways to deal with your children. Parents should expect feedback from the group facilitator about their child's participation in the group and what the professional thinks about the family's needs.

Don't expect that your child will be thrilled about the idea of attending a support group. People usually resist doing something new and children are no exception. Usually, once the child experiences the support and fun a group offers, they are quite eager to participate.

Sometimes parents worry that in a support group, children will learn that people can die from cancer. Most of the time, children know this already. If a child brings this up, the group facilitators will acknowledge that people can die but that the purpose of treatment is to control, and in many cases, cure people of cancer. The emphasis should be on hope for the future. Counselors should also encourage children to talk to their parents if they are worried. The group facilitator will also be available to advise parents about how to deal with their children's fears about the future. Parents should be able to feel confidence in the professional's ability to handle this kind of situation in a way that the child ends up reassured, not frightened.

Should I Consider Complementary or Alternative Therapies?

Complementary therapies are typically those that patients utilize along with their cancer treatments. Examples might be meditation and relaxation techniques, hypnosis, massage, yoga, or changes in diet. Many centers offer "mind/body" groups in which patients are taught how to use these techniques to feel more in control of their fears about cancer or to change automatic "negative thinking" into a more positive way of approaching the cancer experience. These approaches often help people deal with the side effects of cancer treatment and thereby improve their quality of life.

Alternative treatments on the other hand, are usually thought to be those that people utilize instead of standard treatment. Examples might be drugs such as Laetrile, macrobiotic diets, or the use of vitamins, herbal remedies, or faith healers instead of medical treatment. Obviously, the medical community does not support the use of these treatments in lieu of therapy aimed at cure or control of the cancer so if patients talk to their doctors about them, the response can be a negative one. Complementary therapies are more easily accepted as they are thought not to interfere with a person's chance for survival.

There is much written in the popular press about these new or unproven cancer treatments. Some of these treatments are harmless while others can complicate or interfere with your cancer treatment. Some alternative treatments are said to be "natural" substances implying that nothing negative can result from their use. Herbal remedies are sometimes considered to be pretty benign since they're "only herbs" but in fact, there are no clear guidelines about safe dosages so patients are often on their own about how much to take. A strictly macrobiotic diet can seriously interfere with your nutritional status, and if combined with chemotherapy, cause real physical problems. So it is very important that your doctor know if you are using these remedies in the event that complications occur.

Many people are reluctant to discuss complementary or alternative treatments with their physicians because they expect they will get a negative response or jeopardize their relationship with their doctor. Actually, there is more acceptance of these treatments than ever before, especially if patients are not rejecting medical care. If you want to consider adding a complementary treatment to your standard therapy, tell your doctor and ask for his or her advice. Some patients need to do "something extra" in order to feel more in control or to cover all the bases. If this is the case, explain this to your doctor and discuss the pros and cons. Most will be understanding once they see that you are not questioning their medical competence or compromising your chances that treatment will be effective. If your doctor does not understand your need to try a complementary or alternative treatment, it is still your right, as the person in charge of your life, to use it. But we hope that you will not do anything that will interfere with conventional treatments, since they offer you the best chance of a cure or long-tem control of your disease.

The oncology social worker should be able to help you to sort out difficulties you might have with the health care team about alternative or complementary treatments. They can also help you to figure out if the alternative practitioner's credentials are legitimate, whether they practice in an accredited institution, and direct you to research about survival rates. When you hear about alternative treatments, keep in mind that, unless a treatment has been tested scientifically, there is no way to know whether it helps control cancer. Clinical trials are the only way to prove whether treatments are effective.

People sometimes turn to alternative treatments if they have a kind of cancer which is difficult to treat or if it has been established that cure is no longer possible with standard treatment. Well-meaning friends and relatives may suggest that you have nothing to lose by seeking such help. You may be quite eager to pursue this, since the idea that the disease is no longer curable may create a sense of helplessness, depression, and even panic. While these feelings are understandable, a cancer that is not being treated medically can be extremely difficult to live with. Even treatment which is considered "palliative" (to relieve suffering instead of cure), is still important to a patient's quality of life.

There are some excellent materials available to help you to

understand and evaluate complementary and alternative therapies (see list of Reading Materials). We suggest that patients and their families learn as much as possible about these treatments in order to decide if and when they could be helpful. Both the American Cancer Society (1-800-ACS-2345) and the National Cancer Institute (1-800-4-CANCER) can direct you to other sources of information.

WHAT SHOULD I LOOK FOR IN A CANCER COUNSELOR?

In addition to the counselor's education and credentials, the two other important factors to consider when choosing a counselor are a person's experience in helping people deal with cancer and how comfortable you feel with that person. People who work in cancer treatment centers tend to have more knowledge and experience with emotional responses to cancer than counselors who work outside of a medical facility. Their experience with cancer is important because it will give them a way to understand how your reactions and feelings are appropriate to your situation. For example, an experienced cancer counselor will know that a newly diagnosed patient might become depressed after treatment is completed. This is because the medical facility symbolizes safety and that the treatment is fighting against the cancer. Once the treatment is over, patients may find they are more worried than they were when they were "doing something" to control the disease. A cancer counselor will recognize that this is a normal response for many patients and can help you deal with this. If your depression is long lasting or you find that talking about your feelings is not helping, a cancer counselor might suggest a trial of an anti-depressant medication to help you get back on track. An experienced cancer counselor will be able to help you more quickly than someone who does not know what patients normally experience.

Another important factor to consider in selecting a counselor is the person's professional training or credentials. At a minimum people should have a bachelor's degree in one of the counseling fields and often, will have a master's or doctoral degree. Counselors often come from the fields of social work, psychology, psychiatry, psychiatric nursing, or pastoral counseling. While credentials will demonstrate a person's formal education in their chosen field, they ideally should be combined with their experience with cancer. You should not feel shy about checking all of this out. Professionals who are secure in their abilities know that people need to find the most knowledgeable source of help and should not be reluctant to give you this kind of information.

Sometimes people feel that unless a counselor has had cancer or "been there," that they will not be able to help. While a personal experience will certainly add a dimension to the counselor's expertise, it is important not to underestimate the value of experience with other patients and families. Even if a counselor has never had cancer, we have all experienced life crises and losses of one kind or another. Cancer counselors have usually worked with a great number of families and that experience is invaluable in learning how people cope. So a personal experience with cancer is only one criterion to consider in evaluating the suitability of the counselor.

Always consider how you feel with the person you are seeing. Does it feel safe to share your concerns with this person? Do you trust their ability to help you? Do you feel that the counselor is really able to listen to you and understand you as an individual? Do you think your family could relate easily to this person? The suitability of your relationship with a counselor may be hard to understand or describe. However, trust your instincts—if somehow you just do not feel comfortable after a few sessions, it would probably be wise to try someone else. You will know when you have found the right "match."

WILL MY INSURANCE PAY FOR COUNSELING SERVICES?

This will depend on your particular health plan and its coverage for mental health services. Most health plans have some coverage available for counseling but often, this is more limited than it is for medical services. Legislation is being considered to achieve mental health "parity" meaning an appreciation that mental health coverage is as important as coverage for physical illness. However, this is not universally accepted by the insurance industry so you may find that your coverage is inadequate for your needs. Some policies only pay for a limited number of sessions or if it is a managed care policy, it may limit your choices about who you can see. Your insurance may have "contracts" with certain mental health providers, but not with others.

If you are having trouble understanding your coverage, ask the hospital social worker to help. If counseling services are not available free of charge in the hospital where you are being treated, they can usually help you to get accurate information about your plan and what is covered. They also know about services in the community that may operate with a sliding scale adjusted to your income. The hospital billing department may also be able to examine your policy and determine your coverage.

It is important that you get the kind of help you need when you need it. You will learn a great deal about cancer as a result of having the experience. Give yourself the opportunity to learn what you might need in order to manage the impact of cancer for yourself and for those you love.

How Will I Know if Counseling is Needed?

Your feelings about what is happening to you may be a useful yardstick to use in evaluating how you are doing emotionally. In the beginning of a cancer experience, most patients go through a period of turmoil, characterized by feelings of anxiety, sadness, and fear about the future. You may have questions about why this has happened to you, the meaning of life in relation to your illness, your relationship to God, along with worries about your job, finances, insurance, and other practical matters. Gradually, as you move through the first stages of treatment, you will be dealing with these feelings and concerns and figuring out how to begin addressing them. If you have close relationships with other family members or friends, they will play a part in helping you figure out how to manage the experience. If these concerns are not addressed or you find yourself feeling very sad or preoccupied much of the time or unable to make decisions, it may help to talk with a counselor. Your goal will be to gradually feel more in control of the situation and able to devote yourself to managing your treatment along with the concerns of others in your family. Chronic feelings of hopelessness, anxiety, and fear will deprive you of the energy to cope with your current situation. Of course, if you have a history of serious depression, anxiety, or other emotional problems, it would be wise to seek out this kind of help again. Cancer can create significant stress and if you have found the counseling process helpful in the past, it will probably be so again. The advantage in talking with a professional can be to find quicker solutions to the problems you are worried about than you would by continuing to struggle on your own.

Other family members will have their own concerns as a result of your illness. If you are married or in a long-term relationship, your partner will be trying to figure out the meaning of your illness in relation to his or her own life. Sometimes couples have a very difficult time communicating about a new diagnosis. This is usually because of unspoken fears about the future and how life may be different as a result of the cancer. It is normal to want to protect the people we love from difficulty but sometimes this results in people feeling very isolated from one another. It is also to be expected that people will sometimes feel angry about what has happened but be troubled about having such feelings. Gradually people learn ways of communicating and find safe ways of expressing their concerns. If this process seems to be stuck and a patient and partner can't figure out how to meet their needs for support, it can be helpful to talk with someone outside of their relationship to gain some perspective.

These issues can feel more burdensome if you are single or you are in a relationship that was already troubled before the cancer.

Single people may need to identify other ways of getting support. Friends or extended family members may be more important during this time. Or a single person may want to seek out a cancer counselor or join a support group in order to meet others who are dealing with the same issues.

With troubled marriages or relationships, it will be important to find help so that your problems do not interfere with your ability to handle the illness. Dealing with a new cancer diagnosis along with a troubled relationship can feel quite stressful. It will be worth it in the end if you can address the issues that are causing your distress. Sometimes people worry that marital disagreements or unresolved stress will interfere with their ability to get well. There is no evidence that stress causes cancer or interferes with positive treatment results. However, it will effect your quality of life and make it harder to cope with day-to-day challenges.

WHY WOULD PEOPLE BE RELUCTANT TO SEEK HELP WITH EMOTIONAL OR FAMILY PROBLEMS?

For many people dealing with a new diagnosis, just sorting through medical decisions is an enormous challenge. They may not have the energy to cope with much more so dealing with emotional issues gets ignored or put off until later when life feels more settled. This is understandable because people can only cope with so much at one time.

One of the important concerns for people needing support services is how they feel about asking for help. People somehow have the idea that they should know how to handle every emotional problem that comes up, even though they have never been confronted with a crisis like cancer. Sometimes, people see needing help with a problem as a sign of weakness. This is not true—in fact asking for help can be a sign of strength. There is no way you can be expected to know all there is to know about coping with cancer until you have had experience with the disease. Think about what it would take to play the piano—most of us would find a piano teacher. Athletes usually get a coach in order to be really competitive. Learning about what you might expect from yourself and other family members can help you to solve problems quicker than attempting to solve them alone.

There are other reasons to ask for help early. During periods of active treatment, you may feel tired and overwhelmed with all there is to cope with physically. In addition to your physical needs, family members will have their own reactions and worries that you will need to respond to. This takes energy and you will need to preserve yours as much as possible to deal with all that is happening. If family problems are worrying you, it may be harder for you to feel in charge of the situation. Health care professionals want to help families maintain a reasonable "quality of life" in the face of cancer treatment. This means making good choices about managing the illness, preserving your hope for the future, and taking charge of the situation. What you do not want to have happen is to feel victimized by the disease or feel that the disease has taken over your life. You will always have choices about how to feel and think about the situation.

DOES MEDICATION HELP PEOPLE COPE WITH CANCER?

Feeling positive about the future helps many people with cancer get through the bad times. It also helps to enjoy life with those who are important to you. Hope is an essential ingredient in coping with cancer; if people feel hopeless, coping with cancer is very difficult. If you are feeling this way most of the time, you are probably quite depressed and anxious. An antidepressant medication may be what you need to help you get on with day to day living. Antidepressants work better if, at the same time, you are talking with someone about how you are feeling.

Talk to your family doctor or oncologist if you think you are depressed. Sometimes people are reluctant to tell their doctors about depression because they worry that somehow it will take the focus off of getting rid of the cancer. Or that they will be considered "weak" or even emotionally unstable. Doctors are very familiar with human suffering and usually go into medicine to help people. Your doctor will not think less of you if you ask for help—in fact, you are taking active steps to take control of your life. There is a wide range of drugs available and your doctor probably has had experience in using them with other patients. Some of them take a few weeks to work so be patient. Sometimes people need to try a couple different drugs to find the one right for them. If the drug does not seem to be helping, your doctor may refer you to a psychiatrist who is the specialist in using antidepressants. It may be that you need another class of drugs, need the dosage adjusted, or a combination of medications may be the answer. Of course, if you are on chemotherapy, be sure your oncologist knows if a psychiatrist has prescribed drugs for anxiety, depression, or other emotional problems. There may be some incompatibility between drugs and adjustments in the class of drug or dosage may need to be made.

Depression is sometimes the result of chemical changes in the brain related to treatment effects or chronic stress. If this is the case, there will be very little you can do to talk yourself out of it. If your depression is severe and not responding to medication, you definitely should have a psychiatric consultation. The same applies if you are having thoughts about suicide. Occasionally, people dealing with serious medical problems get so desperate that they think about suicide. This is not a usual response to having cancer but can happen to people who may have other stresses in their lives in addition to the cancer. Sometimes people can feel so depressed and hopeless that they can not imagine how the situation will ever get better. If this is how you or a family member is feeling, you need immediate help. This is not the kind of situation that joining a support group will help. A psychiatrist should be consulted who can evaluate the severity of the situation and recommend medications or perhaps a short hospitalization to help the person feel more in control. If you think seeing a psychiatrist would be helpful, ask your oncologist, nurse, or social worker to recommend someone who has experience with people with cancer.

Why Do Some People Need Help and Others Don't?

There are people who need little or no help in dealing with the experience of cancer. These people may be blessed with "good genes," supportive families, resilience in handling stress, generous incomes and insurance resources, superior flexibility and problem solving abilities, strong spirituality or relationship to a higher power, and a history of successful coping over a lifetime. If these people possess accurate information about their cancer diagnosis and treatment, they will probably never seek out counseling services.

For those people that seek or could benefit from counseling, there is a built-in barrier that many need to overcome. This barrier relates to our attitudes about asking for help. As we discussed about help with depression, for many people, the idea of getting help for emotional or family problems is not acceptable. It is thought of as a sign of weakness or even that the person is unstable or "crazy." The American culture puts a high premium on being independent and able to solve any problem that comes along. This cultural norm leads to people suffering more than is necessary when a situation like cancer presents itself. It may seem to you that some people sail through the cancer experience, never revealing any stress or difficulty dealing with a problem. So people make all kinds of judgments about themselves and say things like "what's wrong with me that I can't seem to cope with my problems?" Or, "I should be able to just 'tough it out' until the trouble passes." While we all have this tendency to feel we should be able to manage just about anything, there will be times in this experience that toughing it out just doesn't work.

A person's ability to manage stress depends on a great many things. Some of these are genetic and related to physiologic factors like the influence of hormones on our ability to feel balanced in our reactions to stress. Most people believe that babies come into the world with a predetermined set of characteristics, which are part of our genetic makeup. This "personality" that we are born with does not change a great deal as we grow but is influenced significantly by our life experiences. These life experiences influence whom we become as adults, or our "self image." Other important factors are our relationships with people, especially our parents and siblings, cultural factors, how we were educated, intelligence, relationship to God or a "higher power," career success, finances, gender or sexual identity, and our physical and mental health. So human beings are extremely complex and will vary in their ability to understand themselves and their reactions to stressful experiences.

Your understanding of the cancer itself will also influence your ability to cope. In addition to learning information about your illness and treatment, you will need to understand yourself in relation to the experience. It will take time to absorb what you need to know medically along with what you can expect of yourself and others in your family. Asking for help in understanding cancer and what to anticipate physically and emotionally is not a sign of "weakness" but instead, a smart move to prepare yourself and your family for what is to come. To struggle alone will make the experience more difficult than it needs to be. *People* **learn** *how to cope with cancer; give yourself the benefit of other people's experiences and insights so that you can approach the situation with hope in your ability to manage the illness and get on with your life.*

HOW WILL I KNOW IF COUNSELING IS WORKING?

You will know if counseling is helping you and your family by asking yourself the following questions:

- *Are you gaining more insight into the nature of your difficulty?*
- *Do you feel less anxious or worried?*
- *Is it easier to make decisions?*
- *Can you act on those decisions?*
- *Do you have a clear idea where you are going, or what needs working on immediately and what can wait until later?*
- *Are you more in control over how you are feeling and behaving?*
- *Can you put cancer aside and focus on other things?*

- *Can the counselor give you some idea of how long you will need help?*
- *Could you tell your doctor how counseling is helping?*

Your family should be asked the same questions if they are involved in the counseling sessions. If your answers to these questions seem positive, you are probably on the right track. If you do not feel good about your answers to these questions, discuss them with your counselor. If the relationship with the counselor does not feel comfortable or trusting, the sooner you address that, the better. It may be that your expectations are unrealistic, or you misunderstand the process in some way, in which case, you will need to clarify the situation in order to decide if counseling is helping. Or you may need to find someone who is a better "match" for your personality or situation. This takes work but you and your family's quality of life is well worth the effort.

READING MATERIALS

Books

American Cancer Society's Guide to Complementary and Alternative Cancer Methods. (2000). Atlanta, GA: American Cancer Society.

American Cancer Society. (2001). Cancer Support Groups: A Guide for Facilitators. Atlanta, GA: American Cancer Society.

American Cancer Society. (2000). A Breast Cancer Journey: Your Personal Guidebook. Atlanta, GA: American Cancer Society.

Bostwick, D. G., MacLennan, G. T., & Larson, T. R. (1999). Prostate Cancer: What Every Man--and His Family--Needs to Know. New York: Villard Books.

Cassileth, B. R. (1998). The Alternative Medicine Handbook. New York: W. W. Norton & Co.

Harpham, W. S. (1995). After Cancer: A Guide to Your New Life. New York: HarperPerennial.

Harpham, W. S. (1997). When a Parent Has Cancer: A Guide to Caring for Your Children. New York: Harper Collins. (Includes "Becky and the Worry Cup", an illustrated children's book that tells the story of a 7-year-old girl's experience with her mother's cancer).

Hoffman, B. (1998). *A Cancer Survivor's Almanac*. Minneapolis, MN: Chronimed Publishing.

Houts, P. S., & Bucher, J. A. (2000). *Caregiving: A Step-by-Step Resource for Caring for People with Cancer at Home*. Atlanta, GA: American Cancer Society.

Levin, B. (1999). *Colorectal Cancer: A Thorough and Compassionate Resource for Patients and their Families*. New York: Villard Books.

McCue, K. (1996). *How to Help Children Through a Parent's Serious Illness*. New York: St. Martin's Press.

Morra, M., & Potts, E. (1994). *Choices: Required Reading for Anyone Facing Cancer*. New York: Avon Books.

Moyers, B. (1993). *Healing and The Mind*. New York: Doubleday.

Murphy G. P., Morris, L. B., & Lange, D. (1997). *Informed Decisions: The Complete Book of Cancer Diagnosis, Treatment, and Recovery*. New York: Viking.

Runowicz, C. D., Petrek, J. A., & Gansler, T. S. (1999). *Women and Cancer: A Thorough and Compassionate Resource for Patients and their Families*. New York: Villard Books.

Schimmel, S. (1999) *Cancer Talk*. New York: Broadway Books.

Schover, L. R. (1997). *Sexuality and Fertility After Cancer*. New York: John Wiley & Sons.

Spingarn, N. D. (1999). *The New Cancer Survivors*. Baltimore: Johns Hopkins Press.

Wilkes, G. M., Ades, T. B., & Krakoff, I. (2000). Consumers Guide to Cancer Drugs. Boston: Jones & Bartlett.

Patient Education Materials

Available from the American Cancer Society
(Call 800-ACS-2345 for a free copy, or visit their Web site at: http://www.cancer.org)

After Diagnosis: A Guide for Patients and Families
Breast Cancer Treatment Guidelines for Patients
Caring for the Patient with Cancer at Home: A Guide for Patients and Families

Colon and Rectal Cancer Treatment Guidelines for Patients
Nutrition for the Person with Cancer: A Guide for Patients and Families
Prostate Cancer Treatment Guidelines for Patients
Sexuality and Cancer: For the Man Who has Cancer and His Partner
Sexuality and Cancer: For the Woman Who has Cancer and Her Partner
Understanding Chemotherapy: A Guide for Patients and Families
Understanding Radiation: A Guide for Patients and Families

Available from the National Cancer Institute
(Call 800-4-CANCER for a free copy, or visit their Web site at:
http://publications.nci.nih.gov)
Clinical Trials: A Blueprint for the Future
Facing Forward: A Guide for Cancer Survivors
Pain Control: A Guide for People With Cancer and Their Families
Taking Time: Support for People With Cancer and the People Who Care
About Them
Talking With Your Child About Cancer
What You Need To Know About Cancer
When Someone in Your Family Has Cancer
Young People With Cancer: A Handbook for Parents

Available from other organizations
The Cancer Survival Toolbox™: Building Tools That Work For You. Call
1-877-TOOLS–4–U. Offers free audiotapes and written material
oriented to teaching newly diagnosed patients what they need to
know in order to deal with diagnosis and treatment. It is a collabo-
rative project of the Association of Oncology Social Work, the
National Coalition for Cancer Survivorship, and the Oncology
Nursing Society. Produced with an unrestricted educational grant
from Genentech, Inc.
Hermann, J., Wojtkowiak, S., Houts, P., & Kahn, S. B. (1988).
Helping People Cope: A Guide For Families Facing Cancer. Pennsylvania
Department of Health. Call 800-722-2623 for a free copy.

Web Sites
There are multiple Web sites which can be useful to patients and

their families. Some of these will provide information about cancer and its treatment while others focus on support or advocacy services. In addition to obtaining information, it is also possible to locate an on-line support group or voice messaging system to connect with others who are dealing with cancer. While it is not possible to include an exhaustive listing, the following Web sites may be useful and direct you to others for more in-depth information. In exploring any on-line support group, patients are advised to check out the accuracy of the information you are receiving. Patients will naturally talk about their own experiences with the disease or with their treatment. Check with your physician or health care team about how this information is applicable to your situation. Remember that each person's cancer and response to treatment is different. If you are hearing information that is confusing or frightening, always check it out with your health care team.

Resources

American Cancer Society
1599 Clifton Road, NE
Atlanta, GA 30329-4251
Toll-Free: (800) ACS-2345
Internet: http://www.cancer.org

Description: The American Cancer Society provides educational material and information on cancer, maintains various patient support programs, directs people to services in their community, maintains an online daily newsmagazine, provides advocacy, and funds research. Contact the division office for your state or region to find your local office or call 800-ACS-2345.

Cancer Care, Inc.
1180 Avenue of the Americas
New York, NY 10036
Phone: (212) 221-3300
Cancer Care Counseling Line: (800) 813-HOPE
Internet: http://www.cancercare.org

Publication: *A Helping Hand: The Resource Guide for People with Cancer*

Description: Cancer Care is a non-profit social service agency that provides counseling and guidance to help cancer patients, their families, and friends cope with the impact of cancer. Cancer Care offers support groups; teleconferences for patients, friends, and family members; workshops, seminars, and clinics; a newsletter, and other publications. They also provide a financial assistance program for their local constituents in New Jersey, New York, and Connecticut. The Cancer Care Web site has detailed information on cancer, cancer treatment, clinical trials, services, and links to other cancer-related sites.

Leukemia & Lymphoma Society
600 Third Avenue
New York, NY 10016
Phone: (800) 955-4572
Internet: http://www.leukemia.org

Description: The Leukemia & Lymphoma Society is a national voluntary health agency dedicated to curing leukemia, lymphoma, Hodgkin's disease, and myeloma, and improving the quality of life of patients and their families. This organization was formerly known as the Leukemia Society of America (LSA). They offer patient service programs and resources through many local chapters.

National Cancer Institute (NCI)
Building 31, Room 10A24
9000 Rockville Pike
Bethesda, MD 20892
Cancer Information Line: (800) 4-CANCER
Cancer Fax Service: (301) 402-5874
Internet: http://www.cancer.gov

Description: The NCI provides information on cancer research, diagnosis, and treatment to patients and healthcare providers. Callers are automatically connected to the office serving their region. The service offers free publications and the opportunity to speak directly with a cancer specialist who is trained to provide accurate information on treatment and prevention of cancer and to make appropriate referrals.

National Coalition for Cancer Survivorship (NCCS)
1010 Wayne Avenue, Suite 300
Silver Spring, MD 20910
Phone: (301) 650-8868
Internet: http://www.cansearch.org
Publication: *What Cancer Patients Need to Know about Health Insurance*

Description: The (NCCS) is a network of independent organizations working in the area of cancer survivorship and support. Its primary goal is to generate a nationwide awareness of cancer survivorship. NCCS serves as an information clearinghouse and as an advocacy group. They also publish The Networker quarterly.

National Institutes of Health (NIH) National Center for Complementary and Alternative Medicine (NCCAM)
P.O. Box 8218
Silver Spring, MD 20907-8218
Phone: (888) 644-6226
Internet: http://nccam.nih.gov

Description: NCCAM evaluates alternative medicine practices to determine their effectiveness, to serve as a public information clearinghouse, and to provide a research-training program. The NCCAM facilitates and conducts research, but does not serve as a referral agency for individual practitioners or treatments.

OncoLink
University of Pennsylvania Cancer Center
Internet: http://www.oncolink.com

Description: This Web site provides information on cancer including clinical trials, support groups, educational materials, cancer screening and prevention, financial questions, and other resources for people with cancer.

ASSOCATION OF ONCOLOGY SOCIAL WORK: STANDARDS OF PRACTICE IN ONCOLOGY SOCIAL WORK

Oncology social work is the primary professional discipline that provides psychosocial services to patients, families and significant others facing the impact of a potential or actual diagnosis of cancer. The scope of oncology social work includes clinical practice, education, administration, and research. The standards of practice provided in this document are intended for clinical social workers practicing in the specialty of oncology social work.

The Masters in Social Work degree provides oncology social workers with theoretical knowledge, clinical expertise, and practical experience with patients. In addition, oncology social workers often receive specialized training in cancer care through continuing education, inservice training, and on-the-job experience.

Psychosocial services provided by oncology social workers include individual, family and group counseling, education, advocacy, discharge planning, case management, and program development. These services are designed to maximize the patient's utilization of the health care system, foster coping, and mobilize community resources in order to support optimal functioning.

Source: Reprinted with permission from the Association of Oncology Social Work, Glenview, Illinois.

Oncology social work services are available to patients and families throughout all phases of the cancer continuum, including prevention, diagnosis, survivorship, terminal care, and bereavement. Services are delivered in a wide variety of settings including specialty cancer centers, general hospitals and health systems, ambulatory centers, home health and hospice programs, community-based agencies, and private practice settings.

Oncology social workers are an integral part of the health care team and contribute to the development and coordination of the overall treatment plan. In collaboration with other disciplines, oncology social workers provide discharge planning and case management, linking patients with a variety of services necessary to meet the person's multiple needs.

In addition to services to patients and families, oncology social workers address organizational and community needs through professional practice. Services are provided to institutions, voluntary health organizations, and community agencies with the overall aim of promoting health and improving the delivery of care to individuals at risk for or affected by cancer.

STANDARDS OF PRACTICE

Standard I.
Qualifications

Oncology social workers shall be knowledgeable about oncologic diseases and their treatments, psychosocial implications for individuals and families, appropriate interventions, and available community and governmental resources. Oncology social workers must have knowledge of the usual course of cancer and its treatment so that patients and families can be helped to anticipate and deal with changes in family life.

The oncology social worker shall be masters prepared from a graduate program accredited by the Council on Social Work

Education. It is preferred that the graduate have had prior employment or field placement experience in a health care setting.

Standard II.
Services to Patients and Families

Oncology social work programs shall provide the following clinical and programmatic services:

A. Completion of a psychosocial assessment of the patient and family's response to the cancer diagnosis to include:
      1. stages in human development
      2. knowledge about cancer and its treatment including level of understanding, reactions, and expectations
      3. patient and family psychosocial functioning including strengths, coping skills, and supports
      4. characteristics of the patient's family and/or social and economic environment
      5. ethnic, spiritual, and cultural influences and concerns
      6. the source, availability, and adequacy of community resources.
B. Development of a case plan with patient and family based on mutually agreed upon goals to enhance, maintain, and promote optimal psychosocial functioning throughout cancer treatment and its outcome.
C. Utilization of a wide range of clinical interventions designed to address current and/or future problems as the patient's medical and psychosocial needs evolve.
D. Utilization of high risk screening criteria for case finding and outreach activities.
E. Development of knowledge of cancer, its treatment, and current trends.
F. Maintenance of knowledge of community resources and governmental programs available from local and national health and welfare agencies including expertise in accessing these for

patients and families.

G. Organization and facilitation of patient and family education.

H. Collaboration with other professional disciplines in the planning and provision of services to cancer patients and their families.

I. Advocacy for and protection of patients' dignity, confidentiality, rights, and access to care.

J. Development of research based knowledge that relates to clinical issues, interventions, and outcomes.

Standard III.
Services to Institutions and Agencies

Oncology social work programs shall address institutional and agency needs including the following:

A. Provision of education and consultation to other disciplines and staff regarding biopsychosocial, environmental, spiritual, and cultural factors that affect oncology care.

B. Collaboration with other disciplines and staff in the areas of comprehensive patient and family care, research, and psychosocial education.

C. Provision of services to professional caregivers which are designed to assist staff in the management of stresses inherent in clinical practice.

D. Utilization of clinical documentation, statistical reporting, and evaluation to improve services, assure quality, and develop programs.

Standard IV.
Services to the Community

Oncology social work programs shall address community needs including the following:

A. Identification of barriers to effective service delivery and participation in institutional and community responses to these problems.

B.   Provision of services to at-risk populations, including assistance with access to cancer information, screening, and treatment.

C.   Provision of consultation and volunteer services to institutions, voluntary health organizations, and community agencies to promote health, to provide education, and to develop programs to better serve the community.

Standard V.
Services to the Profession

Oncology social work programs shall address the following needs of the profession and its practitioners:

A.   Provision of the appropriate orientation, supervision, and evaluation of practitioners by clinical social workers, preferably with experience in oncology.

B.   Commitment to continuing professional education.

C.   Promotion of professional practice in accord with the National Association of Social Workers (NASW) Code of Ethics.

D.   Participation in student and professional training and education in the area of oncology social work.

E.   Contribution to oncology social work through participation in professional associations.

ASSOCIATION OF PEDIATRIC ONCOLOGY SOCIAL WORKERS: STANDARDS OF PRACTICE

Association of Pediatric
Oncology Social Workers

Pediatric Oncology Social Work as a specialty discipline is committed to enhancing the emotional and physical well-being of children with cancer and their families. Practice is based upon a unique body of knowledge and expertise in the area of developmental pediatrics and the impact of life-threatening illness on normal child development and family life. Pediatric oncology social workers are clinicians, educators, advocates, and researchers.

The Association of Pediatric Oncology Social Workers, incorporated in 1977 to advance practice, extend knowledge, and influence pediatric oncology policies and programs, endorses the following standards of practice:

Standard I: Qualifications

Pediatric oncology social workers shall be prepared with the Masters in Social Work degree (or international equivalent) from an accredited School of Social Work. The worker shall also be licensed or certified as required by the state or country in which he/she practices. Precious experience in an oncology or a pediatric medical

Source: Reprinted with permission from the Association of Pediatric Oncology Social Workers.

facility will greatly enhance the social worker's ability to work effectively with the pediatric oncology population.

Standard II: Scope of Knowledge

Pediatric oncology social workers shall possess a broad base of social work knowledge and practices specific to the practice of Pediatric Oncology. Such knowledge is obtained through formal education, post graduate training and ongoing professional development. Knowledge, key to all aspects of pediatric oncology social work, is essential in the following areas:

- An understanding of the medical, social, and family dynamics of chronic catastrophic illness and/or disability on the patient and family.
- Knowledge of medical, social, and educational resources essential to promotion of child development and adaptation to illness/treatment.
- A development understanding of loss and death and both functional and dysfunctional grief responses throughout the life cycle.
- An understanding of pediatric cancer, cancer treatment and the late effects of treatment on survivorship.
- An awareness of the special resources available to pediatric oncology patients and families.
- An awareness of the social and religious values of patients/families of culturally diverse backgrounds.
- Theories of normal child and family development; psychopathology; normal and dysfunctional parenting.
- Systems theory as it relates to family functioning, adaptation to medical settings, and utilization of community resources.
- Theoretical framework of clinical interventions including individual, group and family treatment modalities as well as crisis intervention.
- The dynamics of child abuse and neglect and the legal responsibilities of the social worker.
- Knowledge of effective methods of verbal and written communication.
- Knowledge of organizational theory and the dynamics of negotiation.
- Theoretical framework of psychosocial research including processes of planning, conducting, and reporting research findings.

- Knowledge of learning theory.

Standard III: Scope of Skills

The specialty of pediatric oncology requires social workers to possess a number of abilities and skills. Social Workers must function both as generalist and specialist. To provide appropriate interventions in the pediatric oncology setting, social workers shall have skills to do the following:

- Establish and maintain a therapeutic relationship.
- Establish and maintain appropriate interpersonal boundaries with patients/families.
- Tolerate uncertainty and the range of emotions and coping styles of patients and families in crisis.
- Comprehend and promote medical research/treatment and integrate both with social casework.
- Promote patient and family rights to self-determination.
- Enable the family to integrate the medical, social, emotional, and family dynamics of the disease/treatment into the current context of their life situation.
- Provide therapeutic interventions aimed at adaptation throughout the continuum of cancer therapy.
- Plan with families for home care that promotes compliance as well as considers appropriate utilization of resources.
- Negotiate for the needs of patients and families and be proactive on the patient's/family's behalf.
- Utilize other professionals, colleagues, and resource persons on behalf of the patient and family.
- Advocate for appropriate care of children whose parents are unable or unwilling to consent to medical treatment.
- Communicate and disseminate information well in verbal and written form.
- Develop, implement, and evaluate educational goals and objectives.
- Disseminate current knowledge of oncologic and hematologic diseases and treatment protocols and the biopsychosocial impact of the illness experience on patients and their families.
- Collaborate with community organizations and businesses includ-

ing schools, parent groups, and financial institutions regarding childhood cancer and its impact on patients and families.
• Consult and support interdisciplinary colleagues involved either directly or indirectly with the case and treatment of pediatric cancer patients and their families.

Standard IV: Competencies
A. Clinical
The clinical role includes:

1. *Comprehensive Assessment*

   Pediatric oncology social workers should possess the ability to conduct and organize a comprehensive psychosocial assessment. The assessment is the process that assists the social worker in identifying patient and family strengths, copying styles and problem areas within the context of their oncologic, social, financial, cultural, and psychological milieu. Pediatric oncology social workers should be able to assess all issues associated with child and family development as well as adjustment to the diagnosis and treatment of childhood cancer.

   These areas encompass the knowledge base outlined in Standard II and skills in Standard III.

2. *Comprehensive Treatment Planning*

   Pediatric oncology social workers should be able to formulate a care plan that clearly identifies problems and proposes social work interventions. The plan is the critical tool that drives the interventions. It also serves as an integral resource for the medical team in providing continuity of care and case management. Pediatric oncology social workers are expected to implement the plan and subsequently re-evaluate and revise the plan throughout the course of the patient's treatment.

3. *Treatment Intervention*

   Pediatric oncology social workers are skilled at employing a wide range of social work interventions whose use are dependent upon the patient's age, the problem/situation, and its severity. Pediatric oncology social workers should have a repertoire of interventions to draw from including but not limited to:

    a. Pain management and relaxation therapy.

    b. Play therapy and other age appropriate interventions.

    c. Crisis intervention and brief focused therapy (counseling).

    d. Family and group therapy (counseling).

    e. Cognitive, behavioral therapy (counseling).

    f. Grief and Bereavement therapy (counseling).

    g. Financial screening and resource management.

    h. Discharge planning.

    i. Conflict resolution management.

    j. Case management.

B. Educational

Pediatric oncology social workers have the capacity to educate patients, families, colleagues, and the community about the specifics of childhood cancer, treatment alternatives, psychosocial implications of illness and treatment in a variety of formats including:

1. *One-on-one teaching sessions.*

2. *Group educational programs.*

3. *Consultations with colleagues.*

4. *Collaboration with organizations, and professionals including school officials, parent groups, financial institutions, employers, and community groups.*

C. Advocacy

Pediatric oncology social workers are skilled at advocating for patients and families on many levels including:

1. *Promotion of patient/family rights within the medical setting and community to ensure access to care, confidentiality, and critical life resources.*

2. *Reinforcement of informed consent.*

3. *Inclusion of patients/parents in discussions related to treatment changes or ethical issues.*

4. *Promotion of the needs of culturally diverse and socially, intellectually, or physically challenged patients.*

D. Research

Pediatric oncology social workers shall maintain a commitment to initiate or collaborate in research to advance practice and contribute to the body of knowledge specific to pediatric oncology.

Standard V: Professional Development

Opportunities for continued professional growth and knowledge/skill development are recognized as being vital to maintaining high standards of practice. Attendance at national and international conferences/seminars, informal networking, peer review, consultation, supervision, and individual study form the foundation for professional development.

INDEX

B

C

E

F

G

H

I

P

T

U

V

W